OXFORD MEDICAL PUBLICATIONS

Forensic Pharmacology

Forensic Pharmacology
Medicines, Mayhem, and Malpractice

R. E. Ferner
Consultant Physician, City Hospital, Birmingham and Honorary Senior Lecturer in Medicine (Therapeutics), University of Birmingham

with a chapter by

Elizabeth Norman
Barrister-at-Law, Victoria Chambers, Birmingham

and a Foreword by

M. D. Rawlins
Professor of Clinical Pharmacology, University of Newcastle upon Tyne and Chairman, Committee on Safety of Medicines

Oxford   New York   Tokyo
Oxford University Press
1996

Oxford University Press, Walton Street, Oxford OX2 6DP

Oxford   New York
Athens   Auckland   Bangkok   Bombay
Calcutta   Cape Town   Dar es Salaam   Delhi
Florence   Hong Kong   Istanbul   Karachi
Kuala Lumpur   Madras   Madrid   Melbourne
Mexico City   Nairobi   Paris   Singapore
Taipei   Tokyo   Toronto

and associated companies in
Berlin   Ibadan

Oxford is a trade mark of Oxford University Press

Published in the United States
by Oxford University Press Inc., New York

A catalogue record for this book is available from the British Library

Library of Congress Cataloging in Publication Data
Ferner, R. E. (Robin E.)
Forensic pharmacology : medicines, mayhem, and malpractice / R. E.
Ferner, with a chapter by Elizabeth Norman ; foreword by M. D.
Rawlins.
p.   cm. — (Oxford medical publications)
Includes bibliographical references and index.
1. Forensic pharmacology.   I. Norman, Elizabeth, Barrister-at
-Law.   II. Title.   III. Series.
[DNLM: 1. Forensic Medicine.   2. Pharmacology.   W 700 F364f 1996]
RA1160.F47   1996
614'.1—dc20
DNLM/DLC
for Library of Congress   95–38555
CIP

ISBN 0 19 854826 5 (Hbk.)

Typeset by Footnote Graphics, Warminster, Wilts
Printed in Great Britain by Biddles Ltd, Guildford

'I chucked away a lucrative partnership with a Bengali chemist's apprentice, owing to an unfortunate exceeding of the maximum Pharmacopoea-permitted dose of Digitalis on a wealthy woman patient ... as far as I can remember, the shotgun matter this locumwallah gave me to deal out was:

"R_x
Dig. gtt. lxii.
Aquae purae ... viii.
Misce. Signetur, 3ii, Quatris horis,
Syr. Gluc.
Oi!
hh!
$\frac{1}{2}d!$"

In the circumstances, either the lady had a quatris horis (every four hours) dessertspoonful dose of an oi (one pint) of aquae purae (pure water), or an oi of Digitalis, suspended in a gtt. lxii. of pure water. If so, hell, I had certainly helped Dig. her gtt. lxii. grave!'

(G. V. Desani 1972)

'The Attorney-General said he 'could not help saying that it seemed a scandal upon a learned, a distinguished, and a liberal profession, that men should come forward and put forward such speculations as these, perverting the facts, and drawing from them unwarranted conclusions with the view of deceiving the jury".'

A comment on the defence experts at the trial of
Dr William Palmer, quoted by C. Jones (1994)

Foreword

There can be few more disparate disciplines than the law and pharmacology. While lawyers are concerned with the pursuit of justice, pharmacologists are devotees of the effects of chemicals on living matter. Yet in recent years these two disciplines have become entwined in both the criminal and the civil courts. Robin Ferner's brokering of a marriage between them is both timely and necessary. *Forensic pharmacology* will, I know, appeal to lawyers because of the clarity with which he describes even the most complicated pharmacological issues. Equally, *Forensic pharmacology* will appeal not just to pharmacologists but to doctors generally when asked to opine on pharmacological matters. The experience and advice that shines through this book will also help them fulfil Lord Justice Rose's maxim:

The most impressive witnesses before this Court were those whose evidence stemmed from their area of expertise, whose views are in accordance with but not dependent on medical literature, who answered questions clearly and concisely, and whose objectivity permitted them to make appropriate conclusions.

In developing what must now be regarded as both a new branch of law and of pharmacology, Dr Ferner deserves the gratitude of lawyers and doctors alike.

Michael D. Rawlins
Newcastle upon Tyne

Preface

Medicines can do harm as well as good, and doctors, lawyers, police officers, and laboratory scientists have a professional interest in the harm that medicines can cause. So, too, do journalists, crime-writers and others. This book is intended as a help to them in both criminal and civil matters.

The aim has been to make *Forensic pharmacology* sufficiently technical so that an expert will find it helpful, without being so obscure as to be inaccessible to others. The mathematical techniques of pharmacology allow times of administration and doses to be estimated. They have been described in appendices, so the interested reader can use them, while those who are not mathematically inclined are preserved from a tangle of algebra. Practical examples from the literature and from personal experience are given, where possible, to illustrate the points raised, to serve as exemplars for others to use when engaged on similar cases, and to reinforce the variety, excitement, and unpredictability of the subject of forensic pharmacology: the point at which medicines, mayhem, and malpractice meet.

The book owes its genesis to discussions I had over several years with Professor Michael Rawlins, and without his help I should never have learnt much pharmacology, nor would I have written the book. Elizabeth Norman has been a valuable help and a well informed critic. I should also like to thank for their help, encouragement, and practical advice on forensic matters, other friends in Newcastle, particularly Dr Nick Bateman and Dr Jim Smith; and in Birmingham, especially Chris Anton, Dr Stanley Brown, Dr Robin Braithwaite, Dr Anthony Daniels, and Dr Martin Kendall. The staff of Oxford University Press have guided me through the publishing maze. And Dr Celia Moss has been more helpful, supportive, and tolerant than any husband has a right to expect.

While the book could not have been written without a great deal of assistance and support, any errors that it contains are entirely the responsibility and fault of the author. Any comments or corrections would be welcome.

Birmingham   R. E. F.
July 1995

Contents

Introduction

Doctors and lawyers see more and more of each other in these litigious, and legally aided, times.

Sometimes they meet in the criminal courts. Serious crime has become a common-place, and drugs have been used in the commission of rape, manslaughter, and murder. Crime related to alcohol, the most important of drugs in a criminal context, has increased remorselessly as the per capita consumption of alcohol has increased.

Civil actions are also more common now than before. Patients are much more ready to seek legal advice, and doctors more likely to be involved in negligence litigation, where only a few years ago there would have been little more than an acknowledgement that things can go wrong. There was until recently the belief that, while surgical operations were dangerous, drug therapy was safe, and drugs could only do good. Now, there is a belief that drugs can be the cause of any unpleasant occurrence, from a positive breath test for alcohol, or a desire to murder one's wife, to all manner of physical and psychiatric diseases.

In this book, I hope to show some of the ways in which clinical pharmacologists, specialists in the actions of drugs 'at the bedside', can help lawyers in unravelling the truth behind these beliefs. The classification of drugs, their effects, and the way in which their effects are linked to the concentration of drug in body fluid, are all discussed.

By way of illustration, or seasoning, numerous case histories have been included. To provide a background of useful facts, several specific drugs are dealt with in some detail.

Much of the legal discussion is general in nature. Problems that are specific to English law are considered, though, at the risk of appearing sometimes to be parochial. In mitigation, I would plead that the specific examples show how experts need some guidance on the prevailing law in order to formulate their answers to lawyers' questions.

The well-prepared expert wishes to be armed with the relevant texts and learned papers, and references to many of these are provided. It is always wise to return to the original work if time and library facilities allow.

Part 1

General considerations

1

Drugs, their behaviour and their effects on the body

1.1 The different sorts of agent

1.1.1 Some definitions

A *drug* is a single chemical substance or natural product that can be used to prevent or treat disease or to alter the physiological state of the body. This definition of a drug therefore includes those products such as attenuated measles virus which are given to healthy people in the hope of preventing disease. It also includes those substances which alter the physiological functions of the body, examples of which would be contraceptive substances, such as the spermicidal compound nonoxynol-9, and the progestagen used as an oral contraceptive.

The definition encompasses chemical entities which can be taken to alter feelings or thoughts, such as ethanol (ethyl alcohol). Substances like heroin, cocaine, and 'Ecstasy' (methylene dioxymetamphetamine) are included, but the term 'drug' is not synonymous with 'drug of abuse', and its meaning should not be subverted to indicate only that kind of substance.

A *medicine* is a mixture of one or more drug with other ingredients which allow it to be delivered to the patient in a useful, stable, and palatable form. It can contain many components in addition to the active drug. For example, the drug usually constitutes less than half the weight of a tablet. It will also contain an inert matrix, such as starch or lactose, which serves as a vehicle for the drug. There may be *stabilizers* to prevent or retard deterioration of the drug during storage, *colouring* to make the preparation distinctive or appetizing, and *sweeteners* to render it more palatable. These *excipients*, or pharmaceutical adjuvants, can themselves cause adverse effects (Florence and Salole 1990).

The precise composition of the medicine is known as the *formulation*, and different formulations of the same drug can have different properties either by accident or by design. It is now common for drugs to be available in conventional and in 'sustained-release', 'slow-release', 'extended-release', or other formulations. These modified-release preparations are intended to produce the same clinical effects with less frequent dosing than the conventional tablets, or sometimes to overcome the unpleasant effects of a rapid change in the amount of drug in the body.

Serious adverse effects have occurred in the past when new formulations of old drugs have been assumed to share the properties of older formulations. For example, a preparation containing the antiepileptic drug phenytoin was formulated with an excipient of lactose in place of calcium sulphate. Phenytoin was much more readily absorbed from the new preparation, and patients suffered severe toxicity (see Case 6.6).

Pharmacology is the science that is concerned with drugs, their actions and their uses. It is distinguished from *pharmacy*, which is 'the art or practice of collecting, preparing and dispensing drugs, especially for medicinal purposes; the making or compounding of medicines; the occupation of a druggist or pharmaceutical chemist'[1.]

Clinical pharmacology, which means 'pharmacology at the bedside', is that branch of pharmacology which concentrates on investigating the properties and uses of drugs in patients.

Therapeutics is that branch of medical practice which is concerned with *therapy*: treating disease, by drugs or other methods. The practice of medicine usually begins with diagnosis, the process of discovering which disease a patient is suffering from. Therapy is then given for the disease which has been diagnosed. In diagnosis, the discovery proceeds from the history of symptoms, which the patient complains of or admits to on questioning, to the examination for signs, which are the physical manifestations of disease, and the conduct of investigations, which take the form of tests of the blood, radiographs (X-rays) and so forth. Failing a clear diagnosis, the doctor can try to alleviate symptoms, in so-called symptomatic treatment.

By way of example of the practice of medicine, consider a 50-year-old man who complains of chest pain lasting for 1 hour, admits on questioning that the pain was crushing in nature, shows signs on examination of a weak, rapid pulse, and is found on investigation to have changes in the electrocardiogram which are those that occur with myocardial infarction (death of heart muscle from interruption of its blood supply—a 'heart attack'). The diagnosis of myocardial infarction is made, and therapy can be given. This could include drugs to dissolve the blood clots responsible for cutting off the blood supply to the heart, such as the enzyme drug streptokinase. Aspirin and beta-blocking drugs might be given to reduce the chance of further heart attacks. As the patient recovers, he will be likely to have physiotherapy (physical therapy) to encourage him to take gentle exercise and to increase the work that his damaged heart can do.

1.1.2 Systems of therapeutics

Conventional medicine uses a system of therapeutics based at least partly on the scientific knowledge of drugs and diseases. The introduction of new drugs is regulated in such a way that a manufacturer must show some evidence that the drug is effective before it can be marketed. The evidence comes from experiments in which the effects of the treatment are investigated in patients. Evidence would be needed, for example, to show that a drug which was marketed as a hypnotic (sleeping pill) did indeed lead to longer periods of sleep in patients with insomnia.

There are still areas of conventional medicine where therapy relies on the feelings, experience, or preconception of the practitioner, but these are becoming fewer. The Department of Health has tacitly recognized the irrationality of certain treatments by making it impossible for some drugs, such as bitters and tonics, to be paid for under the National Health Service. The *British National Formulary*, which is a list of medicines available for prescription and the indications for their use, is an invaluable source of up-to-date guidance on the prescribing of medicines. It, too, recognizes that it is more reasonable to prescribe some drugs than others, and it lists the latter in print so small that information on them is only available to the seriously short-sighted, or to those far-sighted enough to carry a magnifying glass.

The medicines of conventional medicine are sometimes called *allopathic medicines* and this term is especially used to distinguish them from homeopathic medicines, which are described below.

[1]Oxford English Dictionary, 1st edition (1884–1928).

Drugs used in conventional therapy can be classified in several ways, and there are two main methods. One group of classification schemes relies on the intrinsic properties of the drug, such as its chemical structure. The other group considers drugs by their actions on the body in health and disease. Neither method is perfect. Small changes in chemical structure can lead to large changes in drug action, so the actions cannot be deduced from the structure. For example, the drug propranolol is structurally similar to pronethanol, which was developed as an antagonist to isoprenaline. Pronethanol, but not propranolol, caused cancer in experimental rats, and so only the latter was introduced into clinical practice to treat angina. Most drugs will have a variety of actions as they interact with bodily systems which themselves can manifest a variety of effects. Similar effects can be useful in the treatment of a number of dissimilar conditions. Propranolol is now used to treat hypertension (high blood pressure), anxiety, hyperthyroidism (overactivity of the thyroid gland), portal hypertension (a result of liver disease) and the rare heart disease hypertrophic obstructive cardiomyopathy.

Classification by nature of the drug

Examples are given in Tables 1.1 and 1.2.

Table 1.1 Classification by origin of the drug (after Sneader 1990)

Active principles from plants
Naturally occurring human hormones and their analogues
Other naturally occurring human substances
Natural products from microbes
Inorganic and organometallic compounds
Synthetic organic compounds
Compounds discovered by observation of effects by chance or by systematic study

Table 1.2. The classification of drugs by chemical structure; for example, antimicrobial drugs could be classified as follows:

Aminoglycosides
Cephalosporins
–conazoles
Macrolides
Penicillins
Peptides
Pyrimidines
Quinolones
Sulphonamides
Tetracyclines
Others

Classification by action of the drug

Classifications can be based on the actions of a drug at any level from the inner components of a cell to the whole organism. Examples are given in Tables 1.3 and 1.4

Table 1.3 Drugs acting at specific receptors

Drugs can activate or inactivate many naturally-occurring receptors, such as:

Neural receptors which are involved in the transmission of nerve signals, including:
  adrenergic
  cholinergic
  dopaminergic
  GABA-ergic
  histamine
  opioid peptides
  serotoninergic

Membrane receptors which are on the surface of cells, including:
  ion channels
  calcium channels
  chloride channels
  sodium channels
  hormone receptors
    corticosteroid
    growth hormone
    gonadotrophin
    insulin
    sex steroid
    thyroid

Drugs acting on specific enzymes or co-factors, including the following enzymes:
  angiotensin converting enzyme (ACE)
  carbonic anhydrase
  cholinesterases
  folate
  hydroxymethylglutaryl Co-enzyme A reductase
  monoamine oxidases
  prostaglandin synthetase
  xanthine oxidase

Drugs acting on cell turnover, particularly anticancer drugs

Drugs with membrane effects not mediated by specific receptors

  anaesthetic gases

Drugs active preferentially against infective agents

Table 1.4 Classification by therapeutic action (modified from Duncan 1994; Prasad 1994)

Gastrointestinal system
  antacids and antisecretory drugs
  laxatives
  antidiarrhoeals
  antiemetics
  prokinetic
  pancreatic enzymes
  bile salts

Cardiovascular system
  antiarrhythmics
  treatment for cardiac failure
  antianginal
  antihypertensives
  anticoagulants
  antithrombotics
  fibrinolytics
  haemostatics

Table 1.4 Continued

Central nervous system
  hypnotics
  anxiolytics
  antipsychotics
  antidepressants
  anticonvulsants
  stimulants
  antiparkinsonian
  migraine treatment
  analgesics
Musculoskeletal disorders
  non-steroidal anti-inflammatory drugs
  against gout
  muscle relaxants
  rubs
Respiratory system
  bronchodilators
  anti-inflammatories
  expectorants
  antitussives
  mucolytics
  decongestants
Anti-infective agents
  vaccines
  antiviral
  antibacterial
  antituberculous
  antifungal
  antimalarial
  other antiprotozoal
  antihelminthic
Endocrine and metabolic
  hypoglycaemic agents
  lipid-lowering agents
  gonadal hormones
  contraceptives
  pituitary hormones
  corticosteroid
  thyroid and antithyroid drugs
  drugs affecting bone metabolism
Genitourinary system
  drugs acting on incontinence
  drugs acting on impotence
Nutrition
  vitamins
  iron
  calcium
Neoplasia (cancers and other 'new growths')
  antineoplastic agents
Anaesthesia
  local agents
  systemic anaesthetics
  muscle relaxants
Diagnosis
  radiographic contrast media
  stimulatory hormones
The skin, eyes, ears, nose, and throat

Legal classification of medicines

This is dealt with in Section 1.1.3.

Other systems of therapeutics

Homeopathy

Homeopathy is a system of therapeutics based on the doctrine that the symptoms of disease can be alleviated by administering to the sufferer minute doses of remedies which in larger doses produce similar symptoms. The doctrine was elaborated by Hahnemann of Erlangen at the end of the eighteenth century. He had observed that quinine, which he considered to produce some of the symptoms of malaria, could be used in its cure.

Classical homeopathic remedies are produced by 'potentiation', a process of repeated dilution and succussion (vigorous shaking). For example (Kleijnen *et al.*, 1991), a plant such as *Arnica montana*, mountain tobacco, is macerated and dissolved in ethanol to produce a 'mother liquid' or 'unit preparation'. One part of the unit preparation is then diluted and shaken with 9 parts of ethanol to produce a D1 or first decimal dilution, or with 99 parts of ethanol to produce a C1 or first centennial dilution. The process is repeated to produce a form for administration that can be up to C200, that is, one part of unit preparation in 10^{200}. Since the homeopathic belief is that the medicine becomes more powerful as it is diluted and shaken, the technical term for the dilution is *potency*. It is unlikely that dilutions (potencies) of greater than D24 or C12 contain even a single molecule of the ingredients which constitute the unit preparation.

Therapy is based on finding a *simulium*, a substance that induces symptoms which most closely resemble those that the patient suffers. In classical homeopathy, only a single substance is used, and it is distinct from the causative agent if that is known. Polypharmacy, where many agents are used, or isopharmacy, where the causative agent is given in low dose, are modern adaptations of Hahnemann's ideas.

The efficacy of homeopathic remedies

Homeopathic remedies are not prescribed to treat distinct diseases such as myocardial infarction or tuberculosis,

because homeopathic prescriptions are based on the recognition of a pattern of symptoms and pathology encompassing the whole state of the patient, and are rarely chosen for one specific syndrome. A single medicine may often be used to treat more than one disease in the same patient, for example asthma and eczema. Similarly, different patients with the same diagnosis may require a number of different medicines (Swayne 1989).

This method of choosing a drug differs radically from the conventional method, so attempts to compare the effectiveness of homeopathic remedies with those of conventional (allopathic) medicines, or even to test homeopathic remedies against placebo, have met with limited success.

Kleijnen *et al.* (1991) approached homeopathy as sceptics, but felt that the 107 trials that they reviewed were sufficient to show a need for well-designed, large studies which could adequately test homeopathic remedies.

Reilly *et al.* (Anonymous 1994a; Reilly *et al.* 1994) examined 28 patients with allergies, mainly to house–dust mite, and concluded that a homeopathic preparation containing allergen in a concentration of C30 was more effective than diluent alone in improving symptoms. The trial is notable for its rigour: it was double–blind, randomized and placebo controlled, and sample ampoules of trial drug were examined for possible contaminants such as cortico-steroids. Another well-conducted trial, however, failed to find a benefit from homeopathic remedies (de Lange de Klerk *et al.* 1994).

Hill and Doyon (1990) examined only the 40 trials of homeopathic remedies which they considered to have been conducted with satisfactory randomization of patients. This is an important safeguard of the validity of the trial, though it is only one of several necessary conditions for validity. The review concluded that the trials showed no evidence of effectiveness and that larger trials were unjustified.

The present conventional view of homeopathy might be summarized as:

1. The foundation on which it rests is not 'scientific'.
2. It is unlikely to be harmful, because the doses of active substance used are too low to have any toxic effects.
3. It is unlikely to be beneficial directly, because the doses of active substance are too low to have any therapeutic action.
4. It may be indirectly beneficial, in the way that placebo medicines can be beneficial.
5. Further trials may be warranted, but are unlikely to show a major effect of homeopathic medicines in serious organic disease.

The Medicines Act 1968 deals specifically with homeopathic remedies (Merrills and Fisher 1995), and places restrictions on some preparations which contain potentially toxic ingredients, some preparations with low potency (that is, high concentration) and those preparations which derive from drugs scheduled under the Dangerous Drugs Act 1965 (now replaced by the Misuse of Drugs Act 1971, and the Misuse of Drugs Regulations 1985).

Herbal medicines

Herbal medicine is the oldest form of therapeutics, and curative properties have been ascribed to many thousands of plants by Western, Chinese, African, Native American and other traditional systems of healing.

For example, the empirical use of herbal and other medicines in China dates back over 2000 years, and is based on the need for balance or harmony of the two opposing forces of Yin and Yang. Over 5000 different plants have been used in traditional Chinese medicine.

Mitchell Bruce's *Materia medica and therapeutics: an introduction to the rational treatment of disease* (Bruce 1899) devoted more than twice as many pages to organic materia medica as to inorganic materia medica, and included such remedies as *Oleum Cubebae*, 'the Oil distilled from cubebs, chiefly used in gonorrhoea and vesical affections. It is decidedly less unpleasant than Copaiba, and much less liable to disturb the digestion'. The *National Formulary* (1949), the forerunner of the indispensible *British National Formulary* (Prasad 1994) still contained many remedies such as '*Haustes extracti filicis*', which contained 60 minims of extract of male fern and 120 minims of mucilage of *Acacia* made up to $1\frac{1}{2}$ fluid ounces with cinnamon water. It was used to treat tapeworm infestation.

La thérapeutique en 20 médicaments, by Huchard and Fiessinger (1911), provides an interesting contrast, as it contains only quinine, theobromine, digitalis, opium, belladonna, and ergot amongst its 20 medicaments. These drugs, or their purified relatives, are all still used in conventional therapeutics.

Herbal remedies can be divided into groups, of which the first is those used as conventional medicines. In 1990, 119 identified conventional drugs were still extracted from plants (Farnsworth 1990). These include such important drugs as the heart drug digoxin, the anticancer drugs vincristine and vinblastine, and the opiate pain killers. There are likely to be many more useful drugs to be extracted from plants, but which ones is unclear: the National Cancer Institute in the United States has screened over 32 000 plants in about 30 years, but only isolated 20 compounds of sufficient promise to try in man, and discarded them all as being unsafe or ineffective.

A second group of herbal medicines contains those which have undergone some testing and shown some evidence of efficacy. For example, feverfew, *Matricaria parthenium,* has some action in the treatment of migraine, and a compounded Chinese herbal tea has been demonstrated to help patients with eczema.

Other herbal remedies remain in the realm of folklore and there is no evidence that they possess the curative powers ascribed to them. 'Furthermore, a good deal of magic and superstition of unknown antiquity crept into the herbals, making ... a final hotchpotch of unproved, useless and often absurd information. Amazingly, these alleged medicinal properties have been copied right up to now from the printed herbals of the 15th to 17th century, and they are blandly presented to the present day public by modern writers on herbalism'[2].

The herbal drugs are not in any way exempt from serious adverse effects, and this is as true for those of doubtful efficacy as for those which are known to have some therapeutic action (Zhang and Huang 1988). For example, an epidemic of kidney failure in Belgium was traced to a herbal slimming treatment. Capsules containing germander (*Teuerium chamaedrys L.*) were responsible for an outbreak of hepatitis, in which one patient died; constituents of germander form toxic breakdown products (Loeper *et al.* 1994). The quality of herbal preparations is also suspect, and amounts of active ingredient can vary 100-fold between different samples of the same preparation (Hawkes 1994; de Smet 1995).

A *British herbal pharmacopoeia* is published by the British Herbal Medicine Association (1990). It lists several hundred herbal preparations, their botanical descriptions and their 'indications'. An example is Gileadensis, synonyms Poplar Buds, Balm of Gilead Buds, an infusion of which is specifically indicated for treating laryngitis with aphonia (loss of voice).

A herbal medicine can be made, assembled, sold and supplied without a licence, provided that the remedy is made from a plant or plants only by drying, crushing or comminuting, that the remedy is specified only by the name of the plant or plants and the process by which it is made, that no other name or any written recommendation as to use is made, and that it is not imported (Dale and Appelbe 1989; Merrills and Fisher 1995). This may seem remarkable when compared with the licensing requirements for synthetic products, and there is no reason to assume that 'natural' remedies are benign.

'Herbalists', particularly Chinese herbalists, can use other natural products. 'A number of complete tiger leg bones, cricket-ball sized lumps of congealed bear's blood, a fridge stuffed with the gall bladders of 17 bears, and a stash of 9 inch sections of rhino horn' were recovered by police searching premises from which Chinese traditional medicine was practised in England (*Guardian* 9 February 1995).

---

[2] *Oxford Companion to Medicine* (1991), p. 540.

Ayurvedic medicine

Ayurveda (= 'the science of life' in Hindi) is a discipline or philosophy of healthy living with origins in the second millennium BC, and still widely practised in India and in Indian populations abroad (Anand 1990; Bodeker 1990). Its essential tenet is that bodily health is regulated by the three humours (*doshas*), namely: air (*vayu*), fire (*tejas*), and water (*ap*).Therapy of metabolic and infectious disease aims to restore the equilibrium amongst them. The treatments are vegetable, animal, or mineral, and this last group contains preparations of copper, arsenic, mercury, lead, and antimony, all of which can cause severe toxicity. Cases are well recognized, and have occurred in members of Asian communities born and bred in England (Kew *et al.* 1993; Keen *et al.* 1994; Bayly *et al.* 1995).

CASE 1.1 (KULSHRESTHA *ET AL.* 1994)

A 23-year-old woman of Punjabi origin was admitted to hospital in Birmingham (England) with abdominal pain and vomiting. She and her husband had been undergoing investigation for infertility. She was transferred from the care of the gynaecologists to that of the general surgeons, and she mentioned to the houseman that she had been taking traditional Ayurvedic treatment for infertility. The medicines, obtained from a woman 'healer' in Birmingham but apparently imported from India, were off-white powders wrapped in strips of newspaper. The powders were radiopaque, and contained over 6 per cent lead by weight. The woman's blood lead and zinc protoporphyrin concentrations were raised, as would be expected in chronic lead poisoning. Her symptoms settled with rehydration when she stopped taking the powders. It subsequently transpired that her husband was azoospermic (his semen contained no spermatozoa).

Ethanol

Ethanol (ethyl alcohol, or commonly just alcohol) is a drug in the sense that is a single chemical substance which is used to alter the physiological state of the body. It is also a drug of addiction, and is much more important in this respect than any other abused drug, since its use is widely sanctioned and widespread. It was also until recently recommended as a stimulant in counteracting collapse. *Ballière's Nurses'complete medical dictionary*, 1935 edition (Hitch and Marshall 1935), recommends brandy, by mouth, subcutaneously, or per rectum, for this purpose. Although it might well have been effective, especially by this last route (though not for pharmacological reasons), brandy is no longer used as a stimulant.

The special place of ethanol in forensic pharmacology derives mainly from the effect of ethanol in impairing judgement and co-ordination of movements, a lethal combination when the movements are those of the steering-wheel of a motor-car or the controls of a railway locomotive. The Licensing Act of 1872 laid down the statutory offence of being drunk in charge of a steam-engine and so laid the foundation for current laws on drunken driving. Since ethanol can impair the skills of a driver long before he is obviously drunk to the lay observer, the definition has been refined, and is now based on measuring the concentration of ethanol in the breath, blood, or urine. Such measurements, as we shall discuss, are the basic data for the science of pharmacokinetics, and so their interpretation is very much the province of clinical pharmacologists. This is treated in detail in Chapter 7.

Other drugs of abuse

Drug abuse is the use of drugs for purposes or in quantities which are undesirable. This definition is implicitly subjective, and reminiscent of the definition of an alcoholic as a man who drinks more than his doctor. An example of drug abuse is found in those patients, usually women obsessed by their weight, who take laxatives in such enormous quantities that they lose fluids and essential ions such as potassium from the gut and become ill as a result. No doctor would sanction this excessive use of laxatives.

Drug dependence is a special case of drug abuse where the cardinal features are that the patient craves the drug in question, and withholding the drug from the patient causes an illness with a series of symptoms and signs categorized as 'withdrawal effects'.

The term *drug addiction* is sometimes reserved for that form of drug dependence where the patient's life is dominated by his craving for drugs (Laurence and Bennett, 1992*d*).

Patients who are dependent on drugs or addicted to them can also show a need for steadily increasing quantities of drug to produce the same effect or to stave off symptoms of withdrawal. Addicted patients can, in consequence, sometimes tolerate doses of drugs which would be lethal in subjects who were not habituated. For example, some opiate addicts regularly inject themselves with doses of heroin any one of which would be sufficient to stop the breathing of a non-addicted person. This *tolerance* to the drug is a feature of physical rather than psychological dependence. Physical dependence is a result of adaptation of the body to the habitual presence of a drug.

Although the death rate of intravenous drug abusers is about 40 times that of the general population, addiction is not always a death sentence. Thomas De Quincey acquired his habit of eating opium when an undergraduate at Oxford in 1804, but, in spite of his early addiction, survived over 50 years.

The most commonly abused drugs are those that alter the state of mind, either by depressing and relaxing the central nervous system or by stimulating it. Their effects are not confined to higher animals: spiders spin distorted webs under the influence of cannabis and amphetamines (*Guardian*, 28 April 1995). They are shown in Table 1.5.

Table 1.5 Drugs that are commonly abused

Drugs related to opium alkaloids
    buprenorphine ('Temgesic')
    dextromoramide ('Palfium')
    dextropropoxyphene (a component of co-proxamol 'Distalgesic')
    diamorphine (= heroin)
    morphine
    pethidine (= meperidine in the United States)
Amphetamine and related drugs
    amphetamine
    dexamphetamine
    methyl amphetamine
    methylene dioxyamphetamine (MDA)
    methylene dioxymetamphetamine (MDMA, 'Ecstasy')
    methylene dioxyethylamphetamine (MDE, 'Eve')
Other hallucinogens
    lysergic acid diethylamide (LSD)
    mescaline (from the peyote cactus)
    psilocybin (from the *Psilocybe* 'magic mushroom')
Cocaine and related drugs
    cocaine (cocaine hydrochloride)
    'crack' cocaine (free cocaine base, 'freebase')
Cannabis
    cannabis (marijuana) in various forms, including the leaf and a resin extracted from it

Poisons other than pharmacological poisons

A poison is a substance which in sufficient dose can cause harm. Paracelsus pointed out that it is the dose which determines whether a particular substance is poisonous, '*dosis sola facit venenum*'. Even the most innocuous substance can cause fatal biochemical disturbance.

> CASE 1.2
>
> A 34-year-old patient in a mental hospital drank 6 pints of water in the space of 20 minutes and then died.

For the wrong-doer, a rather more potent poison than water is usually required. As little as 50 milligrams of a soluble cyanide salt can cause death, and so it has been the preferred content of spies' suicide pills. It has also been used for murder.

> CASE 1.3 (DUNEA 1983)
>
> In September 1982, a 12-year-old schoolgirl and a young postal worker died suddenly after minor illnesses. The postal worker's family gathered that evening, and his wife and brother took capsules of 'Tylenol' (paracetamol); both collapsed and died within a few minutes. The 'Tylenol' capsules had been tampered with. Others from the same batch contained 65 milligrams of potassium cyanide. Three more people died before the epidemic was halted. The murderer has not been caught.

In a later case, two people died when capsules of the nasal decongestant 'Sudafed' (pseudo-ephedrine) were contaminated with cyanide (Anonymous 1991a; Logan *et al.* 1993).

The clinical pharmacologist can be confronted with non-drug poisoning, for example, because of the need to interpret laboratory findings or the need to deduce or explain a pattern of illness in terms of the possible agents. The principles are no different from those governing pharmaceutical medicines. In practice it will sometimes be necessary to turn to a clinical toxicologist with special knowledge of, or interest in, the subject in question. It would be a brave clinical pharmacologist who gave an expert opinion on the nature of 'The speckled band', the snake in the Sherlock Holmes story which strikes its owner dead having nearly done the same to Holmes.

1.1.3 Medicines licensed under the Medicines Act 1968

The introduction of new 'conventional' medicines in the United Kingdom has recently been reviewed (Canlin 1991; Wells 1991). The system of licensing medicines has gradually evolved from the Apothecary Wares, Drugs and Stuffs Act of 1540, which provided for four Inspectors to be appointed by the Royal College of Physicians to ascertain the safety and quality of drugs. History does not relate whether penalties were ever exacted under the Act.

The Therapeutic Substances Act of 1921 applied to some, but not all, therapeutic and prophylactic substances. It was superseded by the Medicines Act of 1968. This makes provision for a Licensing Authority, consisting of the Secretaries of State for Health and Agriculture, Wales, Scotland and Northern Ireland. The day-to-day work devolves upon a Secretariat, known as the Medicines Control Agency (MCA). The Licensing Authority receives advice from a body called the Medicines Commission, which is in turn advised by other committees, principally the Committee on Safety of Medicines (CSM), the Committee on Dental and Surgical Materials, and the British Pharmacopoeial Commission.

The Licensing Authority has the right to grant licences in respect of medicines. Manufacturers' licences are granted to those who are considered competent to make a drug; and product licences allow the licensee to market and supply a product for specified indications (reasons for treatment). Product licences are renewable every 5 years.

Since 1 January 1995, the European Union has had a licensing authority, the European Commission, advised by a Committee for Proprietary Medicinal Products (CPMP). The Secretariat, known as the European Medicines Evaluation Agency (EMEA), is based in London. Most medicines can still be licensed in each member state, or they can be licensed through a 'centralized procedure' by the EMEA, or a 'decentralized procedure', in which a licence granted in one member state is ratified for the whole European Community. Products manufactured by genetic engineering can only be licensed centrally (Anonymous 1994b).

Categories of product licence under the Medicines Act

Medicines which are licensed for sale in the United Kingdom are classified according to the restrictions placed on their sale (Appelbe and Wingfield 1994; Merrills and Fisher 1995). The least restrictive category is GSL, that is general sales list, available from pharmacies and other retailers. The presumption is that, GSL medicines are not likely to have serious adverse effects. They are fairly safe if taken in overdosage, or are sold in small quantities which are unlikely to cause severe toxicity. Remedies such as simple antacids and small quantities of the simple analgesics paracetamol and aspirin are in the category GSL; so too are preparations such as 'Labiton tonic', which contains vitamin B_1, caffeine, dried extract of kola nut and a small amount of alcohol. Such a preparation is unlikely to be very toxic, though it is unlikely to have a very wide therapeutic role, either.

Medicines in the category P can only be sold in pharmacies, but a prescription is not required to obtain them. 'Prioderm lotion', a preparation containing malathion, is a current example of a medicine in category P. It is used to treat infestation with headlice. Insulin preparations are also in legal category P, apparently so that there should be no difficulty in maintaining a patient's supply of the drug.

As a matter of policy, the number of medicines classified as P is set to increase, and in particular, many medicines previously classified as prescription-only medicines (POMs) are now available at pharmacies without the need for a prescription. Often, the quantity that can be bought is small, and the licence restricts the promotion of the P medicine more severely than the corresponding POM medicine. It is uncertain whether these changes will be beneficial (Ferner 1994).

Medicines which do not require a prescription, that is, preparations with GSL or P licences, are collectively known as *over-the-counter* medicines. They are listed in reference works (Cooper *et al.* 1992; Reynolds 1992). Many preparations used in conventional medicine can only be obtained against a prescription signed by a legitimate prescriber and presented to a pharmacist or dispensing medical practitioner. Registered medical practitioners can prescribe almost all these *prescription-only medicines* (POMs). Registered dental practitioners can prescribe from a smaller range of products, listed in the 'Dental Practitioners' Formulary' that is published as an appendix to the *British National Formulary (BNF)* (Prasad 1994). Midwives are allowed to administer some POM drugs on their own initiative, provided that they have the requisite training (Dimond 1994) and are now allowed to prescribe under the provisions of the Medicinal Products (Prescription by Nurses, etc.) Act 1992. This act also allows prescribing by certain other nurses. A *BNF* appendix lists drugs that can be prescribed by the small group of district nurses and health visitors who are involved in the nurses prescribing demonstration scheme (Prasad 1994). There may be further extension of prescribing rights, to clinical psychologists, for example (Wardle and Jackson 1995).

Examples of prescription-only medicines run from 'Accupro', a medicine containing the angiotensin converting enzyme inhibitor quinapril, to 'Zyloric', whose active ingredient is the drug allopurinol, used to prevent attacks of gout.

A patient can request an emergency supply of a prescription-only medicine from a retail pharmacist, who may dispense it, providing he (or she) has satisfied himself (or herself) after interviewing the patient that the medicine is needed immediately; that it would be impractical to obtain a new prescription without unreasonable delay; that the patient has previously been prescribed that medicine by a medical practitioner registered in the United Kingdom; and that the pharmacist can establish a safe dose to take. The pharmacist can only provide the patient with 5 days' supply for most drugs, though there are exceptions. The oral contraceptive pill, for example, can be supplied for a month.

Controlled drugs

Further restrictions on the prescribing and dispensing of dangerous drugs are laid down by the Misuse of Drugs Act 1971, and the Misuse of Drugs Regulations 1985 (Prasad 1994). The law requires that prescriptions for *controlled drugs* falling within schedules 2 and 3 of the Regulations as amended be written indelibly in the prescriber's own hand, stating the name and address of the patient, the form and strength of the preparation, the dose, and the total quantity to be dispensed in words and figures. The prescriber must also sign and date the prescription. Pharmacists may only dispense dangerous drugs against a valid prescription, and may not do so in any other circumstances.

The Act lays down five schedules of drugs. The precise arrangements under each schedule of the Act differ. Schedule 1 drugs have no place in therapy, and comprise agents such as lysergic acid diethylamide ('lysergide', LSD). Schedules 2 and 3 include opiates such as morphine and diamorphine, and also synthetic analogues such as pethidine, pentazocine and buprenorphine. Other drugs which can be abused, such as amphetamine and its derivatives, barbiturates, and cocaine, are also included. The principal distinction is that a register has to be kept of schedule 2 drugs, but not schedule 3 drugs. The *BNF* contains a list of drugs which are classified under the Misuse of Drugs Act 1971, or scheduled under the Regulations of 1985.

Limits on National Health Service prescribing

In Britain, only certain licensed drugs can be prescribed under the National Health Service. Other 'black-listed' drugs, or drugs on 'the limited list', must be dispensed against a private prescription. The rules are partly an attempt to limit National Health Service prescribing to preparations which might reasonably be expected to work, partly to reduce the range of drugs available in those classes in which there is a very wide choice of drugs with very similar therapeutic properties, and partly to save money. This last motive is especially clear where preparations can be prescribed under the National Health Service by approved name ('generically') but not by trade name as branded products. This is true for diazepam, known by the trade name 'Valium'.

The limited list can be confusing in action. A general practitioner may prescribe aluminium hydroxide mixture under the National Health Service, and the patient will receive it in the form of 'Aludrox', which cannot itself be prescribed. 'Fefol Z', a tablet containing ferrous sulphate, folic acid and zinc sulphate, is prescribable, but 'Fefol-Vit', which contains B- and C-group vitamins in place of zinc sulphate, is not prescribable under the National Health Service.

Drugs that have not been licensed, or have not been licensed for a particular indication, cannot be marketed for therapeutic purposes, but a practitioner can prescribe them. It would not be wise to do so unless there were reason to believe that they would benefit the patient. A manufacturer can provide drugs for clinical trials if a certificate of exemption ('CTX', clinical trials exemption) has been issued.

Homeopathic and herbal remedies

Homeopathic and herbal remedies are also dealt with by the Medicines Act. They have been considered on pp. 10–12

Disposing of medicines

Unwanted medicines are classified as 'controlled waste' under section 34 of the Environmental Protection Act 1990. The Act imposes duties on the holder, carrier, and disposer of such waste. It must be securely wrapped, and a transfer note has to be signed when the waste is transferred from one agent to the next. The carrier and the disposer are required to hold a licence (Green 1993).

> CASE 1.4 (GREEN 1993)
>
> A general practitioner handed over waste medicines to a pharmacist's assistant, who agreed to dispose of them safely, but simply put them into a local rubbish skip. The general practitioner was charged with failing to transfer the waste to an authorized person, failing to complete a transfer note, and failing to complete a consignment note. The general practitioner was formally cautioned; the pharmacist was fined £1000

1.2 Pharmacokinetics

Pharmacokinetics is the study of the fate of drugs in the body: their absorption, distribution, metabolism and excretion. It describes, for example, changes in the concentration of a drug in the blood or tissues with the passage of time. If the concentration in blood of a certain drug, administered in a specified dose by a given route, is known, it is possible to calculate the time of administration. In the same way, if the concentration in blood and the route and time of administration are known, the dose can be estimated. Here we will discuss and illustrate the terms used in pharmacokinetics.

1.2.1 The dosage of a drug

The effects of a drug on the body depend on how much is present. This relationship is not necessarily linear: twice as much drug does not always produce twice the effect. It may be that drinking a glass of wine makes one more agreeable, but drinking six glasses of wine at once is not likely to make one six times more agreeable.

The absolute amounts of drug needed to produce effects in the body vary over an enormous range. For example, the standard adult dose of the adsorbent activated charcoal, which is given to poisoned patients to prevent the poison being absorbed from the stomach, is 50 grams. By contrast, the starting adult dose of alfacalcidol, a synthetic compound related to vitamin D, is 500 nanograms, which is 100 000 000 times less.

A corollary of this wide range of dosage is that great care needs to be taken in writing and dispensing prescriptions to ensure that the patient is given the correct dose, and not many times too much or too little. Doctors have notoriously bad handwriting, and they, pharmacists, and nurses are often harassed and sometimes careless. Errors in dosage occur and can have serious results. They are the subject of Section 6.2.

1.2.2 Concentration

This simple concept is very useful. The *concentration* of a substance is the amount of it in a single unit of volume. The units of volume usually used in pharmacology are the litre or the millilitre (one-thousandth of a litre).

If the concentration of a compound and the total volume in which it is distributed are known, then the total amount of compound present can be calculated:

total amount = concentration (amount per unit volume) × total volume.

Details of calculations involving concentration are given in Appendix A.

The concept of concentration can be used to determine an unknown volume. A known amount of a substance is introduced into the unknown volume, and mixed so that the concentration is uniform. Measuring the concentration then allows the volume to be calculated. An example is given in Appendix A.

Concentrations are also important in chemical calculations, because chemical reactions take place between molecules in a fixed way. For example, one molecule of hydrochloric acid reacts with one molecule of sodium hydroxide, not two or two and a half molecules. The rate of a reaction also depends on the number of molecules present, so it too depends on the concentration of molecules.

1.2.3 Volume of distribution

It is often important to know the total amount of drug in the body, when the concentration in blood is known; or, conversely, to calculate the blood concentration that results from giving a specified dose of drug. This is possible if the volume of distribution is known.

The *volume of distribution* is the apparent volume which would contain the entire amount of drug in the body at the same concentration as it is present in the blood. It is as if the body were a bathtub. For example, if we inject 40 grams of a drug into the body (the bath), and the concentration of drug in blood (the bathwater) is 1 gram per litre, the volume of distribution (the volume of water in the bath) is 40 litres.

This volume is not the same for all drugs, and has to be found by experiment. Some drugs remain in the bloodstream, while others are distributed widely in the body. If all the drug is in the bloodstream, then the volume of distribution will be the same as the volume of blood in the body[3]. If most of the drug is in other parts of the body, such as fatty tissue, then the concentration in the blood will be low and the volume of distribution will be much larger than the circulating blood volume.

The volume of distribution varies between one individual and another, too, because body size and composition (for example, the ratio of fat to water) vary among individuals. This is partly allowed for by expressing the volume of distribution in litres per kilogram body-weight.

The volume of distribution can also be thought of as the ratio between the total quantity of drug in the body and the amount per unit volume of blood (see Appendix A).

A difficulty in understanding the concept of volume of distribution is that its value is often much higher than any physical volume of the body. For example, the measured volume of distribution of the antidepressant medicine amitriptyline is over 1000 litres in a man of average weight, whereas his physical volume is about 70 litres.

This apparent anomaly arises because many drugs are distributed preferentially to some tissues rather than others. It is as if the bathtub into which dye was poured contained a sponge which soaked up much of the dye, so that the concentration in the bathwater was much lower than if the bath contained only water.

Appendix A, Section A.3.2 gives an example illustrating the forensic value of calculations based on volume of distribution.

1.2.4 Drug disappearance

Drugs after administration usually reach the bloodstream either directly, if they are injected into a blood vessel, or indirectly after absorption from the gut or elsewhere. Exceptions are drugs, such as calamine lotion, whose actions are purely local.

A drug does not remain in the body forever after it has entered the bloodstream, but is subject to processes of removal. The simplest case to consider is the disappearance of drug from the blood after it has been injected directly into a vein.

What happens to the concentration of drug in the blood as time passes after injection? The fall in concentration usually follows one of two patterns. Either the concentration falls by a constant amount in a given time, or it falls by a constant proportion in a given time[4]. These two processes are called *zero-order* and *first-order* elimination, respectively, and we will consider each in more detail.

Zero-order drug elimination

Many drugs are altered in the body by biochemical processes catalysed by enzymes. Most drug-metabolizing enzymes are able to handle much larger concentrations of drug than are ever achieved, even after overdosage. Some, however, have only a limited ability to catalyse reactions, and soon reach their maximum capacity: they become saturated. Then, however much drug is in the bloodstream, the enzyme can only remove a constant amount in a given time, and the graph of concentration against time is a straight line.

The classical example of this pattern is ethanol. The first step in removal of ethanol from

---

[3] That is, about 5 litres in an adult.
[4] These can be compared with simple interest, where the capital investment grows by a fixed amount per annum; and compound interest, where the investment grows by a fixed percentage per annum.

the body is catalysed by an enzyme, alcohol dehydrogenase, which becomes saturated at very low blood ethanol concentrations, and then the amount of ethanol removed is constant. For most people, the rate of removal is between 12.5 and 25 milligrams per 100 millilitres of blood per hour. This means that it takes between 4 and 8 hours for the blood ethanol concentration in a 'standard' adult to fall from 100 milligrams per 100 millilitres of blood to zero (see pp. 121-5).

First-order drug elimination

The rates of many pharmacological processes vary with the concentrations of the substances involved. Usually, the rate of the process depends upon the (first power of the) concentration, and the process is said to follow *first-order kinetics*. When a drug behaves in this way, the rate at which its concentration falls from some high level is initially high, but as the concentration falls, so too does the rate at which the drug is removed, and the process becomes slower and slower. The concentration falls by a constant proportion in a fixed time.

A first-order kinetic process is one in which the rate of change in concentration varies as the concentration itself varies:

rate of change is proportional to concentration.

For example, the concentration of the pain-killing drug paracetamol falls by about 16 per cent per hour.

If the concentration of paracetamol in blood at some time is 100 milligrams per litre, then 1 hour later it will decrease (by 16 milligrams per litre) to 84 milligrams per litre. After a further hour, it will have fallen by 16 per cent of 84 (that is 13 milligrams per litre), to 71 milligrams per litre. When another hour has elapsed, the concentration will be 12 milligrams per litre (16 per cent) less, that is, 59 milligrams per litre, and after a further hour it will be down to 50 milligrams per litre. After 4 hours, therefore, the concentration has fallen by 50 per cent.

The time taken for the concentration of paracetamol to fall by half, the *elimination half-life*, $t_{1/2}$, = 4 hours. This means that if at some time the concentration is 200 milligrams per litre, then after four hours it will be 100 milligrams per litre, after a further 4 hours it will be 50 milligrams per litre, after 4 more hours, 25 milligrams per litre, and so on.

Saturable processes

Processes such as the metabolism of ethanol are considered as zero-order processes because the rate-limiting enzyme is *saturated*: it cannot work any faster even if the concentration of ethanol is increased. However, even the feeblest enzyme system will be able to respond to increases in substrate concentration (the concentration of the substance whose biochemical change is catalysed by the enzyme) if these are low enough: at very low concentrations the system exhibits first-order kinetics, and a gradual transition takes place to zero-order kinetics as the concentration increases. For ethanol, the transition occurs at concentrations well below those usually relevant to forensic work, or to social drinking. However, for some drugs the switch from first- to zero-order kinetics takes place at or near the therapeutic concentration. This is true for the metabolism (biochemical breakdown) of the anticonvulsant drug phenytoin. Saturable enzymes are described as showing *Michaelis–Menten kinetics*.

The importance lies in the effect of a change in dose on the blood concentration. When the enzyme is unsaturated, the kinetics are first-order, and twice the dose produces twice the blood concentration. However, when the system is saturated, a doubling of the dosage produces a much greater than proportionate increase in concentration. Phenytoin is difficult to use precisely because small changes in dosage can cause large changes in the blood concentration. It is correspondingly easy to increase the concentration above the therapeutic value and into the toxic range (see Section 1.3.3).

1.3 Pharmacodynamics

1.3.1 History

Pharmacodynamics is the science that examines the effects of drugs. Drugs do not have effects unless they can interact with the body: however effective a drug in theory, its efficacy while still in the bottle is zero. The mechanisms by which the interactions take place have been clarified over the past 125 years since Crum Brown and Fraser first suggested that for the Amazonian arrow poison curare and its derivatives there was a specific site at which the interaction between the drug and the organism took place. (They were absolutely right.) This work was followed by the observations of J. N. Langley that saliva flowed more freely in the cat in the presence of the drug pilocarpine, and that the flow was reduced by the drug atropine. He deduced that the drugs were able to exert opposite effects at the same site. (He was almost right[5].) By 1934, Sir Henry Dale and others had formulated and tested the theory that there was a specific 'receptive substance' for drugs such as acetylcholine, with which the drug combined according to well-known chemical rules, embodied in the law of mass action.

1.3.2 Sites of drug action

Receptors

Applying the law of mass action to the combination of a drug and its *receptor*, the current term for Dale's receptive substance, we can make a number of important deductions. The relationship between the logarithm of drug concentration and its binding to the receptor is a *sigmoid* (S-shaped) curve, which is straight between about 20 and 80 per cent of the maximum binding. Since the action of the drug is linked to its binding with the receptor, the curve also represents the relationship between log concentration and effect (Fig 1.1). If we are examining responses within the linear (straight-line) part of the curve, then doubling the log concentration causes a doubling of the effect. Note that doubling the log concentration is equivalent to squaring the actual concentration: for example, from 10 to 100 milligrams per litre.

Real receptors

The understanding of receptors and how they work has changed dramatically since the early 1980s. Most receptors are proteins, and many are very similar, with a portion which projects from the cell surface and acts as the specific recognition site for a particular molecule, a por-

---

[5] Pilocarpine prevents the breakdown of the nerve transmitter substance acetylcholine, and so prolongs and intensifies its effect. Atropine competes with acetylcholine at its site of action, and reduces its effect.

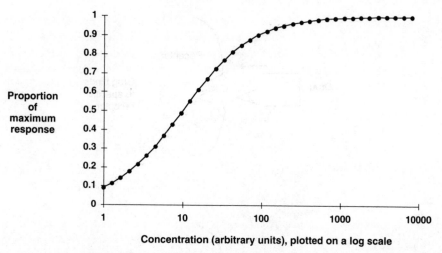

Fig. 1.1 A graph of the response, as a proportion of the maximum achievable response, plotted against the concentration of the drug, in some arbitrary units, on a logarithmic scale. The curve is practically linear between 0.2 and 0.8 of the maximum effect.

tion which sits in the cell membrane to anchor the receptor, and a portion which is inside the cell membrane and signals to the cell some change in the outside environment, such as a change in the extracellular concentration of adrenaline (Fig 1.2).

The number and function of the receptors are not static. In the presence of large quantities of agonist (a drug having a positive action at a particular receptor), the number or activity of the receptors can be reduced, a process called *down-regulation*. In the presence of an antagonist (a drug preventing a positive action at a particular receptor), the number or effectiveness of the receptor can increase, a process called *up-regulation*.

Other sites of action

The analysis of drug actions in terms of specific receptors has been very fruitful, but specific interactions between drugs and the body can occur at other sites.

Table 1.6. Examples of changes in enzyme function brought about by drugs

Enzyme	Drug	Comment on drug action
Angiotensin converting enzyme	Captopril	Inhibits production of aldosterone: lowers blood pressure
C_1-esterase inhibitor	Stanozolol	Induces enzyme activity
Cholinesterase	Neostigmine	Reduces breakdown of acetylcholine
Cyclo-oxygenase	Aspirin	Inhibits platelet function
Dopa-decarboxylase	Carbidopa	Stops peripheral dopa breakdown
Monoamine oxidase-A	Phenelzine	Reduces breakdown of noradrenaline and 5-HT
Monoamine oxidase-B	Selegiline	Reduces breakdown of brain dopamine
Sodium/hydrogen ATPase	Omeprazole	Reduces stomach acid production
Sodium/potassium ATPase	Digoxin	Indirectly increases contactility
Topoisomerase (DNA gyrase)	Ciprofloxacin	Inhibits bacterial reproduction
Xanthine oxidase	Allopurinol	Inhibits urate formation

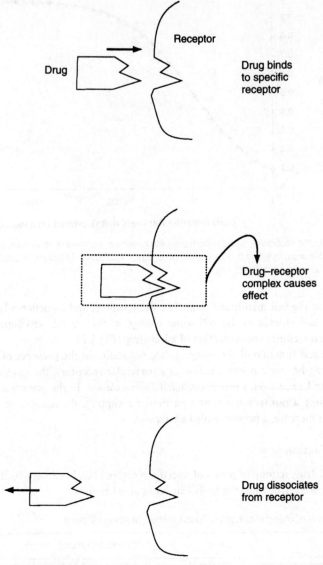

Fig. 1.2 Receptor–drug interactions. The drug fits into a specific receptor site, as a key fits into a lock. The change in the receptor brought about by drug binding causes some change or changes inside the cell. The drug later dissociates from the receptor.

Enzymes (biochemical catalysts) are the key elements in most of the biochemical processes in the body. Their function can be altered by drugs, and changes in enzyme function can have substantial, and sometimes desirable, effects. Examples are given in Table 1.6.

Other sites of action include the ion channels which regulate the movement of ions such as Na^+ and Ca^{2+} into and out of cells. The local anaesthetics, and antiepileptic and antiarrhythmic drugs commonly act at these sites. Some drugs do not have actions directed at specific sites but have rather non-specific physical effects. Osmotic laxatives, which simply carry water with them as they pass through the bowel, are one example. Another is provided by general anaesthetic gases, which appear to act by dissolution in the lipid (fatty) layer of the cell membrane.

1.3.3 Toxicity

Mae West is quoted as saying 'Too much of a good thing is ... wonderful', but this is rarely true for medicines. It is a rule of therapeutics that if a drug has any effect, then it will be capable of causing an undesirable effect. To reiterate Paracelsus's dictum, only the dose makes a poison, and all substances are poisonous in sufficiently large doses. An obvious example would be a beta-blocking drug. Such drugs slow the heart beat. This can be a good thing if the heart has a tendency to beat too fast. Usually, it is of little importance even if the drug is given for some other purpose such as reducing blood pressure or controlling migraine. However, the effect on the heart rate can be so pronounced that the heart is no longer able to pump round enough blood for the body's needs. This, coupled with a tendency for the drug to impair the strength of each heart beat, can cause the patient to develop heart failure.

Exactly the same problem can arise if a previously normal person takes tablets of a beta-blocking drug in an attempt at suicide: it is a problem of dose-related toxicity. This can be usefully represented by dose–response curves for the beneficial and toxic effects of a drug (Fig 1.3).

The greater the separation of the two curves, the safer the drug is in clinical use, because the clinical effect can more certainly be achieved without entering the toxic range. The ratio between the minimum effective dose and minimum toxic dose is called the *therapeutic index*. By their very nature, some drugs have very low therapeutic indices. This is especially true of drugs used to treat malignant diseases such as cancer and leukaemia, since they are required to kill the rapidly dividing tumour cells, but can also kill rapidly dividing normal cells in the bone marrow and gut. Their toxicity is so high that their use is limited by the toxic effects, and not by the dose required for efficacy.

Other treatments, for example treatment with oral penicillin (phenoxymethyl penicillin, penicillin V), rarely, if ever, cause serious dose-related toxicity in normal people, because the toxic dose is enormously higher than the effective therapeutic dose.

1.3.4 Adverse effects

Definitions

All drugs can have unwanted or unintended effects as well as their therapeutic effects, and toxic effects represent one aspect of this. Such unwanted or unintended effects as are due to the pharmacological properties of the drug and occur during or after treatment are called *side-effects*. This definition excludes such mishaps as cutting one's finger on the edge of the tablet box or slipping on a pill and breaking a leg. It might also exclude the potential danger of dextra-nomer beads which are sterile spherical beads of 0.1–0.3 millimetres diameter used to dress wounds. The Data sheet for this product (as 'Debrisan') warns that 'Debrisan spillage can render surfaces very slippery' and spillages should be cleared up promptly (ABPI 1993–4 *H*).

Side-effects are often, but not always, undesirable. An example of a side-effect which poses

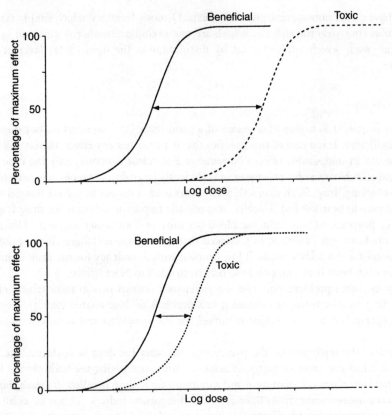

Fig. 1.3 Dose–response curves for a drug with a wide safety margin (above) and one with a narrow safety margin (below). For each drug, two curves have been drawn. One represents the percentage of maximum effect plotted against the logarithm of the dose for the beneficial (therapeutic) effect, and the other the same information for the toxic (adverse) effect. For the safer drug, the two curves are widely separated, but for the drug with a narrow safety margin, they run close together.

no threat to health is the change in colour of body fluids, including urine and tears, to a pinkish-orange colour during treatment with the antituberculous drug rifampicin. A potentially beneficial side-effect is the regrowth of scalp hair in bald men which can occur with the antihypertensive (blood-pressure lowering) drug minoxidil. That effect has now been exploited in the form of a minoxidil lotion promoted as a treatment for baldness. (The results are said to be disappointing.)

Some side-effects may be benign or even desirable, but many are malign and some are potentially or actually lethal. An *adverse reaction* to a drug is defined as 'a response to a drug which is noxious and unintended which occurs at doses normally used in man for the prophylaxis, diagnosis or therapy of disease or for the modification of physiological function' (WHO 1972). This definition is framed so as to include prophylaxis (preventive treatment), for example with vaccines, and diagnostic agents such as the radiopaque (X-ray opaque) dyes used to outline structures such as blood vessels during X-ray examinations. It also includes the oral contraceptive pill, whose function is to modify the normal physiology of women rather than treat them for any disease. It excludes toxic effects which are directly due to use or abuse of a drug in doses higher than those that are normally employed for therapy, and it also excludes undesirable consequences of the non-medical (ab)use of drugs.

Cause and effect

It is often difficult in an individual patient to establish that a particular drug or treatment is the *cause* of an untoward occurrence during or after the drug or treatment. The concept of *adverse event* has been introduced to circumvent this difficulty. An adverse event is any untoward medical occurrence that may present during [or after] treatment with a pharmaceutical product; there is not necessarily a causal relationship between the treatment and the untoward occurrence. This is not very satisfactory for the doctor, who may wish to alter a patient's treatment in the case of a true adverse reaction to it, but leave it as before if there is no causal link between treatment and occurrence. It is worse still for the lawyer who is interested in determining causation.

The difficulty is the result of the identity or similarity of drug-induced disease and naturally occurring disease. Examples of drug-induced disease so severe as to result in the withdrawal of a drug from the market include (Lawson, in Davies 1991*c*) Guillain-Barré syndrome[6] from the antiarthritis drug zimeldine, endometrial cancer from unopposed oestrogen replacement therapy, lactic acidosis from the antidiabetic agent phenformin and heart failure with the cardiac drug xamoterol. All the diseases that occurred with these drugs can also occur spontaneously in nature.

The connection between an agent and an adverse event can be particularly difficult to discover if the agent is used to treat an illness which is itself associated with the event, as is the case with the antiarrhythmic drug flecainide used to prevent sudden death after heart attacks, but which apparently increases the incidence of this very event.

A second difficulty in establishing causation is that adverse reactions are only likely to affect a minority of patients treated with a particular agent. There are both pragmatic and pharmacological reasons for this. The pragmatic reason is that adverse reactions which are both common and severe are likely to prevent a drug from being marketed. The pharmacological reason is that one subject can differ from another both in the handling of a given drug and the response to it. The factors determining these differences are discussed below. An additional problem arises because some adverse reactions occur long after exposure to the agent in question has ceased, and it is also possible for the reaction to be manifest not in the recipient, but in the offspring of the recipient.

It is likely that a drug caused a reaction if:

(1) the event occurred as or after the drug treatment was started;
(2) the event ceased when or after the drug treatment was stopped (known as *de-challenge*);
(3) the event recurred when the drug treatment was restarted (*rechallenge*);
(4) the event is known to occur in association with the drug;
(5) the event is not known to occur as part of the condition for which the drug was given.

However, only the first of these conditions is necessary and none of them is sufficient to prove causation.

---

[6] Guillain-Barré syndrome is an illness of ascending paralysis of the muscles; endometrial cancer is cancer of the lining of the womb; and lactic acidosis is an increase in the acidity of the blood caused by an abnormal build-up of lactic acid.

A series of rules has been formulated to clarify in a particular case whether an adverse event is or is not an adverse reaction. However, the rules are not very robust when applied to real data, and tend to yield different results in different hands, or even in the same hands on separate occasions (Karch *et al.* 1976).

Statistical problems in detecting adverse drug reactions

Important, well-recognized, and serious adverse reactions, such as death from anaphylactic shock after penicillin, are very rare. That particular reaction probably accounts for about 1 death in every 100 000 deaths in England and Wales. If this were not so, then safer alternative drugs would probably be used: chloramphenicol, which was estimated to cause bone marrow failure to one patient in every 50 000, is now used only rarely and for serious conditions such as meningitis (at least in the developed world). At the stage where a drug ceases to be 'experimental' and is granted a product licence, it has probably been tested in about 1500 people (Rawlins 1995). This makes it impossible to be sure at the time of licensing whether the drug can be responsible for a rare but potentially serious reaction: only the observation of much larger numbers of patients will reveal this. The difficulty of detecting an adverse reaction depends also on the background incidence of the event (Anonymous 1981; Stephens 1988). A huge study would be necessary to uncover a reaction such as myocardial infarction (heart attack) in a population treated for angina[7] and therefore at risk of myocardial infarction *ab initio*.

What is an acceptable risk in one disease, for example, meningitis, is not acceptable in another, for instance tonsillitis.

The classification of adverse reactions

It may seem surprising in the light of the foregoing considerations that any consensus has been reached on the existence of adverse reactions, but in practice there is a wide measure of agreement regarding common or severe adverse reactions to drugs which have been in widespread use for a number of years. These reactions tend to fall into a number of defined categories. Rawlins and Thompson (1991) originally designated reactions *type A* or *augmented* and *type B* or *bizarre*. This classification remains important, but can now be extended, as follows.

Type A, augmented, reactions

These are adverse reactions that are the consequence of the known or predicted pharmacological properties of the drug and are therefore dose-related. They represent an exaggeration of the normal response. An example of a type A reaction is the hypoglycaemia (abnormally low blood glucose concentration) that occurs from time to time in most diabetic patients treated with insulin. The blood glucose concentration in diabetic patients is abnormally high without insulin, and the intention is to reduce it to a normal level. The amount of insulin required to produce a satisfactory fall in glucose concentration can vary from time to time in the individual; for example, because of a change in food intake or of exercise. Hypoglycaemia results from overshooting the desired target.[8]

A further important example of a type A reaction is the abnormal bleeding that can occur

---

[7] Angina, more correctly *angina pectoris*, is pain, usually crushing in nature, due to insufficient oxygen supply to the heart.

[8] More details of insulin are given in Chapter 9.

with warfarin treatment (which is used to render the blood less coagulable, or in popular terms 'to thin the blood'). Warfarin is a drug with a low therapeutic index (see Appendix C, Section C.24), and the dose needed to cause catastrophic haemorrhage is only slightly greater than the dose necessary to cause a therapeutic prolongation of the prothrombin time (a measure of how easily the blood clots). Random fluctuation, small changes in the diet of an individual patient, and alteration to the treatment which the patient receives, can upset the balance between over- and under-anticoagulation and so have disastrous consequences, most notably serious haemorrhage.

Type A reactions are, in general, more likely and more serious for drugs that have a low therapeutic index. These include:

1. Anticancer drugs, which kill dividing cancer cells but also other dividing cells, especially the bone marrow cells that produce neutrophils (a type of white blood cell which is necessary to counter bacterial infection) and platelets (small elements in blood which are necessary to stop bleeding). Patients receiving such drugs are therefore prone to infections and to haemorrhage.
2. Anticoagulants such as warfarin, already discussed above.
3. Anticonvulsants, drugs used to suppress or control epileptic seizures, but capable of causing unsteadiness, loss of co-ordination, mental torpor, and other adverse effects related to dose.
4. Digoxin, a drug used to control the rhythm of the heart, but capable itself of causing unstable heart rhythms.

The aminoglycoside antibacterial agent ('antibiotic') gentamicin provides an example of a dose-related adverse effect which is well recognized, but which is not an exaggeration of the therapeutic effect. Gentamicin, and other aminoglycosides, can cause damage to the auditory nerve (responsible for hearing and balance).

Type B, bizarre, reactions

Rawlins and Thompson's type B, or bizarre, reactions are those which are not predicted from the pharmacology of the drug and occur sporadically and in a way that is not (clearly) related to the dose of the drug.

The classical type B reaction is the immediate hypersensitivity reaction in the form of anaphylaxis. This reaction can include sudden collapse, wheeze, urticaria ('hives'—itchy red lumps), and oedema (swelling), especially of the mouth, tongue, and larynx (*angioedema*, formerly angioneurotic oedema). In its most severe form it can cause death in a few minutes. The reaction is an extreme manifestation of allergy, the condition caused by an exaggerated or abnormal immune response to a stimulus that has already been previously encountered. In medicine, anaphylactic reactions are most commonly due to injected drugs, and especially occur with:

(1) penicillin and other antibiotics;
(2) foreign protein such as equine (horse-derived) antitetanus vaccine (now obsolete), equine antirattlesnake serum (still used), egg protein which can be present in certain vaccines, and the thrombolytic (clot-dissolving) enzyme streptokinase which is used to treat heart attacks;
(3) the iodine-containing radiopaque dyes used in radiology.

Type B reactions also include the idiosyncratic and often serious reactions that affect vital organs.

Damage to the liver, kidneys, and bone marrow can occur with, or after, a wide variety of drug treatments. A small number of the most well-recognized dangers is listed in Table 1.7. The standard reference works (D'Arcy and Griffin 1986a; Davies 1991a; Dukes 1992) list many more reactions and many more potential sites of drug-induced organ damage.

Type C, chronic treatment, reactions

The relative immediacy of type A and type B reactions can be contrasted with type C or chronic reactions that become apparent only during long-term treatment. 'Long-term' in this context can mean anything from a few days or weeks to many years. Examples of type C reactions include *iatrogenic* (doctor-induced) Cushing's syndrome. This is a disease induced by weeks or months of treatment with corticosteroid drugs. Features can include: obesity of the trunk, weakness and wasting of the proximal muscles, skin fragility, high blood pressure, diabetes mellitus ('sugar diabetes') and loss of bone density. These features also occur in Cushing's disease, which is due to a pathological oversecretion of the hormone cortisol (hydrocortisone) by the adrenal glands under the influence of an overactive pituitary gland.

Orofacial dyskinesia, a purposeless chewing and grimacing which follows years of treatment with the major tranquillizers such as chlorpromazine ('Largactil' or 'Thorazine'), is another example of a type C reaction (see Chapter 11).

Type D, delayed, reactions

Some reactions only become manifest many months or years after exposure has ceased, or cause illness in the next generation rather than in the patient who took the drugs. Such type D or delayed reactions include carcinogenesis—the promotion of cancers, and teratogenesis— the provocation of congenital malformations in the offspring of the drug-taker.

Cancer due to drugs has been most clearly evaluated in patients who have received anticancer agents for one condition and then go on to develop another malignant disease. The evidence is strongest against the anticancer drugs melphalan and nitrogen mustard (mustine). The anticancer drugs cyclophosphamide and chlorambucil interfere with dividing cells, and can cause chromosomal damage which is the precursor of malignancy. It is likely that they, too, can cause new malignancies.

The drug stilboestrol (diethylstilboestrol, DES) occupies a special place, because it causes a rare cancer, clear-cell carcinoma of the vagina, in the daughters born to mothers treated with it in pregnancy. It therefore exhibits two delayed effects: it provokes cancer, and the effect is seen in the next generation.

The second-generation effects of DES are probably unique, and are only manifest many years after birth. Drugs can also have a devastating effect on the development of the fetus in the womb, and cause malformations in the child.

The most notorious case is that of thalidomide, which led to a heightened awareness of the dangers of drugs in general and the treatment of pregnant women in particular. It also led to an extremely lengthy and acrimonious law suit discussed in more detail in Section 6.1.1 (Sjöström and Nilsson 1972). Briefly, an epidemic of phocomelia (a type of limb deformity in which the limbs are present as rudimentary stumps with malformations of the digits) was

Table 1.7 Some well recognized idiosyncratic (Type B) adverse drug reactions

Liver disease induced by drugs

Drugs that can cause acute hepatic necrosis (liver cell death) include:
amitriptyline, desipramine, and imipramine (antidepressants), chloroform, halothane, and enflurane (anaesthetic gases), isoniazid (an antituberculous drug)

Drugs that can cause jaundice by intrahepatic cholestasis (blockage of bile flow in the liver) include:
chlorpromazine and other phenothiazines (major tranquillizers)
chlorpropamide, tolbutamide and glibenclamide (sulphonylurea oral antidiabetic agents)
erythromycin (an antibiotic) especially as the esteolate ester
flucloxacillin (an antibiotic)
oral oestrogens and androgens, including the combined contraceptive pill and oral anabolic steroids

Drugs that can cause chronic hepatitis (inflammation of the liver) or cirrhosis (irreversible liver scarring) include:
methotrexate (a drug that is used to treat cancer and also psoriasis and arthritis)
methyldopa ('Aldomet', an antihypertensive agent)

Renal disease induced by drugs

Drugs that damage the renal substance directly, to cause acute interstitial nephritis include:
allopurinol (used to treat gout)
mefenamic acid and other non-steroidal anti-inflammatory drugs
penicillin antibiotics (methicillin, the drug most clearly implicated, is no longer used clinically)
thiazide diuretics such as bendrofluazide

Drugs that cause acute tubular necrosis (damage to the microscopically small tubes that drain the urine from the kidney substance) include:
amphotericin (an antifungal antibiotic)
cisplatin (an anticancer drug)
gentamicin and other aminoglycoside antibiotics

Drugs that can block the tubules because they cause muscle breakdown and myoglobinuria (the presence of the muscle protein myoglobin in the urine) include:
amphetamine and its derivatives, including MDMA ('Ecstasy')
bezafibrate, clofibrate and fenofibrate (lipid lowering agents)
cocaine, including 'crack' cocaine

Drugs affecting the blood supply of the kidney include:
captopril and other angiotensin converting enzyme inhibitors (in the presence of renal artery stenosis)
cyclosporin
indomethacin and other non-steroidal anti-inflammatory drugs

Other drugs that cause renal problems include:
analgesic mixtures, such as aspirin, phenacetin, and codeine, which can cause renal papillary necrosis (a condition where the urine-collecting system of the kidney is severely damaged)
methysergide (used to prevent attacks of migraine) can cause retroperitoneal fibrosis (a disease where fibrous tissue surrounds the tubes draining the kidneys, and obstructs the flow of urine)
radiographic contrast media, which can cause acute renal failure
sulphonamide antibiotics, which can cause crystals to form in the urine

Drugs that can damage the bone marrow include:

anticancer agents such as cyclophosphamide and ifosfamide, azathioprine, and methotrexate
carbimazole and propylthiouracil (antithyroid drugs)
chloramphenicol (an antibacterial now usually reserved for the treatment of severe infection)
clozapine (an antipsychotic drug)
co-trimoxazole (an antibacterial) especially in the elderly
gold salts (used to treat rheumatoid arthritis)
penicillamine (used to treat rheumatoid arthritis)

noticed in Hamburg and other centres. Sometimes this was accompanied by other abnormalities. Phocomelia was previously so rare that it was unlikely that any general paediatrician would ever see even one case. Evidence linked the very rare deformity to the drug thalidomide, taken by the mother in the first trimester (3 month period) of pregnancy. The drug was removed from the market, and in 9 months the epidemic had ceased. It now has a very limited place in the treatment of severe reactions in leprosy and certain skin diseases. Cases of phocomelia have been reported recently from Brazil, where supplies of the drug are available for use in leprosy.

Since the thalidomide affair, efforts have been made to prevent unnecessary prescribing to pregnant women and to investigate any new drug for potential *teratogenicity* (the capacity to produce malformation in the baby after exposure as a fetus). Systematic studies in pregnant women have been conducted for only very few drugs, however, and so it is usual to assume that drugs are or may be unsafe in pregnancy. The Data sheet (ABPI, 1993-4*a*) for a licensed product will contain a statement on the safety of the product in pregnancy or lactation, but this is commonly non-committal: 'The safety of this product in pregnancy has not been established'. It is sometimes designed to shift the entire onus for any decision on to the prescriber: 'The product should not be used during pregnancy unless, in the opinion of the physician, the potential benefits outweigh any potential risks'. Since the risks are inevitably unknown, the physician is not in a position to provide an informed opinion.

However, the risks of malformation or disordered development are sufficiently high for some drugs to be accepted as teratogens. These include:

1. The derivatives of vitamin A used to treat skin conditions including severe acne. These cause extremely serious facial malformations in a high proportion of exposed infants, and so no woman taking them should conceive during treatment or for a period afterwards sufficiently long to ensure that all the drug has been eliminated from the body. This is up to 2 years for some members of this therapeutic class, namely etretinate and acitretin.
2. The anticancer drugs, especially the drugs such as methotrexate that inhibit the metabolism of folic acid.
3. Alcohol (ethanol), which is associated with low birth weight, a characteristic facial appearance, and mental retardation, even if exposure occurs late in pregnancy.
4. Cocaine, which has been linked with malformations of the heart and nervous system.
5. The angiotensin converting enzyme inhibitors such as captopril, enalapril and lisinopril, which cause a rare skull defect and can also cause kidney failure in the newborn after exposure in late pregnancy.
6. The anticonvulsant drugs phenytoin, primidone, sodium valproate and carbamazepine, especially in combinations of two or more drugs. The risk is not so high that the treatment should be stopped, but it should be minimized by reducing the number of drugs used as far as possible.

A delayed effect that has only recently become apparent is the transmission of so-called *prion* diseases. These are illnesses due to proteins that have some of the properties of viruses, most notably their transmissibility and their ability to replicate inside mammalian cells. One of the diseases that is likely to be due to such particles is bovine spongiform encephalopathy (BSE, 'mad cow disease'). A human analogue of that disease is called Creutzfeldt-Jakob disease, and takes the form of a rapidly progressive dementia accompanied by increasingly severe and widespread neurological damage leading to death.

Creutzfeldt-Jakob disease has been transmitted to patients treated with products that have come from post-mortem tissue of others who have died undiagnosed. This has been seen in patients having injections of growth hormone extracted from human pituitary glands, of which large numbers are needed to prepare each batch. (Human growth hormone is now made synthetically). It has also occurred after corneal transplantation.

Type E, end-of-treatment, adverse effects

Type E adverse effects are seen at or after the *end of treatment*. They are the result of processes of adaptation to the presence of a drug over weeks, months or years. Withdrawal effects are particularly recognized with prolonged courses of:

(1) clonidine (an antihypertensive medicine), whose withdrawal can cause catastrophic hypertension ('rebound' hypertension);
(2) atenolol and other beta-blocking drugs used to treat angina, whose abrupt withdrawal can cause unstable (crescendo) angina;
(3) diazepam and other benzodiazepines used to treat anxiety or sleeplessness, often causing rebound anxiety and insomnia after treatment ceases;
(4) prednisolone, hydrocortisone, and other corticosteroids, which suppress the production of adrenocorticotrophic hormone (ACTH) by the pituitary gland and so remove the stimulating effect of ACTH on the body's production of hydrocortisone (cortisol); lack of cortisol can lead to collapse and inability to withstand shock;
(5) antidepressants, especially fluoxetine and other selective serotonin-reuptake inhibitors (SSRIs), whose withdrawal can cause a recurrence of depression, or feelings of anxiety;
(6) drugs of addiction, including ethanol (ethyl alcohol), amphetamines, and opiates, where abrupt cessation of intake can cause physical 'abstinence syndromes' and psychological craving.

It would be unwise to stop prolonged courses of any of these medicines suddenly unless the danger was recognized and allowed for.

Susceptibility to adverse reactions

Some individuals suffer adverse reactions to drugs which are innocuous in others. The factors which influence individual susceptibility to drug-induced adverse effects have gradually become clearer.

Some of the differences are genetically determined. Treatments cause different effects in groups with different *phenotypes* (genetically distinct forms which lead to observable differences in form or function). Phenotypic difference is the result of differences in *genotypes* (distinguishable genetic forms), though not all genotypes lead to distinct phenotypes.

One group of such defects causes differences in the metabolism (biochemical breakdown) of drugs, so that the concentrations after a standard dose of drug can differ greatly between groups with different phenotypes.

Oxidative metabolism

CASE 1.5 (LAURENCE AND BENNETT 1992*A*)

A professor of biochemical pharmacology (Professor R. L. Smith) took for the purposes of an experiment the comparatively small dose of 40 milligrams of the antihypertensive agent debrisoquine. His blood pressure fell to 70/50 (about half the normal value) and he was unable to stand for the next 4 hours. His subsequent investigations showed that debrisoquine is usually metabolized (broken down in the body) by an enzyme which he, in common with 10 per cent of the British population, lacked because of genetically determined differences from the remaining 90 per cent.

The particular enzyme deficiency which Professor R. L. Smith suffered is important in predisposing to dose-related drug reactions to debrisoquine, because the blood concentration of the drug is much higher in those who are enzyme deficient than in those who are able to break down the drug effectively.

The specific enzyme involved, one of the cytochrome oxidases whose gene is designated *CYP2D*, is also responsible for the metabolism of drugs such as metoprolol and timolol (beta-blocking drugs used in the treatment of angina and hypertension), and the antidepressant nortriptyline. Slow metabolizers of these drugs are inevitably at risk of dose-related adverse effects.

Acetylation

N-acetyltransferase, the enzyme responsible for the acetylation of drugs, can also be genetically deficient. Drugs metabolized by this enzyme, such as isoniazid (an antituberculous drug), hydralazine (an antihypertensive agent) and procainamide (an antiarrhythmic agent) are all more likely to cause adverse effects that depend on the concentration of parent (unmetabolized) drug in patients who are slow acetylators.

Cholinesterase deficiency (pseudocholinesterase deficiency)

The neurotransmitter acetylcholine carries the stimulus from nerves to muscles to cause contraction. It is destroyed by the enzyme acetylcholinesterase. Related drugs such as succinylcholine (suxamethonium, 'Scoline') are used to paralyse muscles during surgery. They are broken down by an enzyme in plasma called plasma cholinesterase (formerly called pseudo-cholinesterase). The usual form of the enzyme E^UE^U hydrolyses succinylcholine in a matter of minutes. Very rarely, subjects are homozygous for the 'silent' gene, E^SE^S, which codes for a protein without cholinesterase activity, and so unable to break down succinylcholine. The result is that paralysis with succinylcholine in such patients is very long-lasting, and they are unable to breath spontaneously for hours after standard doses of the drug. There is an intermediate form of defect due to the inheritance of one E^S gene and one E^U gene; and certain other forms of the gene are also recognized. These include a form that codes for an abnormally active enzyme that hydrolyses succinylcholine so fast that the drug fails to induce muscle paralysis at all.

These genetic differences lead to changes in the concentration of the drug involved, but others can result in differences in response independent of the metabolism of the drug.

Red cell enzyme defects

Red blood cells contain the oxygen-carrying pigment haemoglobin. It contains iron as Fe^{2+}. Pigment in which the iron has been oxidized to Fe^{3+} (methaemoglobin) is less efficient than haemoglobin at carrying oxygen. The red cell membrane is also liable to disintegrate under oxidative stress. Enzymes inside the red cell protect it from oxidants. The principal enzyme is glucose-6-phosphate dehydrogenase (G6PD), whose inheritance is X-linked (carried through the phenotypically normal mother to the children and affecting on average half the male off-spring, while half the female offspring can transmit the disease to the next generation). There are many distinct genotypes of G6PD: McKusick (1992) lists over 250 forms, from G6PD AACHEN to G6PD ZHITOMIR. There are many phenotypes with different degrees of impairment. Males with the worst forms are liable to suffer episodes of haemolysis (break-down of red cells) when exposed to a wide range of oxidants, including aspirin; quinine and its derivatives, particularly primaquine (used to treat malaria); and dapsone (used to treat leprosy). The deficiencies are most commonly found in Mediterranean, African and South-East Asian patients.

A clinical problem arises when a woman who is (potentially) a carrier of G6PD deficiency is pregnant and requires treatment for malaria: if the fetus is male, then there is a chance that it will manifest the enzyme defect and suffer haemolysis. Primaquine is best avoided in this situation until after the sex of the fetus is known, commonly at birth!

Acute intermittent porphyria

This is an autosomal dominant condition (it can be inherited by offspring of either sex from either parent, and on average half the offspring will be affected). The basic biochemical defect is a deficiency in activity of the enzyme uroporphyrinogen synthase (porphobilinogen de-aminase) which is necessary for synthesis of the red cell pigment called haem. Intermittent attacks of pain, paralysis, and psychosis with hypertension occur when excess porphyrin pre-cursors, no longer metabolized by uroporphyrinogen synthase, build up and also spill over into the urine. The attacks can be provoked by drug treatment with a huge variety of agents, including barbiturates, the oral contraceptive, and the anticonvulsants phenobarbitone, phenytoin, and carbamazepine.

It is unsafe to prescribe any drug to a patient with the condition, but guidance should be sought from specialists, such as the Porphyria Research Unit at the Western Infirmary, Glasgow, as to which drugs are likely to be least unsafe.

Malignant hyperpyrexia (hyperthermia of anaesthesia)

This autosomal dominant disorder is manifest by crises of muscle rigidity, hyperpyrexia (extremely high fever), and rhabdomyolysis (muscle breakdown) in response to general anaes-thesia. The first reported family had 38 members, of whom 11 died after a general anaesthetic. It may affect as many (or as few, depending on viewpoint) as 1 in 15 000.

Emergency treatment with the drug dantrolene, which blocks muscle activity by limiting the transport of calcium into muscle, can be life-saving. In consequence, supplies of dantro-lene should be immediately available where general anaesthetics are given.

These and related genetic differences can be responsible for serious and apparently idiosyn-cratic drug reactions, and the problems are sufficiently well-known that all prescribers should be aware of them. It would probably be negligent to administer a general anaesthetic to a patient whose family history included anaesthetic deaths without further consideration.

SMON

As with genetic differences within a population, so genetic differences between populations can lead to differences in responses to drugs. The drug clioquinol ('Entero-Vioform') was associated with a syndrome (a group of clinical features) which included abdominal pain, tingling in the limbs, and optic atrophy (degeneration of the optic nerve which is essential for vision). The neurological features led to the name *subacute myelo-optic atrophy*, commonly abbreviated to SMON. The drug was used throughout the world, but SMON occurred almost exclusively in the Japanese: over 7000 cases were seen in Japan whereas only 200 were reported from the whole of the rest of the world (Mann 1986) (Section 6.1.5).

Ethanol (ethyl alcohol, 'alcohol') metabolism

Ethanol is metabolized first by alcohol dehydrogenase to acetaldehyde and then by acetaldehyde dehydrogenase to acetate. Oriental groups, notably the Japanese and Chinese, have impaired alcohol tolerance, and about 80 per cent of Japanese develop facial flushing after small quantities of ethanol. This latter feature is thought to be the result of low acetaldehyde dehydrogenase activity.

Differences in age and in sex can also affect responses to drugs and modulate the occurrence of adverse effects. The drug metoclopramide, which is used to treat nausea and vomiting, can cause a bizarre reaction in which the muscles become stiff, trismus (involuntary clenching of the jaw) occurs, the back arches and the eyes turn upwards. This so-called dystonic extra-pyramidal reaction occurs so commonly in children below the age of 15 years that the Data sheet specifically advises against the use of metoclopramide ('Maxalon') tablets in children (ABPI 1993-4 f).

Some adverse effects are by their very nature only manifest in patients of one sex. A classical example is the occurrence of the very rare condition of clear-cell carcinoma of the vagina in the daughters of women who had taken the synthetic oestrogen stilboestrol during pregnancy to treat threatened miscarriage (p. 30).

Susceptibility to adverse reactions can be influenced by disease. This is clearest for liver or kidney disease which impairs the ability of the body to metabolize or excrete drugs, and so increases the likelihood of dose-dependent adverse effects. Other more arcane examples include the high risk of a morbilliform (measles-like) rash if the antibiotic ampicillin is given to patients with infectious mononucleosis (glandular fever); and the risk of worsening myasthenia gravis (a muscle disease) by administration of aminoglycosides.

2

Analyses of drugs and drug concentrations in blood and other body compartments

The forensic pharmacologist is constrained to provide his opinion on the basis of the information he has about a case. The more information, the more he can usefully say. At one extreme, he may be asked whether any drug could possibly have caused a series of events. At the other extreme, there will be several measurements of drug concentration to help in estimating times, doses, and possible effects. Tests to detect drugs, and to measure their concentrations, are extremely important. Their limitations are also important. The methods and their pitfalls are discussed here.

2.1 Samples and sample collection

The volume of blood in the circulation is said to have been first determined by collecting the blood from felons who had been executed by decapitation. It is unusual now to determine the amount of substance in the body so directly.

It is usually necessary to take a sample of the whole and to determine the presence or measure the amount of a drug in that sample. Samples of blood, urine, and breath are all used routinely, and in some circumstances the saliva, the cerebrospinal fluid which bathes the brain, and other fluids or tissues can be used.

The usefulness of an analytical result depends on the nature of the sample, the care with which it is taken and stored, and the skill with which it is analysed.

2.1.1 Blood samples

Blood samples in life are usually collected from the veins of the arm, using a hypodermic needle and syringe or vacuum collecting bottle which attaches to the needle. The skin over the vein is still commonly cleaned with isopropyl alcohol (isopropanol) or sometimes iodine or chlorhexidine. The needles are usually made of stainless steel and the syringe of transparent plastic. This occasionally introduces difficulties, as for example when blood samples are required to test for metals such as chromium or nickel which can be present in the stainless steel. If isopropanol used to clean the skin is not allowed to evaporate, then the sample can be contaminated with the isopropanol. This can subsequently cause problems for the analyst seeking volatile substances, including ethanol (Walls and Brownlie 1985g).

Other difficulties can sometimes be encountered. The antianginal drug nifedipine is very sensitive to daylight, and quantitatively reliable samples can only be obtained in the dark or by the light of a sodium lamp.

2.1.2 Contamination of samples

There are many ways in which samples can be contaminated accidentally at the time they are taken.

A real danger in sampling from patients in hospital is that the blood is taken from a site downstream of an intravenous cannula, a tube which carries fluid used for treatment into the vein. The composition of the blood is bound to be altered by the addition of such intravenous fluid, and accurate results can only be obtained from a remote site. The result from a sample contaminated with intravenous fluid can be misleadingly low, if the drug has been diluted with drug-free fluid, or misleadingly high if the intravenous line has been used to give the drug which is to be analysed.

When post-mortem samples are taken, they can be contaminated by soiling with the contents of hollow organs such as the stomach or bladder, or by the use of unclean instruments, or by contact with disinfectant, embalming fluid, or other extraneous material (Fig. 2.1).

CASE 2.1 (MORITZ 1981)

A woman was splashed with cyanide and died. It was impossible for the prosecution to prove that the cyanide had been absorbed, because tissue samples were taken with the instruments that had been used to dissect the skin that had been splashed with cyanide. The defendant was acquitted. (The events took place in the United States.)

The Association of Clinical Pathologists has published important guidelines on obtaining samples at post-mortem (Forrest 1993).

2.1.3 Blood sampling sites

Blood samples are not all equal, and it will sometimes happen that a sample is inadvertently taken from an artery rather than a vein. The difference between arterial and venous blood is greatest for oxygen content, as might be expected. However, the concentrations of some other substances, such as glucose, also show an arteriovenous difference.

2.1.4 Changes in drug concentrations after death

The difference in drug concentration in blood samples from different sites is a much more severe problem after death, and in general, blood concentrations after death cannot be interpreted from a knowledge of concentrations in life. This is because in life drugs are distributed to different tissues in the body and differences in concentration between tissues can be built up and maintained. Active processes which are responsible for maintaining concentration differences cease after death, and concentrations can change dramatically. For example, the ion potassium, which is predominantly held inside cells during life, leaks out of the cells into the plasma after death (see Chapter 10).

CASE 2.2

A boy aged 7 weeks was admitted to hospital with a severe chest infection, and collapsed. Although he was initially resuscitated, he had apparently sustained irreversible brain damage, and died 10 hours after the collapse. Some 25 minutes after death a blood sample was taken which showed a plasma potassium concentration of 8.2 millimoles per litre, approximately twice normal. Neither prosecution nor defence experts were willing to accept that this was evidence of potassium poisoning, and the time between the collapse and the sampling also made it difficult to argue that the collapse was due to potassium poisoning.

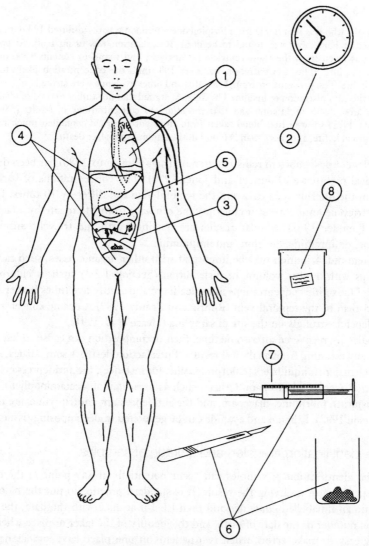

Fig. 2.1 Areas of difficulty with post-mortem samples for drug analysis. 1, the results depend on the sampling site; 2, the time after death is important; 3, gore that collects in the abdominal cavity is not suitable for quantitative analysis; 4, samples of urine and liver tissue can be helpful; 5, stomach contents should be saved in their entirety; 6, contamination of instruments is a source of inaccuracy; 7, volumes of sample should be adequate; 8, samples should be stored in correctly labelled bottles containing the requisite preservatives, securely sealed, and maintained at the correct temperature.

The changes in the blood are not necessarily uniform. Concentrations in venous blood after death are expected to vary according to the tissues whose blood they drain. Blood in the right ventricle (lower heart chamber) drains from the liver and other body tissues and is likely to differ systematically from the blood in the left ventricle, which drains the lungs.

CASE 2.3

A baby girl who was sent home from hospital one afternoon was re-admitted 12 hours later having collapsed at home, but was found to be dead. Resuscitation was to no avail. At post-mortem, blood was taken from the right ventricle for analysis, and found to contain 9 660 milliUnits of insulin per litre. This concentration was over 100 times the concentration likely to have been found in life. The prosecution argued that this and other evidence were strongly in favour of murder by the administration of insulin. The defence argued that no studies existed of insulin concentration after death in infants, and that the study of concentrations in adults (Lindquist and Rammer 1975) showed that blood taken from the right ventricle contained much more insulin than normal in life, and more than is found in the femoral vein after death.

The problem of post-mortem redistribution of drugs (Rouzioux 1980) has been described as 'a toxicological nightmare' (Pounder and Jones 1990). The concentrations of barbiturate in samples from the inferior vena cava and the femoral vein can differ by 10 times. Concentrations of the tricyclic antidepressant amitriptyline can vary from site to site by a factor of four (Jones and Pounder 1987). Similar results are obtained with the tricyclic antidepressants clomipramine, desipramine, doxepin, and imipramine.

Post-mortem redistribution may be important with other organic bases, such as fluoxetine, and for drugs with a large volume of distribution (Section 1.2.3) such as chloroquine and amiodarone. Fluoxetine concentrations after death are apparently five times higher in the pulmonary vein than in the femoral vein (Rohrig and Prouty 1989). Cocaine concentration after death also depends strongly on the site of sampling (Hearn *et al.* 1991).

When bodies are recovered after some time, their decomposition can cause added difficulties in wringing any meaning from analytical results. Putrefaction destroys some drugs, such as the phenothiazine major tranquillizers (chlorpromazine, for instance), the antidepressant dothiepin, and the benzodiazepine nitrazepam. Others, such as paracetamol (acetaminophen), salicylates (including aspirin), morphine, diazepam, and the antidepressant amitriptyline, are much more stable (Paterson 1993). Ethanol and cyanide can be generated in decomposing tissue.

2.1.5 The identification, transfer, and storage of samples

Errors in the identification of samples can occur potentially at any point in the chain from taking the specimen to notifying the result. It is standard practice to put the blood or other specimen into an unlabelled container and then label it at once with the date, the name, the identification number or the date of birth, and the identity of the taker or place where taken. It is especially easy to make errors when two patients in one place have similar names. Self-adhesive pre-printed labels are now widely used, but care is required to make sure that the patient from whom the sample was taken is the patient whose label is attached to the bottle.

The standard blood bottles, which hold 5 or 10 millilitres of blood, can contain a variety of preservatives or anticoagulants for different purposes. Those most commonly used are colour coded to help identify the preservative. Some commonly used codes are shown in Table 2.1.

Table 2.1. Colour codes commonly used to identify blood-sample containers in Britain

White top	No preservative
Orange top	Tube is coated with heparin
Pink top	Crystals of potassium edetate (EDTA)
Yellow top	Crystals of sodium fluoride/potassium oxalate
Purple top	Solution of potassium edetate

There is a danger of inadvertently placing the sample in the wrong container, realizing the error, and then decanting it into the correct container, so that the sample is contaminated or altered by the additive present in the original tube.

CASE 2.4

A laboratory biochemist argued that a blood sample, from a child who collapsed, showing the potassium concentration to be 16 millimoles per litre must have meant that the baby had been given potassium. He was confronted with the result from an apparently healthy child, showing a potassium concentration of 27 millimoles per litre. He explained that doctors who mistakenly put blood for potassium estimation into yellow-topped tubes for glucose analysis then sometimes poured the blood into the correct tube but did not inform the laboratory. The yellow-topped tube for glucose analysis contains crystals of potassium oxalate.

Blood is made up of two principal components, the straw-coloured liquid called plasma, and the red cells. If blood is allowed to clot, the red cells form a mass bound together with the protein called fibrin, and the serum, that is, the plasma less fibrin, can be separated by centrifugation. If an anticoagulant such as heparin is added to the blood, then it will not clot and the plasma can be separated from the red cells without delay.

Drug concentrations can be analysed in whole blood, serum, or plasma, or, rarely, in red cells. The concentration inside and outside the red cells can differ, as we have seen with potassium. This gives rise to a potential error if the separation of red cells from plasma or serum is delayed, because the metabolic processes necessary to maintain the concentration differences gradually wane. The membranes of the red cells are also rather fragile, and can leak as time goes on, releasing constituents of the cell into the plasma. Red cells are able to metabolize (break down) some chemicals, and so delay in separation or assay can give misleadingly low results. Glucose is an example of such a substance, whose metabolism by red cells continues after a blood sample has been taken.

Storage of samples can also introduce errors because of metabolism, or because drug or sample is lost by evaporation. (Brown *et al.* 1973) examined the stability of samples for ethanol estimation under different conditions of storage, and found that samples stored for extended periods were largely protected by low temperatures (1 °C rather than 17 °C) and the presence of adequate amounts of sodium fluoride. Otherwise, losses were considerable.

Blood samples for ethanol analysis kept at room temperature in sealed, evacuated tubes ('Vacutainers') containing fluoride preservative were examined after several years. The median loss was 40 milligrams of ethanol per 100 millilitres of blood, although some samples had lost as much as 80 milligrams per 100 millilitres (Chang *et al.* 1984). The legal limit for driving in the United Kingdom is 80 milligrams per 100 millilitres.

Tubes that are stored in a refrigerator at 4 °C, and contain sufficient fluoride, can be opened several times without appreciable loss of ethanol over 3 months (Somogyi *et al.* 1986).

It cannot be assumed that samples will have been stored adequately.

2.2 Analytical methods

Analytical methods are *qualitative*, that is, they say what substance or substances are present, or *quantitative*, that is, they estimate how much of a substance is present. Qualitative methods implicitly suggest the lowest amount of a substance that could be present, since below some threshold, which is in general a property of the method and of the substance, its presence remains undetected. Qualitative methods are of help in forensic pharmacology if the mere presence of a drug can be taken as demonstrating that something untoward has happened.

CASE 2.5

A 15-month-old girl was admitted to hospital with severe asthma. She collapsed unexpectedly and died in spite of prolonged attempts to restart her heart. A nurse who had been present at this and other similar events was committed for trial[1]. At a late stage in the proceedings, a sample of blood from the child was found to contain the drug lignocaine at a concentration of 1 milligram per litre.

This low concentration suggested that a rather small dose of the drug had been given during the resuscitation. This was feasible because the drug is used to stabilize heart rhythm in just such circumstances. At trial, the consultant paediatrician in charge of the resuscitation and other doctors involved in it all categorically denied using lignocaine. This meant its presence could only indicate a mistaken or murderous injection of the drug.

The nurse was convicted of murdering the child.

Sometimes, the methods can be applied indirectly. A bizarre example is illustrated by the following case:

CASE 2.6 (KINTZ ET AL. 1990)

The putrefied corpse of a man was found in Alsace. The body was infested with hundreds of identical fly larvae. It was impossible to obtain bodily fluids for toxicological analysis but analysis of 100 larvae, thoroughly washed, showed the presence of the psychiatric drugs bromazepam (a benzodiazepine) and levomepromazine (a phenothiazine antipsychotic drug).

Quantitative methods are usually preferred because they may allow the estimation of doses and also some determination of the likely effects. However, the assumptions used to make calculations can be violated if the sampling occurs after death or if the sample is taken or stored with inadequate care. The more data that are available, the more likely it is that useful deductions can be drawn from them, so samples taken from the same site at different times, or from different sites at the same time, are especially useful.

2.2.1 Spectrophotometric methods

A spectrophotometer is an instrument that measures the amount of electromagnetic radiation (for example, visible or ultraviolet light), of a given wavelength or band of wavelengths, that passes from a radiation source, through a sample chamber, to the detector of the instrument. The instrument is able to detect a change in composition or concentration of the sample by a change in the amount of radiation measured by the detector: the more there is to absorb the radiation in the sample chamber, the less radiation is received by the detector.

Such instruments are usually able to scan through a range of wavelengths, measuring absorption continuously, and giving a 'spectrum', really a graph of the wavelength of radiation against the amount absorbed.

The electrons within atoms and molecules can absorb electromagnetic radiation and then store it as an increase in energy, which can be released at a later time. The pattern of absorption of ultraviolet and visible light depends on the way the electrons in the atom or molecule

[1] R. v. Beverley Gail Allitt.

are arranged. The pattern, the spectrum, is characteristic of the compound under test (Fig 2.2). Absorption of infra-red radiation depends on changes in the rotation and vibration of a molecule. These properties depend on the way groups of atoms, the so-called functional groups, behave. Commonly encountered functional groups in organic compounds include the —OH group which is characteristic of organic alcohols, the C=O group which occurs in ketones, and so on.

Spectrophotometric methods are important for identifying pure compounds, since the spectrum depends on the compound's structure, and for measuring the concentration of a

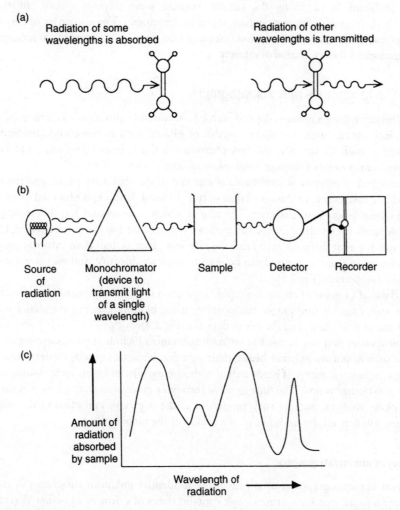

Fig. 2.2 Spectrophotometry. (a) A particular molecule will absorb radiation of some wavelengths, but transmit radiation of other wavelengths. (b) A spectrophotometer examines the transmission of radiation through a sample containing the molecule. The monochromator (which splits a mixture of wavelengths into its components) allows each of many wavelengths to be examined in turn. The signal produced by the detector is proportional to the amount of transmitted radiation. (c) A graph of the amount of radiation absorbed plotted against the wavelength of radiation is characteristic of the compound; and is commonly called a 'spectrum'.

known compound, since the absorption of a solution of the compound is proportional to the concentration of the compound in the solution. This property allows spectrophotometers to be used as the detectors for chromatographic systems that separate the components of mixtures very efficiently, as described below. They are able to make an analysis without damaging the sample, so that another procedure can be used subsequently; and the methods are well-tried, so that the spectra of most compounds of even remote interest will be available for comparison.

Spectrophotometric methods do not work very well with complex mixtures, since it becomes difficult to disentangle the spectra of several compounds measured together. There can be problems in preparing the sample, because some solvents absorb radiation very strongly in the region of interest, and are therefore unsuitable. The sensitivity of conventional spectrophotometric methods can be low, meaning that they can be incapable of measuring low concentrations of the compound of interest.

2.2.2 The techniques of chromatography

All chromatographic techniques depend on the behaviour of substances when they are allowed to come into contact with two distinct media, or phases, such as two immiscible liquids or a liquid and a solid. Commonly, the two phases are a fixed, immobile matrix, the *stationary phase*, over which moves a flowing *mobile phase* of liquid or gas.

A compound or mixture is introduced at one end of the stationary phase, and the distance travelled in a given time, or the time taken to travel a fixed distance, is observed by means of a suitable colour reaction or detector. The rate at which a compound travels through such a system depends on its affinities for the stationary phase and for the mobile phase. Different compounds travel at different rates, and the rate in a given system is an intrinsic property of the substance, so that the method can be used to separate, identify, and measure the concentrations of compounds (Fig 2.3).

The classical example of chromatographic separation is the resolution of black fountain-pen ink into orange, green, and purple components, using blotting paper as the stationary phase, water as the mobile phase, and the eye as detector (Fig 2.4).

The properties that can be used to separate substances include their adsorption on to inert matrices such as porous polymer beads; their partition between aqueous (watery) and organic (oily) phases, using a matrix of beads coated with silicone oils; and their ionic charge, using so-called ion-exchange resins. The time to move through a given stationary phase will vary as the mobile phase changes, because such properties as the degree of ionization of the compound under test will depend, for example, on the acidity of the mobile phase.

Thin-layer chromatography

Thin-layer chromatography is used principally to identify unknown substances or mixtures; for example, to see whether a urine sample contains traces of a drug of addiction. A rectangular glass or plastic plate is coated with a thin, even layer of a suitable stationary phase such as silica or starch. A spot of unknown substance or mixture is put at a known place close to the edge of the plate, and the edge is then dipped into a trough of a suitable solvent mobile phase, which is drawn across the plate by capillary action. As the solvent travels across the plate, the unknown substance is partitioned between the stationary and mobile phases in a way that depends on

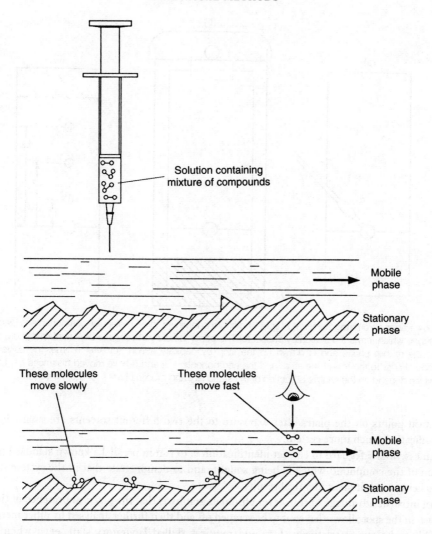

Fig. 2.3 Chromatography. All chromatographic systems consist of a stationary and a mobile phase. Molecules move through the system only if carried in the mobile phase. The speed of a molecule is characteristic, and depends on the relative attraction of the two phases for the molecule. Those molecules which are most attracted to the mobile phase move fastest.

both its physical and its chemical properties. A suitable developer can be applied to the plate to react with the unknown compounds and produce a coloured spot. The retention factor, R_f, which is the ratio between the distance travelled by the solvent front and the distance travelled by a compound under test, is characteristic of the compound under test.

There are some 5 million chemical entities, and a chromatographic spot may be half a millimetre in diameter, so that it is impossible to be certain that a unique assignment has been made by measuring one spot with one solvent system. To overcome this, the process can be carried out twice, using different mobile phases. The chances of two substances occupying

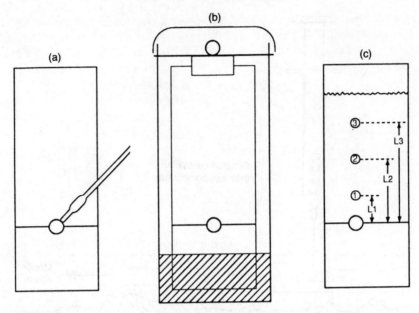

Fig. 2.4 Paper chromatography. (a) A spot of mixture containing three molecular components is placed on the paper, which forms the stationary phase. (b) The paper is held vertically in a tank containing solvent that forms the mobile phase and is drawn up the strip by capillary action. (c) After a time, the solvent has reached almost to the top of the strip, and the components 1,2, and 3 have moved distances L1, L2, and L3, which depend on the relative attraction of the stationary and mobile phases for the molecules.

identical points on the plates after exposure to the two different solvents are small, and the identification much more certain.

An essential safeguard to correct identification is to run in parallel a known standard preparation of the compound which is being sought, and to demonstrate that in the system or systems being used, it gives identical results.

An intrinsic advantage of thin-layer chromatography is that the physical presence of the unknown in the spot allows that spot to be scraped off and then further analysed by other methods.

This technique is relatively slow, and requires skilled laboratory staff, even when using commercial equipment such as the 'Toxi-Lab' system. The separation of opioid drugs by this commercial system has been discussed critically in the literature (Jarvie and Simpson 1986; Nadkarni *et al.* 1987; Dawling and Widdop 1988; Simpson *et al.* 1989). The lowest concentration of drug detected by this method is around 1 milligram per litre. Many drugs, including some drugs of abuse, are pharmacologically active at concentrations lower than this.

Gas chromatography (gas–liquid chromatography)

Gas chromatography depends on the behaviour of volatile substances as they are carried by an inert gas, such as helium or nitrogen, over a stationary phase, of very fine, inert, porous beads coated with a non-volatile liquid such as silicone oil, or over the walls of a coated fine-bore capillary tube.

The beads are packed into a tube, or column, 1-2 metres long, and a few millimetres in diameter. The column is held in an oven to maintain it at a temperature that is high enough to ensure that the compounds under test remain in the vapour state. A solution containing the volatile compound is injected at the head of the column, where it is heated and vaporizes. The sample vapour is swept over the liquid that coats the stationary phase, and dissolves in the liquid, returns to the gas, and redissolves many times during its passage along the column. Typically, the process takes place 6000–8000 times, and so any minor differences in the rate or duration of the dissolution are correspondingly magnified, and very similar compounds can be separated.

On arrival at the far end of the column, the volatile compound can be detected by one of a variety of techniques, which depend on the chemical, thermal and ionic properties of the compound. Most such detectors are relatively non-specific, and many different compounds will produce a signal as they pass over the detector. This is a substantial disadvantage where a compound has to be identified unequivocally. The problems are made worse in forensic work because the mixture applied to the column can contain metabolites (breakdown products) of the parent compound, other drugs and their metabolites, or products of putrefaction.

One way to overcome the problem of rather low specificity is to re-run the chromatogram, using different conditions, and to compare the behaviour of the unknown and an authentic sample of the compound in question.

A powerful method for determining the identity of a compound separated by gas chromatography uses as a detector a device called a mass spectrometer. This is an instrument for separating fragments of molecules according to their mass and ionic charge, by means of a magnetic or electrostatic field. The pattern of fragments, which is deduced from the number, position and size of the peaks on a spectrum, is usually unmistakable. It is also extremely sensitive, and can detect nanogram quantities of a compound. A nanogram is one thousandth of a millionth of a gram. The mass spectrometer is only useful by itself, however, when the substance to be analysed contains just one or a few compounds, otherwise so many fragments are generated that identification is not possible. Combined with the gas chromatograph, it is an extremely powerful analytical device.

High-pressure (or high-performance) liquid chromatography (HPLC)

Gas chromatography requires that a compound or its chemical derivative be stable at the temperature needed to make it vaporize, and this places severe limitations on its usefulness. In HPLC, samples have to be soluble, but they do not have to be volatile, and the system usually operates at room temperature. The mobile phase is a solvent which is pumped under high pressure through a column which is usually about 25 centimetres long and a few millimetres in diameter, and tightly packed with a stationary phase of spherical beads a few micrometres in diameter. It then passes through a detector (Figs 2.5, 2.6). Ultraviolet detectors measure the absorption of ultraviolet light at some pre-set wavelength. Electrochemical detectors are sensitive to the oxidation or reduction of chemicals. Infra-red detectors which allow for absorption by the solvent, and employ the computing technique of fast Fourier transform to analyse signals from a broad band of infra-red frequencies, can also be used.

2.2.3 Immunoassay

Proteins and some other chemicals are able to provoke immune reactions in mammals, and such chemicals are called antigens. The mammalian immune system recognizes antigens as

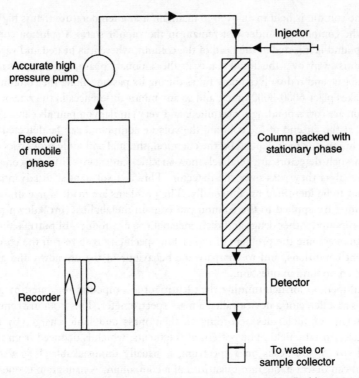

Fig. 2.5 High pressure liquid chromatography (HPLC). The mobile phase is a liquid, pumped at a carefully controlled rate through a thin column packed with the stationary phase. Sample is injected on to the top of the column and molecules in the sample travel through the column to the detector at a rate that depends on the relative attraction of solid and mobile phases for the molecule.

'foreign' to the body by their chemical structure, and a class of white blood cells called B lymphocytes can produce molecules which will bind to the chemically distinct region of a 'foreign' antigen. These molecules are called antibodies. The antibodies have specialized binding domains which are bound to regions of the antigen rather as a lock and a key fit together. The reactions are not altogether specific, since the region of an antigen responsible for binding can be a small or non-specific part of the molecule, shared with other molecules.

Antigen-antibody reactions form the basis for extremely sensitive assays, called *immunoassays*. The classical form of immunoassay is the competitive radioimmunoassay. It requires an antigen which can be made to contain a radioactive atom, usually iodine. This so-called 'labelled antigen' is added in known amount to a system which also contains an unknown amount of the unlabelled antigen, and a fixed quantity of antibody. Both the unlabelled and labelled antigen bind to the antibody, and the extent of binding of labelled antigen is a function of the amount of unlabelled antibody present: the more there is, the more it is bound to antibody at the expense of the labelled antigen, and the more labelled antigen is unbound. The labelled antigen, being radioactive, can be detected at extremely low concentrations.

Techniques exist for separating antigen bound to antibody from unbound antigen. These allow measurement of the bound and unbound fractions of labelled antigen and so can be used

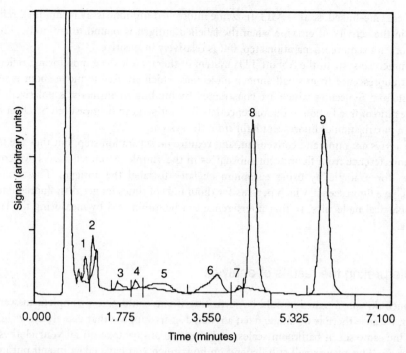

Fig. 2.6 A chromatogram for a complex mixture. The chromatogram was obtained by high pressure liquid chromatography. It represents a graph of the detector signal strength (in arbitrary units) plotted against time from injection. The large peak shortly after injection is the *solvent front*, and the subsequent numbered peaks represent nine components of the sample mixture.

to calculate how much competition there is from the unknown amount of unlabelled antigen, and thence to find the concentration of the unknown antigen.

The measurement of the labelled antigen depends on detecting the radioactivity coming from the label, and so errors can occur if the label does not remain firmly attached to the antigen. The calculation of the amount of unlabelled antigen depends upon an efficient separation of free molecules from molecules bound to antibody, and errors can be generated if the separation is incomplete. The assumption is made that the only species reacting with the antibody used are the labelled and unlabelled antigen. If the antibody reacts with other molecules in the system, such as inactive metabolites, then the results can be distorted.

CASE 2.7 (HAMILTON 1993)

A nurse at the Hospital for Sick Children in Toronto was charged with murder after four babies who died on the cardiac wards were found to have a very high serum digoxin concentrations in the blood, as measured by radioimmunoasssay (digoxin is a drug used to treat heart failure). Grave doubts were raised about the specificity of the assay in babies, who may have digoxin-like substances in the blood even if untreated. The nurse was acquitted.

Other ways of labelling antigen and detecting antigen-antibody complexes can also be used. Antigens can be linked to enzymes which catalyse reactions with coloured end-points. One form of enzyme-linked assay, EMIT (enzyme multiplied immunoassay technique), relies on a change in the activity of enzyme when the labelled antigen is bound to antibody. The technique does not require a separation step, but is relatively insensitive.

A commercial system, the Abbott TDx system of therapeutic drug monitoring, relies on the fact that fluorescence from small antigen molecules which are free to move about is unpolarized, but from molecules which are constrained by binding to antibody is polarized. Therefore, the ratio of free to bound fluorescence-labelled antigen can be measured by observing the degree of polarization of fluorescent light from the system.

Such assays are rapid and convenient, and require no separation step, but they are susceptible to interference from fluorescent substances in the sample. Modified assays overcome this problem, for example by using europium chelates to label the antigen. These rare earth chelates have fluorescence which persists for thousands of times longer than fluorescence from most biological molecules, so that interference can be minimized by measuring the late fluorescence.

2.3 Interpreting the results of analysis

How much do you weigh? It would be surprising if you could give a complete answer to this question because there is no single fixed answer. Let us suppose that you always weigh yourself on the same set of bathroom scales, and that you always take off all your clothes before stepping on. The answer will still depend on how much you have taken in and put out since you were last weighed, so there is an intrinsic variability due to changes in you. It will also depend on how good the scales are at giving the same answer time after time to the same question. They may be old and unreliable, the mechanism could be sensitive to the room temperature and the weather, and so on. The inherent changes in both the state of your body and the state of the scales can be minimized by careful attention to detail, but they cannot be eliminated. There will remain a series of undefined and apparently random perturbations to the reading, so that if you weigh yourself many times, the values will not be identical but will be scattered. This scatter, or *random variation* is the result of *random errors*. It has to be taken into account whenever measurements are made, and is especially important in interpreting numerical results in the biological sciences. There are several excellent standard texts on statistics in medical science (Armitage and Berry 1987; Bland 1987; Altman 1991).

A second type of problem can arise in finding your weight. You may always weigh yourself wearing your dressing gown, or the scales may always show 2 kilograms before you step on because the true zero value has not been set. These difficulties do not alter the way the results are scattered, but they cause a systematic shift away from the true value. They represent the class of *systematic errors*.

The *accuracy* of a result is a measure of how close the measured value comes to the true value, which is in general unknown. The *precision* is a measure of how widely the values of a series of repeated determinations are scattered about the average value. The meaning of a numerical result, then, depends both on its accuracy and on its precision. An equivalent way of expressing this is to say that the accuracy of a given set of repeated measurements is a measure of the difference between the *location* (position) of the average value and the true value. The precision is a measure of the *dispersion* (scatter) of the repeated measures about their average value.

2.3.1 Calibration

Systematic errors in an assay can be reduced or eliminated by ensuring that the assay is set up to give the correct results for samples of known value. The dial of the bathroom scales will have been calibrated initially by placing a known weight, say 100 kilograms, on the scales and marking the dial '100 kilograms' at the point where the needle came to rest. The point where the needle rests when there was no weight on the scales gives the value '0 kilograms'. If we assume that the scales work smoothly, we can then divide the dial between the 0 and 100 marks into equal segments, each indicating 1 kilogram (Fig 2.7).

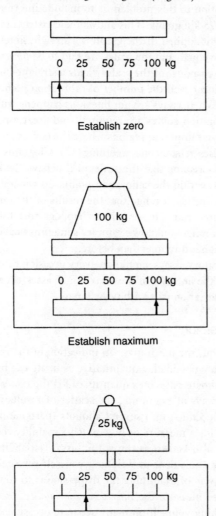

Establish zero

Establish maximum

Establish linearity

Fig. 2.7 Checking the calibration of an instrument whose response is linear, as applied to a set of weighing-scales. The readings for zero and the maximum weight are verified, and the response to an intermediate weight is then checked.

There are three difficulties. We have already described the existence of random errors, which mean that the calibration points could change from day to day or moment to moment. This is not usually important for instruments such as bathroom scales or metre rules, but it is an important consideration in laboratory assays, and means for practical purposes that an assay should always contain calibration samples.

We also have to confront the problem that the springs in bathroom scales are not always perfect. Because of this, the assumption that we can divide the scale between 0 and 100 kilograms into equal 1 kilogram divisions may not be justified. An imperfect spring might cause the needle to move less for the addition of 1 kilogram to a load of 75 kilograms than to a load of 25 kilograms. The most satisfactory solution to this problem is to include intermediate calibration weights, for example at 25, 50, and 75 kilograms. This allows the construction of a graph of needle displacement against the weight applied. If the graph is a straight line, then we are correct to say that the divisions should be equal, and the scales are said to be *linear*: the relationship between the applied weight and the response of the scales yields a straight-line graph. Many laboratory assays are assumed to be linear, and the number of calibration points needs to be sufficient to examine that assumption. When assays are not linear, as happens with radioimmunoassays, for example, then special calibration curves are required, and great care has to be taken in calculating the values of unknown samples in regions where the curves are very 'bendy'.

The third difficulty arises if someone weighing 127 kilograms (20 stones) steps on the scales. We have no right to assume that the scales will behave the same way beyond the last calibration point as they do within the calibration points. In general, laboratory assays should always be calibrated over a sufficient range that the results of the samples being measured fall within the calibration points. Since it sometimes happens that the unknown concentration falls outside the calibration range, unknown samples sometimes have to be re-tested with new calibration samples or at higher dilutions than before.

In summary, then, laboratory assays should on every occasion be calibrated with a sufficient number of samples so that the linearity of the assay can be assessed, and over a sufficient range so that the unknown concentration falls within the range.

2.3.2 Scatter, or dispersion

The scatter of readings about the mean gives an indication of the reliability of the result and, provided several readings are obtained, a quantitative estimate can be made of the precision of the mean reading. This estimate relies on a quantity called the *standard deviation*[1].

There are two distinct ways of examining the scatter of results for laboratory assays. The first is to divide a single specimen into several aliquots (parts) and then assay each of these aliquots together. This yields a measure of how much variability there is within a single run: the *intra-assay variability*, also known as the within-assay variability. Returning to the bathroom scales, this would be equivalent to weighing yourself repeatedly on the same scales on one occasion. The second way of examining the dispersion is to run the separate aliquots in a series of different assays to measure the *inter-assay variability*, or between-assay variability. This is analogous to weighing yourself on many separate occasions. It sometimes happens in experimental work that the intra-assay variability is of more interest than the inter-assay variability because all the samples from a single study are assayed together. This is rarely the case

[1] The standard deviation is the square root of the *variance*, which is itself the sum of the squares of the deviations of each individual measurement from the mean of all the measurements, divided by the number of measurements (see, for example, Altman 1991).

in forensic pharmacology, and the inter-assay variability is usually needed. The difference is important, because the variability within a single assay is necessarily less than the variability between assays, and often considerably so.

If we are told that a laboratory result for a drug concentration is 19.0 milligrams per litre, then we may be able to deduce the likely range into which the true result falls if we know something of the properties of the assay. Suppose that the assay has been checked with a solution which contains approximately 25 milligrams per litre of the drug in question, and that repeated assays give results with a mean value of 24.6 and a standard deviation of 3.1 milligrams per litre. This would usually be written as 24.6 ± 3.1 milligrams per litre (mean ± SD), or 24.6 (SD 3.1) milligrams per litre.

The scatter of the assay results between different assays is such that the standard deviation represents 3.1/24.6 of the mean. This can be expressed as a percentage, when it is known as the (percentage) *coefficient of variation*, or CV

$$\text{coefficient of variation (per cent)} = \text{standard deviation} \times 100/\text{mean}.$$

Here, the inter-assay coefficient of variation is $(3.1/24.6) \times 100$ per cent, or 12.6 per cent.

Provided the properties of the assay do not depend too strongly on the actual value of the concentration being measured, the CV can be applied to the experimental result:

$$\text{experimental result} = 19.0 \text{ milligrams per litre}$$
$$\text{coefficient of variation} = 12.6 \text{ per cent}$$

therefore

$$\text{standard deviation} = 12.6 \text{ per cent of } 19.0$$
$$= 2.4 \text{ milligrams per litre}.$$

There is a 95 per cent probability that the true experimental result lies within ± 2 standard deviations of the mean, that is, in the range 19.0 ± 4.8, or 14.2 to 23.8 milligrams per litre. The range is known as the *95 per cent confidence interval*. The values 14.2 and 23.8 milligrams per litre are the *lower* and *upper* bounds or *confidence limits* of this interval.

An inter-assay coefficient of variation for analytical work would often be less than 12.6 per cent, and so the probable value of the measured sample would often be more clearly defined, but this is by no means always the case. The interpretation of results should allow for the possibility that the true value lies close to one extreme or the other.

In calibrating the equipment used to analyse breath for ethanol in the United Kingdom, a calibration sample specially prepared by the National Physical Laboratory is used. The breath-testing equipment is accepted as sufficiently accurate if the reading for the calibrant is between 32 and 38 micrograms per 100 millilitres of breath (Walls and Brownlie 1985*b*). These values are ± 8 per cent of the mean, and so, to the same degree of accuracy, any measurement made by the machine will have a confidence interval of approximately ± 8 per cent around the observed value. This may explain why the police in Britain do not prosecute drivers whose readings are below 40 micrograms per 100 millilitres, even though the legal limit is set at 35 micrograms per 100 millilitres.

2.3.3 Accuracy and quality control

Repeated measurements on an unknown sample can give a clear picture of the dispersion of the results in terms of the SD. However, the location of the mean cannot be assessed from internal evidence of this sort. For example, a systematic error in which the calibration samples were only 50 per cent of the intended concentration would remain completely undetected. The calibration curve would remain a straight line, and the random errors (and therefore the SDs or CVs) would be unchanged, but the results would be wildly wrong. For this reason, it is good practice to include in laboratory assays a specimen whose concentration is determined independently. Such samples are known as *quality control* samples, or QCs. A good assay will obviously give values for the QCs close to their true values. *External* QCs are prepared in another laboratory, and their concentrations are unknown to the analyst. They allow the performance of one laboratory's assay to be compared with that of others.

2.4 Summary

The results of a laboratory assay should be carefully scrutinized. Before they are interpreted, it should be clear what assay was used, how specific it was for the compound of interest, how it was calibrated, and whether it was linear. The value for the sample should fall within the calibration range. The coefficient of variation for the assay should be known, and the accepted and measured values for QCs should be sought to confirm that the assay is accurate. Using these data, the likely confidence interval for the experimental result can be derived. It will often surprisingly wide, and the deductions to be made from a value at one end of the interval may be very different from those to be made at the other extreme.

3

Legal considerations

Elizabeth Norman

3.1 'What am I doing here?'

The function of the expert witness within the English legal system is the same whatever the area of expertise. The problem faced by the would-be expert in identifying the nature of that function may vary, depending on the nature of that expertise. The doctor, for example, is accustomed to diagnosing and treating illness, but may be less comfortable in saying what percentage of a patient's disability is attributable to a particular injury, the very issues that the legal system may want addressed. It is very important to understand the basics of how the legal system works, in order to see what it actually requires of the expert. In that way, a lot of time (on behalf of the doctor) and frustration (on the part of the lawyer) can be saved. It is also important to understand how lawyers function in court.

Many experts will never actually have to stand up and defend their views in the courtroom, either because the case or their part in it is decided by agreement beforehand, or because what they have to say (while very useful for the lawyer who has to question the opposition witness, for example in destroying the basis of the particular views being expressed) could in some areas prove embarrassing to their 'own' side. However, the possibility is always there, and some thought needs to be given to life under the spotlight of the witness box. Equally, the lawyer needs to make sure that the expert understands what is required.

The legal process may be seen as contrived and unreal by many. Others may be in the unfortunate position of believing that they understand what is happening, based on reason, logic and experience of life—none of which, unfortunately, are reliable guides to those who unexpectedly find themselves in the witness box. No one who has not been adequately briefed can be expected to do a good job. For lawyer and expert to get the best out of each other, each must understand the other's language and assumptions, and have a clear idea of their respective objectives. In particular, experts need to know why they are there, what their role is and what questions need to be answered.

3.2 Proof

The English legal system is adversarial. There is an umpire, whether it be judge, tribunal, or magistrates, and two or more sides. The side that brought the proceedings is the side that carries the 'burden of proof'. The implication of this is that if for some reason no evidence, or inadequate evidence, was called, the side that brought the proceedings would lose and the other side(s) would win.

3.2.1 Who needs to prove what?

There are basically two types of legal process, criminal and civil.

Proof in criminal cases

In the criminal courts the prosecution bring the case, and carry the burden of proof. If the prosecution evidence is not good enough to prove the case beyond reasonable doubt, the defence need not call any evidence; the prosecution will have failed to prove their case and will lose and the defendant will be acquitted. The danger of the defence calling evidence in those circumstances is obvious: something said by a defence witness might inadvertently lend support to the prosecution case and allow them to succeed where otherwise they would have failed. It is obvious from this that a defendant need not be innocent as such to be acquitted.

Where, for example, there has been a robbery at a petrol station and the cashier was too shocked to remember clearly what the assailant looked like, the prosecution may seek to rely on a security video recording of the incident to identify the culprit. The expert may be asked to compare photographs of the suspect with the video films to see if the two are of the same person. Comparisons can be made, for example, with the general shape of the features, the line of the jaw, and especially the shape of the ear, which is particularly distinctive. Depending on the quality of the images, the expert may only be able to say that there is nothing inconsistent with the two sets of images being of the same person. That is not, of course, to say that they are the same person.

If the jury have the opportunity to study the defendant in the course of the trial and get to know him, they may be able to recognize him as the man in the video. The way that people recognize each other is not fully understood, but it does not seem to depend on the objective calculations of the expert, as those quiz programmes which show partly concealed pictures of sportsmen for the panel to recognize indicate. If the jury are thus sure the defendant is the man in the video, he will be convicted. If, however, he unsportingly remains below in the cells throughout the trial, the jury will not have the opportunity to recognize him and he will be acquitted even though he was in fact there, because the prosecution evidence is not good enough.

In the criminal courts the defendant will face one or more charges, allegations that he has committed particular offences, and all the various elements of those charges must be proved. If the charge is murder, for example, the prosecution must prove that the accused caused the death of the victim and in so doing intended to cause death or really serious bodily harm, or should have realised those were likely consequences of his actions (see below).

Proof in civil cases

In the civil courts the burden of proof is on the plaintiff, the person bringing the case, who claims to have suffered some injury or wrong at the hands of the defendant. The area most likely to involve the doctor as expert witness is that of negligence. Negligence is one of a variety of actions grouped together under the title of 'tort'. Torts are civil wrongs which do not depend on the pre-existence of any contractual relationship between the parties.

Negligence

Negligence requires the existence of a duty of care owing by one party to the other. A supermarket, for example, has reason to suppose that people will walk around its aisles to do their shopping, and so has a duty to make sure it is reasonably safe for them to do so. Negligence then requires a breach of that duty of care, for example allowing a large pool of spilt yoghurt to lie on the floor unattended. It usually requires that breach of duty has foreseeable adverse consequences such as a shopper slipping on the yoghurt and being injured. The 'tortfeasor', the party responsible for the commission of the tort, is only responsible for reasonably foreseeable consequences, not for remote effects such as not being able to attend a theatre production because of a broken leg.

Sometimes the case seems so clear that lawyers talk about *'res ipsa loquitur'*, 'the thing speaks for itself'. The law student's favourite case is that of the patient who went into hospital to be cured of two stiff fingers (he had Dupuytren's contracture) and came out with four stiff fingers[1]. In a clear case like that it would be for the hospital staff to provide an acceptable explanation, if they could, because on the face of it the medical treatment must have fallen far below the required standard.

The defendant can sometimes provide an explanation, even when the facts on the surface strongly suggest negligence.

CASE 3.1[2]

Patients who underwent spinal anaesthesia were paralysed and sued the hospital. The hospital showed that the ampoules of anaesthetic were kept in phenol solution, as was then the practice. Undetectable flaws in the glass of the ampoules allowed phenol to enter the anaesthetic solution, and was the cause of the paralysis. Since, at that time, the possibility of this danger was completely unforeseen, the defendants could not be expected to avert it, and the court found for the defendants.

It is not necessary to be perfect in order to avoid negligence. In the field of medical negligence, for example, it is well recognized that doctors cannot be expected to know everything (though some like to give the impression that they do). The duty of care is a duty to take reasonable care, not to be infallible. Thus, a doctor was said to be required to act 'in accordance with a practice accepted as proper by a responsible body of medical men [sic] skilled without particular art' in a 1957 case which is still a good guide[3].

A person may be negligent, but may escape being held liable to pay damages by way of compensation because no loss has in fact been caused. A GP who, over a period of 4 weeks, prescribed co-codamol, 'Distalgesic', and 'Tylex' to a woman in an attempt to cure various pains, to no avail (so that she went of her own accord to a chemist and obtained paracetamol in desperation) was doubtless negligent in not explaining to her that these products all contained paracetamol and, if taken together, might result in overdosage, but fortunately for him no damage resulted and so there were no legal consequences.

---

[1] *Cassidy* v. *Ministry of Health* [1951] 2 KB 343, 365. Lord Denning put the plaintiff's case thus: 'I went into hospital to be cured of two stiff fingers. I came out with four stiff fingers and my hand is useless. That should not have happened if due care had been used. Explain it if you can.'
[2] *Roe* v. *Minister of Health* [1954] 2 QB 66.
[3] *Bolam* v. *Friern Hospital Management Committee* [1957] 1 WLR 582, 586.

3.2.2 The standard of proof

The standard of proof is a crucial concept, and is a major difference between criminal and civil proceedings. The party on whom the burden of proof falls must prove the case to the required standard. Anything less means the case is lost. Generally, in the criminal courts the standard of proof is 'beyond reasonable doubt'.

The jury or magistrates must be sure that the crime has been committed and the defendant is responsible before they can convict. This is something which must be kept in the forefront of the expert's mind. If the prosecution cannot produce the appropriate evidence, they will lose. This does not mean necessarily that a prosecution expert must be certain, depending on the nature of the evidence. The expert who could only say that there was nothing inconsistent in a video being that of a defendant if used to corroborate another witness who thought he or she recognized the defendant, would be of great assistance to the prosecution. It is the totality of the evidence which must be considered, not any particular evidence in isolation. The defence need not prove that the prosecution expert is wrong, only that the expert might be wrong, or cannot be sure.

In the civil courts, the standard of proof is the balance of probabilities, that it is more likely than not that a particular situation came about or existed in a particular way. It is thus easier to make out a case in the civil than in the criminal courts.

3.3 The expert witness

3.3.1 The role of the expert before trial

As has already been said, many cases never get to court. This is especially so in civil cases, where an early exchange of documents, expert reports and other evidence may well lead to a matter being settled by agreement between the parties in the light of the mutually anticipated outcome if a trial were to take place. However, criminal cases can also be determined on occasion without the intervention of the court.

For example, in an alleged rape, penetration was said to have taken place from behind, and all significant acts to have taken place out of sight of the victim. An expert report from the defence showing that the finding of semen in the vagina could be explained by insertion of a finger, after external ejaculation (the defendant's account), if not rebutted by the prosecution expert, might well lead to the prosecution deciding not to proceed with the rape allegation, since rape requires there to have been penile penetration. Of course, the charge of rape might be replaced by one of indecent assault, but that carries a lesser maximum sentence.

3.3.2 Expert advice

Whether advice is sought in the criminal or civil arena, the expert is likely to be asked initially to provide a written report. There may then be occasion for advice in conference with the lawyers.

The expert has a duty to advise impartially, so far as possible. There will inevitably be an awareness of the interests of the instructing party, but this should not be allowed to lead to a misrepresentation of opinion. There is, of course, the question of professional integrity. There is also the possibility that evidence will have to be given on oath. On a more pragmatic level, the expert who does not alert the instructing party to any weaknesses or potential weaknesses in the forensic evidence is a liability.

The most impressive expert, whether on paper or in the witness box, is usually the one who carries an air of objectivity, and is able to provide reasoned justification for any views that are expressed. It should be remembered that the law is a small world, and experts who allow themselves to be identified too closely with a particular position (for example, always supporting the prosecution, whatever the strengths of the evidence) are likely to carry less weight than those with more balanced reputations.

Experts have two major functions: first, they have to explore the strengths and weaknesses of the case made out by the instructing party, and also, so far as it can be determined, the case of the opposition. Secondly, they may be used to express views on behalf of the instructing party, by way of a written report, or possibly by giving live evidence in court.

Assessing the case; communicating conclusions

In order to carry out the task of assessing strengths and weaknesses in a case, the expert must insist that all relevant information is made available, and if it appears that necessary information is lacking, it should be requested. For example, in acting for the defence in a criminal case, it will usually be helpful to see any prosecution statements relevant to the issue in question, and any statements regarding it made by the accused. The expert can then take a view as to whether these accounts are consistent or not with the relevant objective evidence.

Just as sometimes an expert witness may be tempted to tailor views to please those issuing instructions, so sometimes legal advisers may be tempted to withhold troublesome evidence from their expert. This can lead to considerable discomfort under cross-examination in the witness box, should the other side introduce such gremlins.

The expert is awarded no prizes for offering a firm opinion outside his or her area of expertise. Lawyers often have no idea where the boundaries lie between one discipline and the next. The expert may have to recommend seeking the views of others, and it is better for all concerned that the lawyers are notified at an early stage that others may have to be brought in, not least because if the case is legally aided, the approval of the Legal Aid Board may have to be sought, and may not arrive speedily (or at all, but that is another problem). The expert will inevitably be asked 'Who do you recommend?' and the lawyer is likely to be eternally grateful for the provision of suggested candidates.

Experts should remember when advising on a case, whether orally or in writing, that lawyers and others are likely to have little or no technical knowledge. A balance must therefore be struck between presenting oneself as an 'expert's expert', commanding respect amongst one's peers, and actually being understood by lay people as well. Unfortunately, some lawyers wish to appear to have universal knowledge and complete understanding, so the expert must ensure that the issues have been correctly understood by the recipients. Equally, lawyers must not be ashamed to admit confusion and ask for clarification of matters that are only straightforward in the light of 5 years' training at medical school.

The written report

Written reports follow certain conventions. The report begins with information on who wrote it, about what, for whom. The relevant case and file number should be given, and then the name of the instructing party, usually a solicitor but sometimes the coroner, the police, or an insurance company. The writer needs to state name, professional address, and qualifications, with a brief description of his or her expertise in the subject of the report.

It is generally important to establish next the basis on which the report has been written. This involves identifying any documents considered, such as prosecution papers (or 'depositions'), defence statements, laboratory notes, hospital case notes, and so on, and to list any material supplied and any tests carried out on the material. This may be done either in the report itself or in a covering letter. The potential importance of the covering letter will be referred to later.

The purpose of identifying the evidential basis is twofold. First, if some vital papers, for example, have been inadvertently omitted from the documents supplied by the solicitors, that omission may be noted and remedied on receipt of the report. Secondly, in making clear what information has been supplied and what procedures have been carried out, the expert is able to identify the parameters of relevance of the report.

A brief summary of the facts as they are understood is usually helpful, not only to put the report in context and make it more readily comprehensible, but also in case those facts have been misunderstood, so that the lawyers can detect that the report has been based on a false premise.

An explanation of any techniques used or referred to should be given in clear language and in sufficient detail to enable the future advocate to understand the processes involved, both to assist in ensuring that any court understands, so far as possible, what is involved, and to assist in cross-examination of opposing experts, if appropriate. It can be helpful to keep various 'explanatory paragraphs' on record (these days, in the memory of a word processor) so that they can be recycled from report to report as appropriate.

When considering the contents of the main body of the report, it is important to realize that expert reports are frequently exchanged between the parties as part of the legal process. This can come as a great shock to doctors, particularly, who may write 'Confidential' on a report they have been asked to supply, and then find its contents being referred to in open court, quite possibly by the other party.

It may be that what the expert wishes to say is simple and uncontroversial, and can be put down in writing in the initial report for all to see. It may, however, happen that although the views to be expressed are genuinely and legitimately held, the expert is aware that there is a body of opinion, for example, which would disagree, or that there are aspects of the case, which, if explored further might lead to adverse conclusions. In those circumstances, or where there is any query about what should be covered by the report, it might be prudent to set out any concerns or potential areas for investigation in a covering letter clearly marked 'Not for disclosure'.

Similarly, an expert might be asked to re-write a report to exclude certain topics. In considering the final contents of a report, the expert must always have regard for the professional duty to give an honest and justifiable opinion. This does not mean, however, that it is necessary to alert the opposition to any potential areas of attack, if those are not, in fact, fatal flaws in the expert's own case. In other words, the expert should not express an opinion which is untenable on the known facts.

Exchange of reports

In criminal cases where either party intends to call expert evidence the relevant reports must be exchanged with the other side, generally some time before trial. This is to avoid the necessity of seeking an adjournment which would otherwise arise if an advocate were un-expectedly to be faced with assessing surprise expert evidence without assistance. The prose-cution have a general duty of disclosure, which may extend to revealing the contents of expert reports on which they do not in fact propose to rely in proving their case. They may have difficulties where a report, for example, does not support the contentions of the prosecution.

3.3.3 The expert in court

In the witness box

The courtroom is a completely comfortable environment for the advocate, full of old friends (and sparring partners) and familiar in jokes and rituals. Even a lawyer who does not regularly attend court will recognize much of what is happening and know whom to ask about the rest. It can be difficult for lawyers to remember what a strange and alien environment it is to 'normal' people, including expert witnesses[4].

The watchword for the expert witness who is an inexperienced witness is 'ask'. Do not fear that you will lose face: the lawyer would be unlikely to operate your gas chromatograph with any great success, and probably thinks that a mole is small and furry, with sharp teeth and a ferocious temper (see Appendix A, Section A.1).

If you are needed as a witness, you may be lucky enough to know the date well in advance, but this is not certain. Court listing of cases, particularly in the Crown Court, can be one of life's more impenetrable mysteries, so ask your instructing solicitor to tell you when you are likely to be needed. Sometimes a case appears on what is alarmingly called the 'warned list', and you will know that the case might be heard during the period covered by the list, but will not know the actual day until the afternoon before. You should therefore make sure that you are well-prepared, with all your notes in order, and any articles or publications you might want to refer to gathered together. The advocate may well have been given the papers the day before and have to work all night to master the case, but there is no reason why you should suffer as well.

It is important to make clear from the outset those dates on which you will be unavailable. The court can issue a witness summons, which you must obey, whatever you were supposed to be doing, but usually efforts will be made to accommodate you. Make sure you know during which parts of the case you will be required, and which other witnesses your solicitor wants you to listen to (so that you can comment on their evidence, for example). Sometimes you will not be required to give evidence yourself, perhaps because some of your views might not assist the lay client's case, but you might still be asked to sit in court to help the advocate with cross-examination.

Dramatis personae

Advocates can be solicitors or barristers. The courts in which they appear may deal with a mixture of criminal and civil cases (for example, Magistrates' and Crown Courts), or just with civil cases (for example, the County Court). In the Magistrates' Court, the advocate is usually a solicitor, and no wigs or gowns are worn. In the Crown Court, you may come across a solicitor advocating a case, although it will more often be a barrister. The barrister is the one in the

---

[4] There is a clear parallel with doctors and hospitals.

wig. All barristers are 'juniors', unless they are Queen's Counsel (QCs), also called 'silks' or 'leaders'. These important beings, who appear in more weighty cases, wear a version of court mourning dress, and squarer gowns than juniors. A leader, if instructed, will normally be accompanied by a junior who is more involved in the preparation of the case than in its presentation.

The advocates sit facing the judge or magistrate. If a barrister is the advocate, the solicitors' representatives will sit behind, and you will probably be asked to sit there too, so you can communicate with the advocate. The defendant in a criminal case will be in the dock. In a civil case, your client may very well sit beside you.

Depending on the forum, the case will be presided over by lay magistrates, or a stipendiary (professional) magistrate, or a judge, alone, or with a jury, or (if hearing an appeal from the Magistrates' Court) with magistrates.

Magistrates are referred to either as 'Your worships', or 'Sir' or 'Madam'. Solicitors more often use the first form, and barristers the second, but they are equally acceptable. Judges pose more difficulties. In the County Court, a district judge is addressed as 'Sir' or 'Madam', and a circuit judge as 'Your Honour'; a High Court judge is 'My Lord'. At the Central Criminal Court in London (the 'Old Bailey'), all judges are 'My Lord'. Judges of different sorts wear different coloured robes, but in practice it is easiest to ask.

Most hearings are open to the public, so if you are to give evidence for the first time, it would be sensible to go to the local court of the appropriate kind and listen to someone else give evidence. Try to view the performance of witnesses with detachment, and analyse those ways of behaving, speaking and dealing with questions which seem to you impressive, and those which you find irritating or unconvincing, and learn effective witness strategies!

When your turn comes, you will be asked to go into the witness box. The usher, who wears a black gown and appears to be organizing everyone, will ask whether you wish to swear or affirm. If you wish to take the oath[5] on a particular holy book, it is prudent to have a quiet word with the instructing solicitor or the usher before you are called. It may take a little while to locate a Koran or an Old Testament, for example, in some parts of the country.

You will be asked to stand to take the oath or affirm. Evidence is normally given standing up, but if you are disabled or infirm, you can ask whoever is presiding whether you may sit. Wheelchair users should discuss court layout in advance, so that the most appropriate arrangements can be made.

You should take all your papers into the witness box with you, but ask permission before you refer to them, because the rules of evidence which govern what can and what cannot be used in court are complex. Normally, however, you will be allowed to refer freely to your notes.

At the start of your evidence, 'your' advocate will ask you to give your name, professional address and qualifications. Don't be shy! Tell the court how well-qualified you are, speak clearly, and speak up. Your advocate will then question you to obtain your *evidence-in-chief*.

While the questions come from the advocate, you should turn to face the *tribunal* (the magistrates or judge) and direct your answers to them. This can be disconcerting, and is more so if counsel keeps reminding you to speak up and address your answers to the judge. The judge will be making hand-written notes of your evidence, so speak at dictation speed.

Some experts, and some advocates, like there to be a metaphorical 'start button'; it is

---

[5] 'I swear by Almighty God that the evidence I shall give shall be the truth, the whole truth, and nothing but the truth.'

pushed and the expert is free to give the body of their evidence uninterrupted. Other experts or advocates prefer to go through the evidence step by step. If you get the opportunity, discuss this with the advocate in advance; if not you will have to go with the rhythm that the advocate sets. The opposition are unlikely to question you according to your own preferred pattern.

The tribunal can interrupt and ask questions. Resist any temptation to bite their heads off for interrupting your flow—now is your opportunity to look them in the eye, and impress them with your experience, common sense, and reasoned objectivity.

It may be at the end of your evidence-in-chief you feel your advocate has forgotten something. This omission may in fact have been by design rather than accident, and you should try in advance (particularly if you have a conference with the lawyers) to establish an understanding of how the case is to be presented, and what the relevant issues are.

You hope during your examination-in-chief to have set out your opinions clearly, and explained your reasons in a way that has been understood by the judge and jury. It is difficult to be certain in relation to the latter, because they are not entitled to speak to you, so look at them from time to time when giving your evidence, and seek for signs of bewilderment or joyful comprehension. Now comes *cross-examination*, when the opposition can question you.

Cross-examination, if viewed from outside the spotlight of the witness box, can be a fascinating exercise in psychoanalysis. The advocate may look at you as if considering the nature of your relationship with your mother, or your response to peer-pressure. He or she probably is. One element of your evidence is made up of the facts and opinions you have presented, and how they stand up to detailed consideration. The other element is your personal character. The latter can completely destroy the former.

There are many types of witness, and the experienced advocate will waste little time in establishing which you are. The opposing expert will have relayed your reputation among your peers to the person cross-examining you. You may have revealed much by your demeanour during examination-in-chief. The rest can be established by a little probing. This means you should assess your personal Achilles heel (by asking your nearest and dearest if you dare) and learn to recognize when the advocate has come close to finding it, or, worse, has found it. You then need to have developed a strategy for dealing with it.

Is this you?

The most common weakness in the expert (I say nothing of the barrister) is arrogance. The arrogant witness responds badly to being patronized, and foolishly to being flattered. A combination of these approaches can push arrogant witnesses into making more and more extreme statements, because they become involved in a personal battle with the advocate. Suddenly, they look round and find themselves out on a very long limb, with the advocate merrily wielding a saw at the other end.

Often associated with arrogance is dogmatism, though some are dogmatic from fear rather than conceit. The game, and for the advocate there is probably an element of game-playing going on, is to get the witness to be dogmatic about apparently small and unrelated matters in circumstances where there is not really any simple answer. A series of dogmatic statements is built up, but on close examination they are unsustainable. The statements may appear to have no individual substance, but joined together they are suddenly revealed as a net in which the witness has been treading, the advocate pulls on the net, and the witness realizes that he or she is entrapped.

The nervous witness facing cross-examination will worry how to avoid any traps that the advocate might lay. This type will become more and more unassertive under pressure, giving concessions at every turn, whether they are justified or not, simply as a short-term relief from the feeling of stress. The firm ground established in evidence-in-chief becomes more and more uncertain and insubstantial until (with a faint gurgling sound, no doubt) the witness's original opinions sink into the quagmire. You can, no doubt, think of several other types.

Now consider how you would deal with your own evidence. Have you prepared your case thoroughly, having your authorities at your fingertips, or are you hoping that no one will think to ask you those difficult questions that you are not sure you completely understand? (They will.) Are you at risk of letting your temper or your fear run away with you? Learn to face not only the strengths and weaknesses of your case, but also your own strengths and weaknesses; so, for example, recognize when someone is pushing you to assert that something is absolute which is really only a matter of conjecture, and hold yourself back. Beware, if you are very experienced, of being so casual that you appear to be sloppy. This raises the issue of pace. Your opponent will try to dictate the pace and rhythm of your evidence in cross-examination. If you feel you are being hurried, consciously slow down. Take time to consider your answers if you need to. Do not allow yourself to become angered by constant interruptions—a courteous look at the judge may well bring relief. The courtroom may be an arena, but it is not your fight. You are there merely to present your views to the best of your ability, to assist the court in coming to a conclusion. Thoughts of victory and defeat should be for others, not for you, though a little quiet gloating may be permitted if, whether the case was won or lost, your contribution was as impressive as it possibly could have been. In court, you have the privilege of saying whatever you believe to be true and relevant. Outside court, the line between legitimate criticism and defamation can be a fine one. When the defamation is widely disseminated, the consequences can be serious.

CASE 3.2 (*THE TIMES*, 28 MAY 1994)

An acrimonious action for libel concerned an eminent expert on sleep disorders and the drug manufacturer Upjohn. Professor Ian Oswald claimed in a television programme, 'The Halcion nightmare', that Upjohn had deliberately hidden from regulatory authorities the results of a trial on the drug triazolam ('Halcion') which it manufactured. The results showed a higher incidence of adverse effects than expected. The company contended that the information was not passed to the regulatory authorities because of administrative errors.

The judge held that Upjohn had indeed made serious errors when it informed the authorities about 'Halcion', but that these 'were not made intentionally and dishonestly'. He therefore found for Upjohn, and the British Broadcasting Corporation and Professor Oswald had to pay substantial damages and an even more substantial bill for the legal costs of both parties.

There was a further twist in this case: Upjohn's vigorous response to the programme was found to be libellous of Oswald, who was also awarded damages.

3.4 Homicide and related matters

It often happens in the criminal field that an expert is asked to advise in relation to a death. It may be helpful, therefore, to consider the legal framework within which the facts of the case should be considered.

3.4.1 Murder and manslaughter

Murder can be summarized as the unlawful killing of a person with malice aforethought. At present, death must occur within a year and a day of the causative event, although this provision is likely to be altered in the light of modern medical techniques, where persons can be kept alive by mechanical ventilation.

Malice aforethought is the intention to kill or cause grievous bodily harm. This is known as the *mens rea* of the crime. The *actus reus*, the thing that is done, is unlawful killing. Killing a person in self-defence, where no more force than was necessary was used, would not be murder, because the killing would not be unlawful.

A person may be acquitted of murder, but found guilty of some lesser offence, such as manslaughter. The *actus reus* of manslaughter and murder is the same, but the *mens rea*, the intention behind the act, differs.

A person may be convicted of manslaughter, though charged with murder, where one of three special defences to murder exists. They are: provocation, killing in pursuance of a suicide pact, and diminished responsibility (see below). A person may be charged with manslaughter as a specific charge where the necessary mental element for murder is lacking, or may be charged with murder but convicted of manslaughter where the prosecution fail to prove the mental element at trial. Manslaughter as a result of the successful raising of one of the special defences to murder is known as *voluntary manslaughter*, to distinguish it from other forms of manslaughter, known as *involuntary manslaughter*.

The most common examples of involuntary manslaughter involve the killing of someone by an act which was both unlawful and intended to cause some bodily harm; and killing recklessly.

If a person commits an act which he or she deliberately intends to kill another, but the act does not result in death, then the person can be charged with attempted murder.

CASE 3.3[6]

A respected consultant rheumatologist had cared for a patient for 13 years up to the time that she was terminally ill and in great pain. She implored him to put her out of her misery, and he administered a potentially lethal intravenous dose of potassium chloride. She died a few minutes later. The consultant was charged with attempted murder and convicted. He received a suspended sentence.

The prosecution may have been unwilling to bring a charge of murder, since the patient was anyway terminally ill and so there might have been great difficulty in proving beyond reasonable doubt that she died from the potassium injection. The prosecution was, however, able to establish beyond reasonable doubt that the consultant had given the potassium with the express intention of causing his patient's death.

3.4.2 Diminished responsibility

By virtue of the Homicide Act 1957, section 2, it is a defence to murder to show that the defendant's mental responsibility for the relevant acts or omissions was substantially impaired because 'he was suffering from such abnormality of mind (whether arising from a condition of arrested or retarded development of mind, or any inherent causes or induced by disease or injury)' as to cause that impairment.

Although the burden of proof in a criminal case is normally on the prosecution, this is one of those exceptions which, if raised, has to be proved by the defence. As is always the case

[6] *R. v. Cox* [1993] 1 MedLRev 232.

when the defence has to prove something, the standard of proof is the lower one of 'on the balance of probabilities', as in civil cases.

Since the introduction of the defence of diminished responsibility, it has become rare for the defence to take refuge in the old defence of insanity, which has the inherent drawback that the sentence is certain to be incarceration in a mental institution without limit of time. However, the Criminal Procedure (Insanity and Unfitness to Plead) Act 1991 made a wider variety of sentencing options available. Insanity as a general defence, not just applicable to homicide, is dealt with below.

For a defence of diminished responsibility to succeed, medical evidence will be necessary, though the jury is not bound to follow it slavishly but may consider all the circumstances of the case. Abnormality of mind may involve not only perception of physical acts and matters and the formation of a rational judgement of right and wrong but also the ability to control physical acts as a result of that judgement. The test is whether the ubiquitous 'reasonable man' would consider the defendant's state of mind to be abnormal[7].

Acceptable causes of abnormality of mind have included depression, postnatal depression, and premenstrual syndrome, but not simple intoxication with alcohol or drugs of abuse. Intoxication is only relevant where it is associated with an actual disease, alcoholism for example, which has caused permanent damage to the brain. In those circumstances, it is not the intoxication as such which diminishes the responsibility, but the underlying disorder.[8]

3.4.3 Some general defences

The special defences referred to above relate only to murder. There are, however, a number of general defences to various crimes, some of which arise in the context of forensic pharmacology and are discussed here. These are insanity, automatism, and intoxication.

Insanity

The M'Naughten rules, called after the 1843 case of the same name, set out the criteria that have to be fulfilled to prove insanity. It must be proved that, at the time of committing the act, the accused party was labouring under such a defect of reason, from disease of the mind, as not to know the nature and quality of the act he was doing, or, if he did know it, that he did not know what he did was wrong[9]. This is another example of where the burden of proof rests on the defence, and so the standard of proof is only the balance of probabilities.

CASE 3.4 (TATTERSALL 1986)

Daniel M'Naughten shot and killed Sir Robert Peel's private secretary in January 1843 because ' ... the Tories have compelled me to do this. They follow and persecute me wherever I go and have entirely destroyed my peace of mind ...,'. He was plainly mad. At his trial, the judge directed that M'Naughten be found not guilty of murder by reason of insanity. The verdict caused an outcry, and in its wake a group of Law Lords formulated rules by which to judge whether an accused could be acquitted of a crime by reason of insanity. The M'Naughten rules demand that it be shown that 'the accused was labouring under such a defect of reason, *from disease of the mind,* as not to know the nature and quality of the act he was doing'.

[7] R. v. *Byrne* [1960] 2 QB 396.
[8] R. v. *Tandy* [1989] 1WLR 350; see Case 4.4 Section 4.1.3.
[9] *M'Naughten's Case* [1843] 10 Cl and F 200f.

It is the state of mind at the time of the offence, not at the time of the trial, which is relevant here, though a person may in any event be found unfit to plead at trial. There must be an actual defect of reason, rather than simply a failure to act rationally because of emotional turmoil. The defect of reason must flow from a disease of the mind, which may or may not be organic. Doctors often find it difficult to accept that it is for the judge to decide whether there is an operational disease of the mind, but this is a question of law. The judge will listen to medical experts as to whether there was damage to the mental faculties, and if so, why; but it is the judge who must decide whether what he has heard described constitutes a 'disease of the mind' in law.

CASE 3.5[10]

A diabetic man developed hypoglycaemia (a low blood glucose concentration; Chapter 9) as a result of injecting his prescribed dose of insulin, taking little lunch, and drinking alcohol. While hypoglycaemic, he allegedly committed assault. He was convicted, but appealed. It was held that 'such a malfunctioning of his mind as there was, was caused by an external factor, and not by a bodily disorder in the nature of a disease which disturbed the working of his mind'.

In another case[11], a man whose behaviour was due to hyperglycaemia (a high blood glucose concentration) from untreated diabetes mellitus was held to have an internally generated condition that constituted a disease of the mind.

Automatism

A person who is unconscious of his actions may be able to rely on the defence of automatism, because it cannot generally be said he intended to carry out the acts amounting to the offence. However, if the condition is brought about by self-induced intoxication, then the defence would not normally be available (see below).

Self-induced consequences might still allow a defence of automatism to be raised if, for example, the defendant did not appreciate that the likely consequence of his action would be to induce automatism. A diabetic patient would be unlikely to be held responsible for his actions if he had not be instructed that failure to take regular meals might result in hypoglycaemia and abnormal behaviour, whereas a diabetic who was aware of the consequences of missed meals would be expected to take appropriate precautions.

CASE 3.6[12] (MAHER AND FRIER 1993)

A man who had had insulin-dependent diabetes for 30 years went, armed with an iron bar, to the home of a rival lover and attacked him. Ten minutes before the attack, the accused asked his victim to fetch a sugary drink because he felt unwell.

The accused accepted that he had attacked his rival, but argued that he was hypoglycaemic at the time and was acting as an automaton. The trial judge directed that self-induced intoxication could not be a defence to a crime.

The appeal court later held that there was a distinction between taking alcohol or hallucinogenic drugs and taking therapeutic drugs which had unexpected side-effects. In the case of insulin, however, provided that the patient appreciated that failure to take food could lead to aggressive or uncontrollable behaviour, then (voluntary) failure to take food could constitute

---

[10] R. v. *Quick* [1973] QB 910.
[11] R. v. *Hennessy* [1989] 1 WLR 287.
[12] R. v. *Bailey* [1983] 1 WLR 765.

recklessness. More generally, if a defendant were aware that a drug taken as therapy could have a dangerous side-effect that would result in harm to others, the jury would have to decide whether the defendant was responsible for the outcome if harm did result.

In this case there had been clear evidence of intent and little indication of hypoglycaemia. The conviction was upheld (Samuels 1987).

The following case shows again that the mere fact that a crime was committed in an abnormal state of mind which was brought about by drugs is not necessarily a defence.

CASE 3.7 (TATTERSALL 1986)

An orderly at a psychiatric hospital who suffered from diabetes took his morning insulin, but substituted whisky and quarter of a bottle of rum for his lunch. He then assaulted one of the patients. He had a history of severe hypoglycaemia from taking insulin and ethanol, and had often been violent as a result. It is likely that on this occasion, too, he was hypoglycaemic when he became violent.

He was convicted, and at appeal it was held that the effect of hypoglycaemia was not a defence because it was induced by his own recklessness.

Intoxication

A person who deliberately takes drugs known to have an intoxicating effect, such as alcohol, cannot generally take refuge in the old (but non-legal) excuse 'I only did it because I'd been drinking'. However, when an apparently safe drug leads to criminal behaviour, then whether or not the effect of the drug can be relied on as a defence will depend on whether the defendant was aware of, or reckless as to, the possible existence of potential adverse effects.

CASE 3.8 (BRAHAMS 1985B; WELLER AND SOMERS 1991)[13]

A man was charged with arson and recklessly endangering life and property. Before the offence he took about five diazepam tablets 'to calm his nerves', having been told that it was 'old stock' and could do him no harm. He was not himself prescribed the diazepam by a doctor. The jury were directed to disregard the possible effects of self-intoxication.

There was no evidence in this case that the defendant knew that diazepam could cause aggressive behaviour or alter the perception of risks. Diazepam was a soporific or sedative, and so it was different from alcohol or other stimulant drugs whose taking involves a degree of recklessness that might not exist when diazepam was taken. That would depend on the circumstances, since taking a soporific might not excuse a subsequent episode of dangerous driving. The conviction was quashed on appeal.

Some offences, such as murder and wounding with intent, require 'specific intent', that is, the intent, or a specific state of mind, forms part of the definition of the offence. Self-induced intoxication can provide a defence to a crime of specific intent, if it is of such a nature as to prevent the intent being formed. It cannot provide a defence to crimes requiring only 'basic intent', since they do not require any specific intent or foresight. A man was charged with manslaughter. His defence was that at the time of the killing, he was suffering from drug-induced hallucination which caused him to believe that he was defending himself against snakes at the centre of the Earth. He was nevertheless found guilty[14].

[13] *R.* v. *Hardie* [1985] 1 WLR 64.
[14] *R.*v. *Lipman* [1970] 1 QB 152.

3.5 Summary

Expert evidence is of great importance in civil and in criminal cases, and the lawyers will be best helped by honest, straightforward, and carefully-considered views. They need to be expressed clearly in writing and in speech. It is usually easier to provide what is needed when the expert has an inkling of what the lawyer will wish to know, and how the expert advice is to be used. The expert should seek clarification from the lawyer if there is any doubt about what is required.

Part 2

Specific problems

4

Effects of drugs on behaviour

It is common experience that chemical substances can alter one's state of mind. Many people have tried to 'drown their sorrows' in ethanol, which provides the most familiar example of the phenomenon. There are prescribed drugs used specifically to treat anxiety, depression, psychosis and other psychiatric ('mental') diseases. These drugs are intended to alter the subject's feelings or state of mind therapeutically. Many more drugs can cause psychiatric disturbance as an adverse effect. The pleasurable feelings engendered by some drugs and chemicals can also lead to their non-medicinal use and abuse.

The interaction between drugs and the mind is important in forensic pharmacology because the expert can be asked to say whether a defendant committed a crime, or confessed to it, while in an abnormal state of mind, and whether that was due to a drug or a disease. These matters are considered here.

Experts can also become involved when criminals use drugs to reduce the ability of their victims to resist them, or where a complainant who is legitimately given a drug has been led by its effects to believe that some crime has taken place after the administration of the drug and against the complainant's will. These matters are considered in Chapter 5.

4.1 The defendant's behaviour

Experts will sometimes be faced with problems that hinge on how the actions of a defendant have been altered by drugs. This is discussed in Section 3.4.3, and some further examples are given here to illustrate the pharmacological problems.

CASE 4.1 (MILNE 1979)

A 35-year-old man was treated for depression with the tricyclic antidepressant maprotiline. He was also receiving 'Mandrax' (a mixture of the sedative drugs methaqualone and diphenhydramine) and the benzodiazepine drug lorazepam. One night the man attacked his widowed mother, who later died. He had no memory of the events. There was no prior history of epilepsy, but an electroencephalogram (brain-wave tracing) did show signs of temporal lobe epilepsy, a form of the disease associated with complex seizures. The man was charged with murder.

Drugs such as maprotiline can lower the threshold at which people with a predisposition to have epilepsy actually manifest epileptic phenomena. The phenomena that characterize epilepsy affecting the temporal lobe of the brain can take the form of bizarre behaviour, and it was possible that the defendant was suffering from an attack of temporal lobe epilepsy, due to structural brain disease, but only brought out by the maprotiline, at the time he killed his mother.

He was acquitted.

4.1.1 Drug-induced hypoglycaemia

Treatment for diabetes mellitus ('sugar diabetes') can result in hypoglycaemia (a condition occurring when the blood glucose concentration falls below normal). It is well recognized that hypoglycaemia can cause abnormal behaviour, including aggressive and irrational behaviour. This is not surprising since the brain relies on glucose to provide cellular energy. Section 3.4.3 deals with the legal issues and Chapter 9 deals more fully with the scientific issues regarding hypoglycaemia. Sometimes a person's behaviour is, or may have been, modified by hypoglycaemia.

CASE 4.2 (TATTERSALL 1986)

A man with insulin-dependent diabetes mellitus was interrogated at work for 4 hours by a manager and a security officer. He had taken his usual insulin, and was due to eat a main meal, but had no food during his interrogation. At the end of it, he 'confessed' to theft, and was then taken to a police station and questioned for a further 2 hours before he was able to eat. The case came to trial.

Tattersall explained to the Jury that the defendant's diabetes was usually well controlled, and his blood glucose concentration had previously been low. The missed meal would have made hypoglycaemia likely, and in Tattersall's view hypoglycaemia would have so altered the defendant's state of mind that he became unusually suggestible, and could have confessed to a crime which he had not committed.

A confession, to be admissible in evidence, has to be both voluntary and reliable. The defendant was acquitted.

4.1.2 Other drug-induced mental changes

An American case illustrates the chaos that can result when a suspect confesses under the influence of drugs.

CASE 4.3 (CURRAN 1969)

The mutilated body of a woman was found in her caravan after a man called Cameron told a friend that he had killed her. All three had been drinking together at the caravan site earlier that evening, and Cameron was arrested. A physician examined him and took a blood sample which showed the concentration of ethanol in his blood to be 180 milligrams per 100 millilitres. (The permitted limit for driving a motor-car in the United Kingdom is 80 milligrams per 100 millilitres.)

The doctor nevertheless declared that the suspect was fit to be questioned. Cameron broke down during the interrogation, and asked to be shot. He was transferred to a psychiatric hospital where he was given an injection of the major tranquillizer chlorpromazine in the large dose of 300 milligrams. The next day he was further interrogated in the presence of two more psychiatrists and made at least three confessions.

Two juries failed to agree on the defendant's guilt in the subsequent murder trials, but a third jury convicted him of murder in the first degree. Nine years after the crime, the Supreme Court of California held that the conviction was unsafe, because the chlorpromazine and ethanol could have destroyed the defendant's will to resist suggestions that he confess, and the case was returned to the lower court for a fourth murder trial.

As the *New England Journal of Medicine* stated, 'if any case illustrates the need for better medicolegal handling of criminal cases, this is it'.

4.1.3 Is the behaviour due to a disease or a drug?

Experts can sometimes become embroiled in arguments over the difference between a disease and a temporary, drug-induced state (Section 3.4.3).

CASE 4.4[1] (TROTT 1992)

An alcoholic mother drank nine-tenths of a bottle of vodka and then strangled her 11-year-old daughter. There was no doubt that she was in an abnormal state of mind when she killed her daughter.

The legal arguments, which went to the Court of Appeal, hinged on the medical issues. If the crime had been committed as a result of a disease, that is, brain damage caused by alcohol, the abnormality of mind would have constituted a defence. It would also have been a defence to show that, at the time of the crime, the defendant's addiction to alcohol had gone so far that she was incapable of resisting the urge to drink: 'if her drinking was involuntary, then her abnormality of mind at the time of the act of strangulation was induced by her condition of alcoholism' (Lord Justice Watkins). If she had voluntarily drunk the first drink of vodka on the day of the crime, however, and the abnormality of the mind was a result of her temporary intoxication, then that was no defence.

In the event, the Court of Appeal upheld her conviction for murder.

The question sometimes arises whether a drug other than alcohol has caused brain damage or intoxication.

CASE 4.5 (TROTT 1992)

A man with no history of psychiatric disease voluntarily took LSD and cannabis and then committed an apparently motiveless and bizarre killing. After the killing he made off with some of the deceased's belongings and hid them. At his trial the medical experts argued as to whether the accused was suffering *brain damage* from the drugs at the time of the killing. The judge invited the jury to decide whether there was a disease or intoxication.

The defendant was convicted of murder.

4.1.4 Pathological intoxication

Ethanol (ethyl alcohol) may cause a very unusual and rather ill-defined form of *pathological intoxication*, or *mania a potu*, in which the consumption of ethanol is followed by senseless violence, then prolonged sleep; the subject loses his memory for the events occurring for several hours after drinking (Coid 1979). The difficulty of using pathological intoxication as a defence is underlined by Coid's observation that the evidence '…tends to suggest that courts are not the testing grounds where many British psychiatrists will attempt to defend such a diagnosis'.

4.2 Drugs that cause aggression

Drugs that have been linked with aggressive behaviour are listed in Table 4.1, and the list includes a number of drugs usually thought of as sedatives. These drugs are supposed to impair the mechanisms that normally inhibit violent or antisocial behaviour (Sheard 1984). Ethanol is the most important agent from a practical viewpoint, and is often a factor in crimes where other agents are also involved (Turner 1987). Common wisdom has it that a drinker becomes 'fighting drunk' before collapsing into a coma.

Anabolic steroids and several other drugs can increase or cause aggression, and therefore catalyse violent crimes which might otherwise not have been committed. Cases are discussed in Section 15.5.

[1] The case is reported as *R. v. Tandy* [1989] 1 WLR 350.

Table 4.1 Drugs linked with aggressive behaviour (after Sheard 1984; Turner 1987)

---

alcohol (ethanol)
amitriptyline
amphetamines
anabolic androgens such as testosterone
barbiturates such as quinalbarbitone ('Seconal')
benzodiazepines such as diazepam ('Valium')
cocaine
ethanol (alcohol)
fenfluramine (an appetite suppressant related to amphetamine)
hallucinogens such as lysergic acid diethylamide (LSD)
opiates such as diamorphine (heroin)
phencylidine ('Angel dust')
propranolol

4.3 Drug-induced depression

Drugs can cause depression (Table 4.2), which can itself result in violence either against the sufferer as suicide or against others. The depression can occur during treatment or as an effect of drug withdrawal.

Table 4.2. Some drugs that can cause depression (D'Arcy and Griffin 1986d; Davies 1991e)

Drugs that can cause depression include:
  clonidine (an anti-hypertensive drug)
  corticosteroids such as hydrocortisone (cortisol)
  indomethacin (a non-steroidal anti-inflammatory drug)
  L-dopa (used to treat Parkinson's disease)
  methyldopa (an anti-hypertensive drug)
  oral contraceptive pill
  phenothiazine tranquillizers such as chlorpromazine ('Largactil')[a]
  propranolol and other beta-blocking drugs (used to treat hypertension and angina)

Drugs whose withdrawal can cause depression include:
  amphetamines
  anabolic androgens such as testosterone
  anorectic drugs such as fenfluramine

---

[a] Although depression appears to be part of the schizophrenic illness for which the drugs are given, so the role of the drugs is disputed.

4.4 Hallucination

Hallucination is sensory experience without a corresponding sensory input. It can be visual or auditory; more rarely it is olfactory or tactile. Patients can hallucinate as a result of psychiatric disease, notably schizophrenia, but sometimes also in severe depression. The interest for forensic pharmacology is that a number of drugs can induce hallucination, either during treatment or on withdrawal. The former effect is sought by those who take *hallucinogens*, also known as *entactogens*, drugs that are abused because they can cause hallucination: 'mind-expanding drugs', in the naïve or cynical phrase of the 1960s. Ethanol withdrawal, with 'spiders crawling up the wall' and 'pink elephants', provides a paradigm for the latter.

CASE 4.6

A 42-year-old solicitor had drunk about 16 units of alcohol (equivalent to 8 pints of beer) a day for many years. He was persuaded by his girlfriend to join Alcoholics Anonymous, stopped drinking at once and had a series of fits due to ethanol withdrawal. As he was recovering from his fits, he developed terrifying visions (delirium tremens; 'the DTs'); believing that he was being pursued by a giant dentist's drill, he threw himself out of a first-floor window, breaking the bones in both ankles.

Illusion, in contrast to hallucination, is the misinterpretation of sensory input:

CASE 4.7

A staid lady in her fifties had alopecia totalis (which results in complete baldness). She underwent an operation to remove her gall-bladder. While recovering from the anaesthetic, she ran round the surgical ward throwing her wig in the air under the impression that it was a hedgehog.

Table 4.3. Examples of drugs that can induce hallucination or psychosis (D'Arcy and Griffin 1986*d*; Olson, 1990; Davies, 1991*e*)

Abused drugs causing hallucination or psychosis:
  amphetamine and its derivatives (including Ecstasy)
  bufotenine (from licking the skin of the toad *Bufo vulgaris*)
  cannabis (marijuana)
  cocaine (including 'crack' cocaine)
  datura (*Datura stramonium* - Jimsonweed, thornapple; and other species)
  khat (*Catha edulis*)
  lysergic acid diethylamide (LSD)
  mescaline (from the peyote cactus)
  myristicin (from nutmeg)
  phencylidine
  psilocybin (from the *Psilocybe* 'magic' mushroom—the Liberty cap)

Therapeutic drugs causing hallucination or psychosis during treatment:
  anorectic drugs such as fenfluramine ('Ponderax')
  antibiotics, including benzyl penicillin, ciprofloxacin and nalidixic acid
  anticholinergic drugs such as atropine and benzhexol
  anticonvulsants such as phenytoin
  anti-inflammatory drugs, particularly indomethacin
  antimalarials, especially chloroquine
  beta-blocking drugs such as propranolol
  corticosteroids such as dexamethasone and prednisolone
  dopamine agonists, such as L-dopa and bromocriptine
  isoniazid (used in treating tuberculosis)
  opioids, such as pentazocine and diamorphine

Drugs causing hallucination or psychosis on withdrawal
  benzodiazepines, such as diazepam ('Valium')
  ethanol
  opioids

Delusion is mistaken but unshakable belief, and can take the form of *paranoid* delusion, a mistaken belief that the sufferer is being persecuted.

Hallucination, illusion, and delusion can all form part of a drug-induced psychosis. Examples of drugs that lead to this are given in Table 4.3.

The features of drug-induced psychosis can be indistinguishable from those of schizophrenia. This is particularly the case for amphetamine psychosis (Creese 1983), where the only distinguishing features are evidence of amphetamine intake and recovery after the last traces of amphetamines have gone (from the urine). The distinction is forensically important, because a psychosis due to disease might constitute a defence, whereas a psychosis induced by drug abuse would not.

4.5 Summary

Drugs can so alter a person's state of mind that they lead to an act which would not have occurred in their absence. Where the person voluntarily took the drug and should have known the consequences, this will not usually provide a defence; though it might in some circumstances diminish responsibility for a criminal act. Where the drug was a prescribed drug, and the patient was not reckless in its use, then a defence of involuntary self-intoxication may subsequently be available.

5

Effects of drugs on the victims of crime

5.1 Some history

Poison is a particularly evocative agent of crime; '…incensed at the most cowardly of crimes [the private individual] regards with horror the execrable assassin and demands his punishment' (Orfila 1814, quoted in Morrison 1930). The secret poisoner was regarded with such abhorrence that a statute of Henry VIII (1531) prescribed that convicted poisoners should be boiled alive:

CASE 5.1 (WROITHESLEY'S CHRONICLE 1542 QUOTED IN MORRISON 1930)

'This year, the 17th of March, was boyled in Smithfield one Margaret Davie, a mayden which had poysoned three households that she dwelled in.'

Article 301 of the Napoleonic Code Penal defined the specific crime of '*empoisonnement*' (poisoning) as the crime of making an attempt on the life of another by administering a substance capable of causing death. Article 302 laid down that 'tout coupable d'assassinat, de paricide, d'infanticide et d'empoisonnement, sera puni de mort'[1] (Orfila 1852).

The forensic problems which face a pharmacologist today in a case of murder are little different from those that confronted Orfila, the foremost nineteenth century medicolegal toxicologist. 'To *affirm* that poisoning has taken place, the expert has to demonstrate the presence of poison by rigorous chemical methods or by certain botanical or zoological characteristics. If he is unable to do this, he can establish the *probability* of poisoning if he has been able to observe symptoms, signs and organic changes consistent with those produced by poisonous substances … Without definitive analysis, then the physician should always be reserved in his conclusions, no matter how probable it appears to him that poisoning has taken place.'

Modern methods of chemical and biochemical analysis are incomparably more sensitive than those available to Orfila, but the principles hold true. The sensitivity of the assays for poisons actually increases the difficulties, in the sense that mere presence of a poison may not be enough to say that it was administered in sufficient quantities to be capable of doing harm. This is especially true for drugs that can be used therapeutically.

The case of William Palmer is an example of the principles in action. The jury were convinced by the experts for the prosecution that the symptoms and signs in the dying man were unequivocally due to poison, and the accused had the motive, opportunity, and means to commit murder. The prosecution managed this in spite of being unable to demonstrate the presence of the suspected poison by chemical means.

[1] All found guilty of murder, paricide, infanticide, and poisoning shall be punished by death.

CASE 5.2 (LATHOME BROWNE AND STEWART 1883)

William Palmer was a general practitioner in Rugeley, Staffordshire. He was a gambler, indebted to an acquaintance called John Parsons Cook, and to a money-lender. Cook was taken ill after a drinking session with Palmer and another man called Fisher. At one point, Palmer had given Cook a glass of brandy and water, which Cook drank. Within a minute, he exclaimed 'There's something in it; it burns my throat dreadfully'. Cook began vomiting, and became progressively more ill. The next day Cook at first improved, but after treatment from Palmer his condition deteriorated. Despite Palmer's ministrations, Cook suffered from continued vomiting and convulsion and then died in dreadful agony. A post-mortem examination was held. Palmer behaved in extraordinary fashion, nudging the operator's elbow so that some of the stomach contents were spilt, and remarking 'They won't hang us yet.' It was also suspected that he had tried to steal the viscera (entrails).

Traces of antimony but not strychnine were found in the body. Palmer was tried for murder. A succession of the most eminent medical men gave evidence for the prosecution to the effect that the symptoms were inconsistent with any natural illness, and must have been due to strychnine poisoning. More experts described unequivocal cases of strychnine poisoning, which were strikingly similar to Cook's demise.

The defence pursued the argument that the illness of vomiting and convulsion was tetanus (a result of infection with *Clostridium tetani*), syphilis, epilepsy, or apoplexy. His private physician averred that Cook had 'no venereal taint'.

Dr Taylor, the prosecution expert, then explained how, in his view, death was certainly due to strychnine poisoning even though he had been unable to detect any of the drug in the remains of the deceased. A Guy's man, he maintained this view in the face of fierce cross-examination, and other experts concurred.

Palmer was proved to have bought strychnine shortly before the death.

Defence experts stated that minute quantities of strychnine could be detected. However, the non-discovery of strychnine 'was foreign to the merits of the case, inasmuch as the evidence… tended to prove, not that there was no strychnia (strychnine) in Cook's body, but that Dr Taylor ought to have found it if it was there' (Mr Justice Stephen, quoted in Lathome Browne and Stewart 1883).

The authors point out a difficulty for the defence over Taylor's evidence: he failed to detect strychnine, but could find no other explanation for Cook's death. If he was incompetent, then the defence was implying that strychnine *might* have been present. If he was competent, then the jury would take due note of his view that Cook's death could only have been due to strychnine.

The upshot of this was that Palmer was found guilty even though there was no analytical proof of the administration of strychnine, and the experts agreed that the antimony which was detected had not been responsible for Cook's death.

He was hanged at Stafford Gaol.

It seems unlikely that the prosecution would have succeeded today, when the methods for analysis are sufficiently sensitive and specific that failure to find a drug usually makes it improbable that it was the cause of death.

The Victorian poisoners favoured aconite (Dr Lamson and perhaps Dr Warder), antimony (Dr Pritchard, Dr Smethurst, and Thomas Waislow), arsenic (Mary Lennox, Madelaine Smith, Florence Maybrick), cyanide as 'prussic acid' (John Tawell, George Ball, and Peter Walker), and strychnine (Dr Cream, Dr Palmer, William Dove, Eliza Edmunds and Silas Barlow). Adelaide Bartlett was found not guilty of murdering her husband with liquid chloroform.

Medical men were heavily over-represented. Poison has become a much rarer method of murder, though doctors still have recourse to it. This century, opiates have figured in two medical murder cases: Dr Bodkin Adams was acquitted, and Dr Clements committed suicide before he could be arrested. The *soi-disant* 'nurse' Dorothea Waddingham also resorted to opiates. Dr Paul Vickers of Gateshead was convicted of murdering his mentally ill wife with the anticancer drug lomustine (CCNU). Dr Crippen, an American dentist working as a salesman in London, poisoned his wife with hyoscine.

Non-medical poisoners in the earlier part of the twentieth century continued to use the old favourite, arsenic (Henry Armstrong, Edward Black, Charlotte Bryant, John James Hutchinson, Frederick Henry Seddon). Strychnine, too, has found favour (Thomas Mathieson Brown, Ethel Major, and Jean Pierre Vaquier) (Shew 1960).

More recent poisoners have used the barbiturate mixture 'Seconal' (John Armstrong was convicted; his wife was acquitted), yellow phosphorus (Louisa Merrifield was convicted; her husband was acquitted), thallium (Graham Frederick Young), insulin (Kenneth Barlow), lignocaine and potassium chloride (both used by the nurse Beverly Gail Allitt), and the opioid drug etorphine (the veterinary surgeon David James). The Bulgarian exile Georgi Markov was jabbed in the back of the thigh with an umbrella while crossing Westminster Bridge, and then became ill and died. A small metal pellet with holes drilled in it was discovered in his thigh. The holes had apparently contained the deadly but rather slow-acting poison, ricin, derived from the castor-oil plant. Ricin has subsequently been used, attached to specific antibodies, in experimental treatment of cancer.

5.2 Crime and death by poisoning

Poison is still sometimes used to kill people. Forensic pharmacologists are usually faced with the same problem as in the nineteenth century case of William Palmer, that the prosecution wishes to show that the victim has received a potentially lethal dose of a drug.

Sometimes the features of poisoning are distinctive enough to suggest the diagnosis, and this is confirmed by laboratory analysis.

CASE 5.3 (*THE TIMES* 2 FEBRUARY 1995)

The family of a consultant anaesthetist became ill after drinking tonic water, and he suspected from their symptoms that they had been poisoned with atropine[2]. Several days later, a woman was admitted to hospital seriously unwell with similar symptoms after drinking gin and tonic. Remnants of the drink contained much more atropine than the tonic water used to mix it. The woman's husband had tried to kill her, and had adulterated bottles of tonic in a supermarket to make it appear that she was the random victim of the 'tonic water poisoner'. He was convicted of attempted murder of his wife, and of endangering the lives of seven other people, and imprisoned for 12 years.

In an interesting inversion of the usual circumstances, the following case illustrates how the Defence argued that the concentration of a drug in a post-mortem specimen might have been sufficient to cause death.

CASE 5.4

A 27-day-old baby boy was admitted to hospital collapsed, and died after a spell on a ventilator ('life-support machine'). He had evidence in life and after death of severe brain damage of the sort caused by shaking. His father was committed for trial, accused of his murder. He maintained that

[2] Anaesthetists use atropine to dry up secretions, and it also dilates the pupils, speeds the heartbeat, and makes the skin hot and dry.

he had simply shaken the boy because he was deeply asleep, and he could not rouse him. He also said that his common-law wife, the boy's mother, had given the boy some medicine to keep him quiet.

The defence found that blood samples taken after death contained a measurable amount of the sedative antihistamine promethazine. This is used to quieten children, but is not recommended for use in children under one year old, and has been linked to apnoeic spells (cessation of breathing) in young infants. It was argued in defence that it was likely, or at least possible, that the mother had given enough promethazine to cause sedation and possibly respiratory arrest, and that the father's story was corroborated by the finding of promethazine in the blood.

The prosecution experts argued that the concentration in the blood was too small to be regarded as toxic. The defence experts were of the opinion that any dose in a child below 12 months was an overdose in the sense that the drug was not safe at that age. Furthermore, if all the delays were taken into account, the concentration was likely to have decreased substantially from the peak value, and that was likely to have been toxic in the conventional sense (Appendix A).

In the event, the defendant pleaded guilty to manslaughter, and was gaoled for 3 years.

Reckless or deliberate acts short of murder can result in charges of, or conviction for, manslaughter. Medical negligence can be so great and the behaviour of the doctor concerned so foolhardy as sometimes to justify a charge of manslaughter. This is discussed in Chapter 6. Such charges can arise in other circumstances. One example is discussed in Section 12.3.

Murder requires that the victim die within a year and a day of the crime, and that the perpetrator intended to cause death or grievous bodily harm. Sometimes the necessary intent is lacking, and then there may be a conviction for manslaughter.

CASE 5.5 (MALTBY 1975)

A general practitioner, addicted to amphetamines and ethanol, gave his drunken mistress a rectal injection of the short-acting barbiturate thiopentone; and also intramuscular injections of morphine, pethidine (an opioid related to morphine), chlorpromazine (a major tranquillizer) and promethazine (a sedative antihistamine, related to chlorpromazine). He then took obscene photographs of her in bizarre positions. During this session, his mistress was asphyxiated, and died. The general practitioner was charged with her murder.

There was no evidence that the general practitioner intended to kill his mistress, and she died of asphyxia, so that the drugs he administered were not the direct cause of her death. He was, however, reckless in administering them without guarding against asphyxia.

He was convicted of manslaughter.

Occasionally, the intended victim is not human. A prize-winning Rottweiler dog needed urgent treatment with vitamin K after it had been poisoned with a mixture of tranquillizers and an anticoagulant rat poison (Pike 1994).

5.3 Child abuse by poisoning

Child abuse is any treatment which is injurious to a child's physical or emotional health. The classical picture, the 'battered baby syndrome', is of children beaten so badly that they suffer broken bones, brain damage, and death. Sometimes children are deliberately injured by chemical rather than physical agents.

A particular and bizarre form of child abuse is called Munchausen's syndrome by proxy, a term coined by Meadow (1977) to describe cases where mothers, or occasionally other carers, cause factitious[3] disease in a child with the intention of deceiving doctors and other medical

[3] factitious: made artificially; fictitious: imaginary.

staff. The syndrome represents a variant of 'Munchausen's Syndrome', a condition first named and described by Asher (1951), consisting of factitious disease, often accompanied by fabulous and exaggerated stories of illness, and without any discernable motive. Baron Heironymous Karl Frederich von Munchausen (1720–97) was famed for his fabulous adventures.

The syndrome has also been called Polle's syndrome, after the daughter of Baron Munchausen. She died in infancy (Burman and Stevens 1978). It is sometimes known as Meadow's syndrome after the professor who wrote the definitive description.

One of the earliest documented cases of the syndrome was described by Dine:

CASE 5.6 (DINE 1965)

A 19-month-old boy was admitted for the fifth time in 4 months with sleepiness, convulsion and fever. The mother explained the illnesses as due to a head injury, and denied that the boy could possibly have ingested any medicines, other than phenobarbitone which he had lately been prescribed for the fits. However, the mother's doctor was contacted, and said that she took the phenothiazine tranquillizer perphenazine, after a psychotic illness which she suffered when the boy was born. The child was kept in hospital, recovered, and remained well for seven days. Half an hour after he had eaten an ice-cream given to him in hospital by his mother, he became unconscious.

His urine showed the presence of phenothiazines. The mother continued to deny that she had administered it, but agreed to psychiatric treatment.

This is a paradigm of Munchausen's syndrome by proxy.

Rogers *et al.* (1976) published an early series of cases and outlined some of the features. They wrote that 'regrettably the first requirement for diagnosis is a low threshold of suspicion. Bizarre symptoms and signs with no apparent pathological explanation should lead to the consideration of pharmacological causes … A full drug history of all members of the child's household may show the availability of appropriate drugs. A history of parental drug abuse or overdose should heighten suspicion.' In several of their cases, too, the child's condition improved at first but deteriorated while the child was still in hospital after an intervention by the mother. The features that should arouse suspicion have been tabulated (Guandolo 1985; Pickford *et al.* 1988). Relevant features are listed in Table 5.1. The validity of empirical criteria for diagnosing Munchausen's syndrome by proxy has been questioned (Morley 1992).

Table 5.1 Clues to the diagnosis of Munchausen's syndrome by proxy due to drug administration (after Guandolo 1985; Mahesh *et al.* 1988; Pickford *et al.* 1988)

The illness involves neurological signs, 'biochemical chaos', bleeding, diarrhoea, or chemical burns in the mouth or oesophagus

Seizures can be resistant to standard therapy

There is unexplained recurrence (or persistence) of illness

The symptoms do not correspond to the signs

A rare or unique disorder is suspected; that is, 'a differential diagnosis consisting of a disorder less common than Munchausen's syndrome by proxy'

The features are absent when the mother is absent

The mother is reluctant to leave the child's side

The mother is less concerned at the illness than might be expected

The mother has been a nurse or other hospital worker

The mother has suffered from Munchausen's syndrome or other mental disorder

To prove that a sick child has been abused with drugs, it has to be shown that a drug has been administered, that the administered drug has caused the illness, that the drug was administered deliberately to cause harm, and that it was administered by a particular individual. The apparent difficulties of diagnosing Munchausen's syndrome by proxy once it is suspected are diminished by the bizarre nature of the illness involved, the relatively small number of drugs that babies could reasonably be given, and the remarkable persistence of the perpetra-

Table 5.2 Substances that have been used in the chemical abuse of children (Rogers *et al.* 1976; Schnaps *et al.* 1981; Dine and McGovern 1982; Tenenbein 1986; Meadow 1989; Proudfoot 1989)

Analgesics	Aspirin
	Dextropropoxyphene ('Darvon')
	Dihydrocodeine
	Paracetamol (acetaminophen)
Anticoagulants	Warfarin
Anticonvulsants	Carbamazepine
	Phenytoin
	Sodium valproate
Antidepressants	Amitriptyline
	Imipramine
Antidiabetic agents	Phenformin
	Insulin (given directly)
	Insulin (mother gave glucose + added acetone to the urine)
Antipsychotic drugs	Chlorpromazine
	Perphenazine
	Promethazine
Diuretics	Frusemide
	Chlorthalidone
Drugs of abuse	Cocaine
Household products	Common salt (NaCl)
	Ethanol
	Lye (caustic soda, NaOH)
	'Naphtha' (petroleum distillate)
	Peppers (capsicum)
	Pine oil
	Rat poison (anticoagulant)
	Water
Hypnotics	Barbituates ('Tuinal')
	Benzodiazepines (e.g. alprazolam, diazepam)
	Chloral hydrate
	Glutethimide
	Methaqualone
Laxatives	
	Phenolphthalein
	Epsom salts (magnesium salts)
Other drugs	Vitamin A

tors. The most difficult part in the process is to suspect that a 'good' mother could be harming her own child.

Dine and McGovern (1982) described seven cases and found references to 41 more. Tenenbein (1986) was able to find 75 cases in the medical literature in which children had been abused by administration of 'drugs, chemicals or other exogenous agents', though these included three cases of material contaminated with bacteria, and three of water deprivation.

Neither author distinguishes clearly between Munchausen's syndrome by proxy, with its essential component of deception, and other forms of abuse. For example, Dine and McGovern (1982) describe a child who, having been given chilli peppers, was beaten so hard that he suffered a subdural brain haemorrhage and died; the chillies had apparently been given to punish the child, not to mislead doctors into believing that he was suffering from organic illness. Table 5.2 lists some of the agents that have been incriminated, and some of the common ones are considered here in more detail.

5.3.1 Common salt (NaCl)

One of the cases reported by Rogers *et al.* (1976) had been poisoned with common table salt, prefiguring the second case described in Meadow's classical paper:

CASE 5.7 (MEADOW 1977)

A baby boy had recurrent illnesses manifest as sudden attacks of drowsiness, vomiting and hypernatraemia (a high sodium concentration in the plasma), with high concentrations of sodium in the urine as well. The plasma sodium concentration was in the range 160–175 millimoles per litre on admission. (The normal range is 135-143 millimoles per litre). He was very carefully investigated in three centres without a diagnosis being made. On one occasion, his mother's breast milk was found to have a high sodium concentration, though on a second occasion, when the specimen was taken at once to the laboratory, the concentration was normal. The attacks only occurred at home and their frequency increased as he grew older. His mother had been a nurse. He recovered during a prolonged stay in hospital when his mother was excluded, but relapsed after she had visited. He was allowed home but was readmitted with extreme hypernatraemia and died at the age of 14 months. The mother attempted to kill herself.

Meadow hypothesized that the mothers in these cases fabricate their stories 'to get themselves into the sheltered environment of a children's ward surrounded by friendly staff.'

In a later series of 12 cases, the median serum or plasma sodium concentration was about 170 millimoles per litre (range 150–228 millimoles per litre) and the urine sodium concentration was in the range 150–360 millimoles per litre (Meadow, 1993). In these and other cases (Chesney and Brusilow 1981) it is unclear how much of the hypernatraemia was due to excessive salt intake, and how much to water deprivation.

5.3.2 Medicines used in psychiatry

Minor and major tranquillizers, antidepressants, and sleeping tablets have all been used to induce illness in infants.

CASE 5.8 (WATSON *ET AL.* 1979)

A boy aged 7 years 10 months was admitted to hospital unconscious and twitching. He had episodes of apnoea (spells without breathing). Investigations were normal and he recovered over the next 48 hours. The parents said he had been prescribed amitriptyline for enuresis (bed-wetting), but denied any possible poisoning. He was sent home after 14 days, but vomited repeatedly after discharge, and was again admitted with drowsiness 1 month later. During his time in hospital he was intermittently drowsy and had twitching of his limbs. There were episodes of jerking and drowsiness during his admission, but he recovered without treatment. He was admitted for a third time 12 days later, unconscious with twitching limbs and ventricular tachycardia (a serious abnormality of heart rhythm). Blood and stomach contents contained the antidepressant imipramine[4] and its metabolite (breakdown product) desipramine. The mother was receiving imipramine, and confessed to administering it to the child.

    This case was unusual, but not unique, in so far as the child was old enough to move about and to understand if harm was obviously being done to him.

CASE 5.9 (LORBER 1978*A,B*; LORBER *ET AL.* 1980)

A 2-year-old boy was admitted to hospital deeply unconscious. He recovered, but over the next 14 days had nine further episodes of unconsciousness, including two cardiorespiratory arrests (his heart-beat and breathing ceased). The episodes were accompanied by a rash. Investigations failed to provide a diagnosis and the paediatrician wrote to the *Lancet* to ask if any reader could help. An Australian doctor suggested deliberate barbiturate poisoning, which had by then been diagnosed. The mother, who herself had Munchausen's syndrome, was subsequently sentenced to 3 years in prison.

    The characteristic clues in these cases of psychotropic drug poisoning are neurological symptoms or signs, such as drowsiness, unconsciousness, fits, twitching, or incoordination, together with a history that the abuser has access to the medicine and the opportunity to give it. The presence of treated psychiatric illness in the mother (usually) provides both the opportunity for and an explanation of the abuse. The diagnosis, as with other chemical causes of Munchausen's syndrome by proxy, rests on toxicological analysis of the appropriate samples at the appropriate time.

CASE 5.10

A 5½-year-old girl was admitted to hospital after a fit. She had previously been admitted with fits witnessed by her mother. A CT brain scan[5] and electroencephalogram (brain wave recording) were normal on this as on previous admissions. There were episodes of drowsiness while on the ward, and one event when the girl became stiff and had dilated pupils. A urine drug screen 5 days after admission was negative, although the specimen was very dilute. Ten days after admission, the ward clerk interrupted the mother administering a white medicine to the girl from a shampoo bottle. The girl's subsequent urine specimen contained imipramine and its metabolites. It transpired that the general practitioner had prescribed the drug to treat bed-wetting. The mother denied administering any drug when questioned by the hospital social worker, but later confessed to the police.

    The defendant's solicitors asked for an explanation of the nature of the various medicines involved in the case, discussion of the nature of the witnessed fit, and comment on the part played by imipramine in the child's illness.

    Imipramine can cause drowsiness in therapeutic doses, and the detection of imipramine and metabolites in the urine means that imipramine must have been given, but does not indicate

---

[4] Dilated pupils, coma, convulsion, a fast heart rate, and ventricular tachycardia are the typical features of poisoning with a tricyclic antidepressant such as imipramine or amitriptyline.

[5] A CT (computerized tomographic) brain scan is a radiological study of the brain in which a series of images (slices) is reconstructed by computer from many measurements of X-ray absorption.

whether the dose was excessive. Imipramine in overdose usually causes classical tonic–clonic fits with shaking of the limbs, which were never seen in this girl. The stiffness would be consistent with imipramine poisoning, but not diagnostic of it. The medical evidence was therefore not sufficient, by itself, to indicate that the girl's illness was unequivocally due to imipramine poisoning.

5.3.3 Laxatives and emetics

Babies often develop diarrhoea or feeding difficulties, and can fail to thrive. These problems have, in rare instances, been the result of deliberate administration of laxatives (Forbes *et al.* 1985).

CASE 5.11 (FENTON *ET AL.* 1988)

A 7-month-old girl was investigated for diarrhoea and failure to gain weight. She passed up to 10 loose stools a day. She improved rapidly but briefly when her feeds were changed to soya milk. She subsequently became severely ill with dehydration and collapse. Stool osmolality was measured, and the result (284 milliosmoles per kilogram) was at odds with the very low sodium concentration (less than 5 millimoles per litre). Stool and urine magnesium concentrations were measured, and found to be 10 times normal. The mother then admitted to administering Epsom salts[6] to her baby, 'so that the doctors would take her more seriously'. The child gained weight dramatically over the next 3 months.

Another laxative, phenolphthalein, becomes red in alkaline conditions, and the baby can appear to have blood in the stool or urine. The colour disappears if the sample is acidified (Fleisher and Ament 1977).

The diagnosis of laxative abuse should be considered in cases of unexplained diarrhoea or failure to gain weight in infants.

The emetic ipecacuanha (ipecac) has been recommended for the emergency treatment of children who have ingested poison. In the United States, a supply is commonly kept at home. Repeated administration causes vomiting and diarrhoea, and has been recorded as a form of Munchausen's syndrome by proxy (Sutphen and Saulsbury 1988).

5.3.4 Insulin

CASE 5.12 (MCSWEENEY AND HOFFMAN 1991)

A 5-year-old boy suffered from 'seizures'. For 2 years his 'diabetic' mother had treated him with insulin for diabetes that had been diagnosed in another town by a doctor whose name she could not remember. The boy was investigated in hospital, and found to be completely normal. 'Insulin-dependent diabetes mellitus is so readily recognized that once a child has been assigned this diagnosis, it is rarely questioned...His mother may also have [had] fictitious diabetes...'.

5.4 Effects of drugs on the state of mind of the victim

There are two important considerations:

1. A victim of crime can be induced by a drug to take part in an act or to fail to resist an act to which no consent would have been given in the absence of the drug

[6] Epsom salts contain magnesium sulphate, which is a laxative. They originally came from natural springs in Epsom, Surrey.

2. A complainant who has taken or legitimately been given a drug may be led by the drug to believe that some crime has taken place after the administration of the drug and against the complainant's will.

5.4.1 Administration of a drug to alter the victim's behaviour

The drug can be administered deliberately to induce in the victim a state of mind in which she (usually) will agree to an act which would not otherwise have had her consent, especially sexual intercourse. No doubt ethanol has been widely used for this purpose.

Rape consists of a male having sexual intercourse with a female when he knows that at the time of intercourse she does not consent to it, or he is reckless as to whether she consents or not.

Section 4 of the Sexual Offences Act 1956 specifically makes administering a drug to facilitate intercourse a crime. Drugs other than ethanol have sometimes been used.

> CASE 5.13
>
> A 17-year-old girl worked part-time as a doctor's receptionist. One evening the doctor took the girl with him in his motor-car and gave her a handkerchief to sniff, saying that it smelt of his new after-shave. She recalled little else until she woke up naked in a bedroom with the doctor and another man. The doctor again held a dampened handkerchief to her face and she again became unconscious.
>
> When she was examined later, it appeared that the girl had been raped. She also had marks on the skin of her face consistent with chemical burns. It subsequently transpired that the doctor had ordered chloroform through the local pharmacist shortly before the events.
>
> Simpson, the Scottish Professor of Midwifery who pioneered the use of chloroform as an anaesthetic in the nineteenth century, wrote that a little chloroform on a pocket-handkerchief held over the mouth and nostrils 'generally suffices in about a minute or two to produce the desired effect.' Chloroform is also an irritant to the skin capable of causing chemical burns.
>
> The doctor was committed for trial, and in due course convicted of rape and sentenced to 10 years in prison.

In this case, the victim was forced to inhale the anaesthetic agent. Where the victim has taken drugs such as ethanol (ethyl alcohol) voluntarily the situation can be different.

> CASE 5.14 (TURNER 1987)
>
> A 45-year-old woman accused a man whom she had voluntarily accompanied to a flat of having sexual intercourse with her without consent. She was at the time treated with phenobarbitone for epilepsy, and methyldopa and bendrofluazide for hypertension. She had also received treatment for alcoholism, and admitted that on the evening of the alleged rape she had drunk brandy and several pints of beer. She could not recollect giving consent.
>
> An expert would be able to say that ethanol and phenobarbitone, together or separately, might have resulted in her having forgotten that at the time she did consent.

> CASE 5.15 (PILKINGTON AND BUNTING, GUARDIAN 20 OCTOBER 1993)
>
> A 21-year-old man was accused of raping a fellow university student. The prosecution alleged that she was so drunk that she was incapable of consenting or resisting, but did not argue that she withheld her consent. There was evidence that she was in fact so drunk that she mistook the accused for another man. She could not recall whether or not she had consented.
>
> The man was acquitted.

5.4.2 Drugs lead the complainant to perceive that a crime has been committed

Drugs can also so alter the patient's perceptions of what has happened that the patient believes that a crime has been committed where this is not the case. For reasons which are unclear to the author, this is a particular hazard in dentistry. Jastak and Malamed (1980) described nine such cases associated with dental anaesthesia using nitrous oxide (N_2O) gas, although the details that they provide are sketchy. Dundee described 41 cases of fantasy during sedation with the benzodiazepines midazolam or diazepam, given intravenously. Sixteen of these occurred during dental treatment and three led to spontaneous complaints of sexual indecency: 'none of these events ever happened'. The fantasies most commonly involved oral sex (Dundee 1990*a,b,c*). It can, of course, be difficult to determine whether an event has been real or imaginary.

CASE 5.16 (BRAHAMS 1990*A, B*)

A 21-year-old university student was treated in a (Canadian) hospital emergency room for hyperventilation, and the treatment included intravenous diazepam. She alleged that while she was sedated she was sexually assaulted by the physician attending to her. He claimed that she had been befuddled and thus misinterpreted his action in asking her to 'squeeze [his two fingers] hard', a test of her ability to respond to commands. He was acquitted at a criminal trial, but subsequently had his licence to practise revoked on the grounds that he denied the offence, that the victim's account was likely to be correct, that therefore he refused to face up to his failings, and that he as a result required psychiatric help.

5.5 Summary

Drugs can be used to kill or injure people. They can also be used to so alter the victim's perception that the victim agrees to an act, or fails to resist an act, when in other circumstances consent would have been withheld. Rarely, drugs can induce the delusion that a crime has taken place when it has not.

6

Negligence and medicines

Errors in prescribing and giving medicines can be fatal. Such errors accounted for 10 deaths over a period of 6 years in the jurisdiction of the Coroner for Birmingham and Solihull. In the same period, 36 deaths were recorded as the result of adverse reaction to drugs (Ferner and Whittington 1994).

To prove that someone has been negligent, it is necessary to show that they have failed to fulfil a duty to exercise care, that this failure has caused an effect in the plaintiff (complainant), that the effect was reasonably foreseeable, and that this effect has harmed the plaintiff (see Chapter 3). Harm can arise at any stage of the therapeutic process, from drug development to drug administration.

The cause of an illness or injury can be difficult to decide, since natural disease and drug-induced disease can result in identical clinical pictures (see Section 1.3.4). Certain facts can at least help to establish that a drug may have been responsible:

(1) the injured person had been exposed to the medicine;
(2) the exposure took place before the beginning of the illness or injury ascribed to the medicine;
(3) the time between exposure and illness or injury was neither so long nor so short that the exposure could not have been responsible for the injury;
(4) the extent of the exposure was sufficient to account for the illness or injury, that is, a sufficient dose was given for a sufficient time to cause the illness or injury;
(5) where the illness or injury is temporary, that it remits after exposure ceases, and recurs after it recommences;
(6) the illness or injury is known to occur with the medicine in question; and
(7) the illness or injury can best be explained by exposure to the medicine, and not to some other cause such as underlying or intercurrent disease.

Causation is important for medicolegal reasons, and it has been studied extensively in the context of adverse drug reaction monitoring. The conclusions of scientific studies are not very encouraging, since they demonstrate that even if experts use guidelines such as those above, they often disagree amongst themselves on the likelihood of a given agent causing a given illness or injury (Karch *et al.* 1976). The medicolegal consequence is that decisions on causation may depend on expert evidence which itself cannot be reliable, since agreement amongst experts is so poor.

The expert can also be asked to assess whether reasonable care has been taken. In the professional sense, reasonable care is the care that an average practitioner of the seniority and specialty concerned would have exercised, or which at least has the backing of other reputable practitioners.

If this seems disheartening, some comfort comes from the standard of proof required: it is only necessary to show that it is more likely than not that the facts are as the plaintiff alleges for the case to succeed.

The scope for error at each stage of the therapeutic process is illustrated here, and serves to show how each party to the process can be liable. Not all cases where harm results are due to negligence, and not all careless acts lead to harm, or litigation. The cases discussed below illustrate how harm can occur.

6.1 The manufacture of medicines

The law relating to the manufacture of medicines (outlined in Section 1.1.3) has, to a degree, been driven by the need to avoid repeating errors that have been made by drug manufacturers in the past. Dukes and Swartz (1988b) discuss the legal aspects in detail.

6.1.1 Testing a new drug or formulation

The manufacturer of a medicine should be careful to see that it is, as far as possible, safe for its intended purpose by testing it.

The testing of new drugs in human subjects now proceeds in a series of stages, from the judicious administration of small, single doses, and then repeated doses, to healthy volunteers (a Phase I study), via similar tests in patients (Phase II), to carefully controlled clinical trials (Phase III) and then surveillance of treated patients after the drug has been marketed (Phase IV).

The first Phase I study of a new chemical entity in human subjects is always a cause for anxiety, however thorough the prior laboratory testing in animals has been. Reassuring data from such studies in 'normal prison volunteers'[1] identified only 64 significant events in experiments on 29 162 subjects studied over more than 600 000 subject–days. Allergic phenomena, including angioedema (swelling of the soft tissues of the face and mouth, sometimes leading to breathing difficulties); haematuria (blood in the urine); and hepatitis (inflammation of the liver) were among the reactions seen. One man died of a brain haemorrhage when receiving inactive placebo, and one was left with permanent hip damage after infection complicated his experimental treatment (Zarafonetis et al. 1978). Deaths do occur, however rarely (Darragh et al. 1985).

It must be rare, and may be unknown, for a volunteer to bring an action for negligence against a manufacturer. A volunteer did sue the Canadian university that employed two research workers responsible for a study that went wrong:

CASE 6.1 (KENNEDY AND GRUBB 1994)[2]

A university student agreed to take part in an experiment to investigate the response of the heart and circulation to a general anaesthetic. He was told that a tube would be inserted into a vein in his arm, but not that it was a cardiac catheter which would then be advanced along the vein until it reached his heart.

He consented, the catheter was introduced, and he was anaesthetized. He then suffered a cardiac arrest (his heart effectively stopped beating) and was resuscitated by open cardiac massage

---

[1] Here are two possible contradictions and one ambiguity in a single phrase.
[2] The case referred to is *Halushka* v. *University of Saskatchewan* [1965].

(his chest was split open so that his heart could be squeezed to pump blood round his body). He recovered but required 10 days in hospital.

He was subsequently awarded damages, partly because the research workers had failed to tell him facts (that the experiment would entail cardiac catheterization) which might have materially affected whether or not he consented.

The failure to exercise due care in testing drugs can lead to harm when patients are treated, and that in turn can lead to charges of negligence. The 1938 US Food Drug and Cosmetic Act was the direct result of an error in manufacture of an antimicrobial.

CASE 6.2 (GEILING AND CANNON 1938)

A sulphonamide antimicrobial drug called sulphanilamide was originally formulated as a tablet. A liquid preparation was also desirable, for example, in treating children. An 'elixir' was made up in a 10 per cent solution of ethylene diglycol (diethylene glycol). Elixir is, in this context, a technical term meaning a medicine made up into a solution with ethanol (ethyl alcohol), though this product did not contain ethanol. Massengill, the firm making the 'elixir', failed to carry out any tests of the product's toxicity before it was marketed. Had such tests been carried out they would have shown what was already well known: that ethylene diglycol is highly toxic. As a result, over 100 people died. This tragedy was the stimulus to effective drug regulation in the United States (Wax 1995).

CASE 6.3 (D'ARCY AND GRIFFIN 1986B; DAVIES 1991B)

An unfortunate error in testing a French antiseptic, 'Stalinon', containing an organic compound of tin called diiodoethyltin, had rather similar results. The form prepared for toxicity testing was intended to contain 50 milligrams of the tin compound, but in fact contained only 3 milligrams per capsule as the result of a dispensing error. This low dose did not cause toxic symptoms. The marketed preparation contained 15 milligrams per capsule. One hundred and two people died from organotin poisoning from the 15 milligram capsules, and many more suffered permanent brain damage. The pharmacist responsible served 2 years in prison and his company was held liable for damages.

The sleeping tablet and anxiolytic, thalidomide, was not tested in pregnant animals prior to marketing, but was none the less promoted as being safe in pregnancy. Several thousand children were born with deformed limbs and with other congenital malformations. It is as a result of the thalidomide tragedy that manufacturers are now obliged under the 1968 Medicines Act to satisfy the drug regulatory authority of the safety of any product before it can be licensed (see p. 15).

The legal demonstration that a manufacturer has failed to carry out adequate tests is often difficult. It is necessary to show that the manufacturer did not carry out the tests prescribed by law or that he failed to conduct such tests as an averagely prudent manufacturer would do. Now that medicines have to be licensed under the Medicines Act 1968, the testing procedure is both explicitly laid out and rigorously examined. The historical examples show how necessary the legislation was.

It was not possible to prove that testing was inadequate in the case of Massengill's 'elixir' of sulphanilamide, since at that time there was no legal requirement for any test of toxicity before a medicinal product was offered for sale. The company was, however, pursued for misrepresenting their product as an elixir when it contained no ethanol. This semantic argument cannot have brought much comfort to the bereaved.

It is also necessary to demonstrate that the failure to carry out satisfactory tests has led to harm.

CASE 6.4 THE THALIDOMIDE CASE, (SJÖSTRÖM AND NILSSON 1972; D'ARCY AND GRIFFIN 1994) (SEE ALSO P.95).

This case shows that it can be difficult to prove that a medicine caused a specific adverse effect. The case led to litigation in several countries, notably Germany, where the drug had been manufactured by Chemie Grünenthal; Britain, where it had been licensed by Grünenthal to the Distillers Company; and Sweden, where Astra held the licence. In the United States, W.S. Merrell Co. were unable to market the drug as the Food and Drug Administration was not satisfied by the company's evidence that the drug was safe. However, there were North American cases of thalidomide embryopathy, as the drug was used for clinical trials in the US, and was granted a licence by the Canadian Food and Drug Directorate.

Nine senior members of Chemie Grünenthal were tried in the Criminal court in Aachen, as a prelude to eventual civil proceedings. Even causation was disputed. It had previously seemed impossible that anyone would contradict the evidence: the malformation allegedly caused by thalidomide (phocomelia, in which the limbs are rudimentary and the hands and feet can be vestigial) is otherwise extremely rare. The incidence of the malformation rose in proportion to the sales of thalidomide and declined rapidly in the months after thalidomide ceased to be sold. The abnormality occurred in a high proportion of children whose mothers had taken the drug in the sixth to seventh week of pregnancy, when the limbs develop their usual form. Exposure later in pregnancy did not cause limb abnormalities.

None the less, Chemie Grünenthal assembled experts to dispute the causal link between thalidomide and phocomelia. By this time, experiments had demonstrated a very similar teratogenic effect in rabbits, so that even those who argued that only a planned scientific experiment could demonstrate an unequivocal relationship might have been satisfied. The criminal trial dragged on for about 2 years, and was eventually abandoned. The civil cases were settled out of court between the firm and the representatives of damaged children for 114 million Deutschmarks. No verdict was ever reached on civil or criminal proceedings in Germany. Liability for damages in a series of actions against the Distillers Company (Biochemicals) Ltd was assessed in court in England (Nelson-Jones and Burton 1990a).

New preparations of old drugs can have very different bioavaliability from previous formulations. Standard preparations of a number of drugs are poorly absorbed from the gut, but the absorption can be enhanced.

CASE 6.5 (JOHNSON ET AL. 1973)

Wellcome, the major British manufacturers, changed the manufacturing process for the heart drug digoxin, sold under the brand name 'Lanoxin'. The new preparation complied with the quality standards that then existed (and there was not, therefore, a question of negligence). However, many patients suffered digoxin toxicity when given the new preparation in place of the old. Experimental studies in healthy volunteers showed that the peak plasma concentration after a given dose of digoxin was over twice as high with the new preparation as with the old.

CASE 6.6 (TYRER ET AL. 1970)

An outbreak of poisoning from the anticonvulsant, phenytoin, occurred in Australia when the excipient (filler) in the phenytoin capsule was changed from calcium sulphate to lactose and this caused an unpredicted increase in oral bioavailability. Fifty-one patients in Brisbane, who had taken the anticonvulsant for some time without ill-effect, developed symptoms of phenytoin poisoning when they took the new preparation.

Other problems can occur with new preparations of old drugs.

CASE 6.7 (COMMITTEE ON SAFETY OF MEDICINES 1983)

A formulation of indomethacin was devised in which the drug together with an electrolyte was contained within a semipermeable tablet shell. A laser-drilled hole allowed the drug to be expelled gradually by osmotic force. The drug was released at a constant rate and this prolonged its effective duration of action. Unfortunately, if the tablet lodged in the small bowel, a jet of indomethacin impinged on a very small area of bowel wall, and caused intestinal perforation.

Even if manufacturers conduct rigorous tests, difficulties might occur. Suppression of the results of tests on a new drug which have given unfavourable results, or inadvertent failure to reveal them, would pose potential problems for a company if they subsequently became known (see Case 3.2.3)

6.1.2 Making medicines

When the nature of the drug and its precise formulation have been fixed, then the manufacturer has a duty to make it according to that formulation, within specified tolerances. 'An extremely high standard of care is required because of the nature of drugs and the drastic effect which even slight faults can have' (Breuning *et al.* 1981; Dukes and Swartz 1988*a*).

The tolerances are sometimes laid down by the pharmacopoeia. For example, insulin preparations that are nominally made in a strength of 100 Units per millilitre are obliged to contain between 90 and 110 Units per millilitre. Tolerances can also be laid down in the product licence or elsewhere. Sometimes the matter is clear-cut and no recourse to technical standards is necessary.

CASE 6.8 (BINIMELIS *ET AL.* 1987)

A preparation of the thyroid hormone thyroxine contained 100 milligrams and not 100 micrograms. The patients who took the defective product therefore received 1000 times the intended dose, several became extremely ill, and some died.

CASE 6.9 (GRAVES 1994)

Thirteen children with leukaemia or cancer were treated in hospital with vincristine, an anticancer drug. Most of the children developed 'short-lived but unpleasant' symptoms, such as hair loss, abdominal pain, and nerve pain in the hands and feet.

The batch of vincristine delivered to the hospital was found to contain double the stated amount of vincristine, when the pharmacy noticed that the volume of drug was incorrect. The manufacturers offered to compensate the children for any ill-effects they suffered.

The manufacturer must also ensure that the product is not contaminated with other drugs, or chemicals or particles, or with unintended infectious agents or agents of unintended virulence.

CASE 6.10 (DUKES AND SWARTZ 1988*E*)

Errors in making a vaccine resulted in live virus particles being present in Salk 'killed' poliomyelitis vaccine, and the manufacturers were sued as a result.

Proof that manufacture has been defective is likely to come from analysis of the product to demonstrate that it contains more or less of the intended constituents, or that a contaminant was present. It might also come from process records indicating that some defective equipment had resulted in an unsterile, contaminated, or otherwise defective batch of product.

6.1.3 The packaging and storage of medicines

The manufacturer has to ensure that the product he supplies will remain active and safe for as long as specified provided his instructions are followed. Outdated products are sometimes unsafe, and an outbreak of Fanconi's syndrome (a form of kidney damage) has been linked to the use of old tetracycline which had become chemically degraded (Mavromatis 1965).

6.1.4 Failure by the manufacturer to provide information on medicines

The manufacturer has a duty to make known how his product can be used to best effect while minimizing the risk of harm. This duty exists towards the regulatory authorities, the professional people who dispense, prescribe, and administer the drug and (particularly in the United States) the patient who receives it.

> CASE 6.11 (SJÖSTRÖM AND NILSSON 1972; D'ARCY AND GRIFFIN 1994)
>
> An aspect of the thalidomide case which has understandably received less emphasis than the damage to embryos is the damage to peripheral nerves in children and adults. This can be severe, and is usually irreversible. Although the manufacturers became aware that this was the case in 1959, they suppressed the information, and later admitted that a neuropathy could occur, but described it as 'reversible' in spite of strong evidence to the contrary.

The manufacturer should also amend the information he provides to physicians so that it reflects current knowledge of the medicine's adverse effects. Dukes and Swartz (1988c) refer to three cases in the United States where companies were found liable for failing to provide information in accordance with current knowledge, so that patients were injured. In one case a woman successfully sued for loss of sight in one eye related to oral contraceptive use, because it was held that the information provided to her physician was inadequate. In another, visual loss, a well-recognized effect of the drug chloroquine, was not mentioned in the manufacturer's literature; and in the third case, the manufacturer had failed to warn adequately of the serious aplastic anaemia that can complicate treatment with chloramphenicol ('Chloromycetin').

Current knowledge in this context might include references in standard textbooks, or editorials in widely available medical journals. It might not include articles in obscure or inaccessible foreign medical journals to which the relevant practitioner is unlikely to have access.

6.1.5 The monitoring of adverse effects of medicines by the manufacturer

Adverse reactions to drugs do not necessarily become manifest in the clinical trials which precede its licensing and marketing. This is because relatively few people are exposed to the drug at this stage. A typical drug will have been tested in at most a few thousand people, and so the chance of detecting a serious reaction occurring with a risk of, say, 1 in 10 000 is very small.

Rare but serious complications can be manifest many years after a drug is introduced. Reye's syndrome of encephalopathy (brain disturbance) and liver failure after aspirin was only recognized 65 years after the drug's introduction. The manufacturer should monitor his licensed products to ensure that they do not cause unpredicted adverse effects. This was explicitly recognized in a Japanese case.

CASE 6.12 (D'ARCY AND GRIFFIN 1986c; DUKES AND SWARTZ 1988c; DAVIES 1991D)

Between 1955 and 1970, an epidemic occurred in Japan of an illness of peripheral neuropathy (nerve damage), optic atrophy (degeneration of the optic nerve) and encephalopathy (brain damage). The condition became known as *subacute myelo-optic atrophy* (SMON) and was linked to the drug clioquinol which was used as a gut anti-infective agent in the product 'Entero-Vioform' (see p. 36). The manufacturers were found liable for damages, and the Japanese court explicitly mentioned the continuing responsibility of a manufacturer for [the safety of] his drug even after it has been licensed.

6.2 The prescriber

No physician is perfect, and so no physician can guarantee cure without risk of incidental harm. The patient has a right to expect that the physician will exercise reasonable skill and care in his interests, and in this context reasonable means that the care should be that of 'an ordinary skilled man exercising and professing to have that special skill'. The skill expected of a general practitioner will be different from that of a neurologist or an orthopaedic surgeon. Each will be judged by the average standard of his group, and not by the theoretical or even the attainable best.

This is little consolation for those whose carelessness or lack of thought leads them to harm their patients. Obvious errors recur with sufficient frequency for them to seem inevitable. A survey of over 7500 prescriptions written for in-patients at a teaching hospital showed that more than 30 per cent of prescriptions contained some error. While many of the 'errors' were lapses in practice that would not have harmed patients, some were potentially lethal. For example, the heart drug digoxin was prescribed in a dose of 0.5 grams, which was 1000 times the intended dose of 0.5 MILLIGRAMS, in any event better written as 500 micrograms (Tesh *et al.* 1975).

Common errors in prescribing have been reviewed, with examples (Ferner 1992; Table 6.1). The American Society of Hospital Pharmacists has also published a nosological[3] list of medication errors, as part of a report on the subject (Anonymous 1992). The report contains guidelines on the prevention of medication errors[4].

There are many examples of most of the errors, a rich source being the annual reports of the medical defence organizations. Recent changes in the arrangements for medical protection (malpractice insurance) in Britain have made these reports less useful.

Prescribing the wrong drug or writing illegibly

This involves a conspiracy of error between the doctor and the pharmacist. Pharmacists are expected to cope with doctors' often appalling handwriting (as part of the pharmacists' 'culture'). It is hardly surprising that errors occur.

Good practice in writing prescriptions is described in the *British National Formulary*, which is provided to every prescriber in the United Kingdom.

---

[3] Nosology is the branch of medical science concerned with the classification of disease.
[4] The guidelines contain both very general statements, such as 'Sufficient personnel must be available to perform tasks adequately', and very detailed recommendations; for example, to write the word 'units' in full on prescription charts. Whether the guidelines are useful or workable remains to be seen.

Table 6.1. Errors in prescribing (adapted from Ferner 1992)

Prescribing the wrong drug
   writing illegibly
   confusing the name of one drug with that of another

Prescribing the wrong dose of drug
   calculating the dose incorrectly
   giving the adult dose to a child
   prescribing the wrong dose for a particular route of administration
   writing the wrong dose
   writing the dose in such a way that it is wrongly interpreted
   prescribing with insufficient knowledge of the prior
   concentration of the drug in blood
   prescribing the wrong dilution

Prescribing the wrong formulation of a drug

Prescribing the duration of treatment incorrectly

Prescribing wrongly for a given individual
   making an error in the name or identity of the patient
   failing to take account of pre-existing disease or idiosyncrasy
   failing to take account of concurrent therapy

Prescribing with inadequate or incorrect instructions

Prescribing without the informed consent of the patient

Prescribing outside or against currently accepted practice

CASE 6.13 (LUDMAN *ET AL.* 1986; BRAHAMS 1989; NELSON-JAMES AND BURTON 1990B)[5]

A doctor wrote a prescription for the antibiotic amoxycillin as 'Amoxil', but the pharmacist read it as 'Daonil', which is glibenclamide, a drug used to lower the blood glucose concentration in diabetic patients. It also lowers the blood glucose concentration in normal subjects. The man was not diabetic, but took the tablets three times a day in the belief that they were antibiotics, developed severe hypoglycaemia (the condition in which the blood glucose concentration is abnormally low), and suffered severe brain damage as a result.

    Bad handwriting can lead to erroneous prescribing when doctors communicate with each other.

CASE 6.14 (FERNER AND WHITTINGTON 1994)

A woman who was treated with lithium injured herself and required admission to hospital. The handwritten referral letter stated that she was being treated with lithium carbonate tablets 600 mg daily, but was interpreted by the hospital doctor as 600 2 daily, and as a result the patient was given twice her previous dose of lithium carbonate, a drug with a very narrow therapeutic range. She died.

Confusing the name of one drug with that of another

Drugs can have rather similar names, and confusion can easily result. Lists of potentially confusing pairs of names have been published (McNulty and Spurr 1979; Anonymous 1985).

[5] *Prendergast v. Sam & Dee Ltd and others.*

CASE 6.15 (ANONYMOUS 1987A)

A doctor wrote a repeat prescription for 'chlorpropamide 25 milligrams one to four tablets each night'. Chlorpropamide is a drug used in the treatment of non-insulin-dependent diabetes mellitus, and is available in 250 milligram tablets. It is usually prescribed once daily, and in a fixed dose. The doctor had in fact intended to prescribe the tranquillizer chlorpromazine, which is available in 25 milligram tablets and might perhaps reasonably be prescribed for use as needed for sedation. The pharmacist realized that the drug and dose were inconsistent and without enquiring of the doctor what was intended dispensed chlorpropamide 250 milligram tablets. The son of the patient for whom the drug was prescribed queried the change of tablets with a district nurse, who wrongly reassured him that the tablets were the same as previously. The son gave the patient the anti-diabetic tablets, which lowered his blood glucose concentration so far that he suffered irreversible brain damage. The error in prescription was compounded at each subsequent stage by trained staff, even though it had been spotted by the patient's untrained son.

Prescribing the wrong dose of drug

Calculating the dose incorrectly

Errors can occur whenever arithmetical calculations are made, and this is especially true when they are carried out hurriedly, by tired people, in stressful situations, and without others to check them.

The calculation of doses for children is especially fraught with potential danger, because the incorrect doses might seem 'reasonable' as they would be appropriate in a larger child or adult, and because the effects of overdosage are likely to be proportionately more severe.

Nomogram charts which allow doses to be read off by weight, age, height, or a combination of these or other factors can be less prone to error. Guides to paediatric prescribing (such as Davidson 1982; Insley 1990) are also extremely helpful.

CASE 6.16 (ANONYMOUS 1988)

A paediatric registrar (a middle-grade doctor) correctly calculated that a 5-week-old baby should receive a dose of 0.06 milligrams of digoxin. It is good practice to prescribe doses as whole numbers rather than decimal fractions, and the registrar converted the calculated dose in milligrams to a dose of 600 micrograms, not 60 micrograms, an error of a factor of 10 (as 1 milligram = 1000 micrograms). A typical initial dose of digoxin in an adult would be 500 micrograms.

The tenfold error in calculation of doses for children is sufficiently common that Koren *et al.* (1986) described it as 'a neglected iatrogenic disease'.

Giving the adult dose to a child

This is an error which arises through thoughtlessness: the smaller the size of the patient, the larger the concentration that results from a specified dose of drug.

Prescribing the wrong dose for a particular route of administration

Some drugs are absorbed slowly and incompletely from the gut into the bloodstream, and so much higher doses of the drug are needed if it is given by mouth than if it is given directly into a vein. There is a consequent risk of overdosage if the two different doses are confused or are not appreciated. For example, the vasodilator drug isosorbide dinitrate would often be given as an intravenous infusion of 2 milligrams per hour, whereas the oral preparation is available in 10 and 20 milligram tablets.

The volume of blood circulating in the body of an average adult is about 5 litres, but the volume of cerebrospinal fluid, (the fluid that bathes the brain and spinal cord), is only about 150 millilitres, about 4 per cent of the circulating blood volume. Consequently, the most serious errors in dosage come when drugs are injected into the spinal canal, which contains the cerebrospinal fluid, in quantities appropriate for intravenous use.

CASE 6.17 (ANONYMOUS 1978, 1986A)

A four-year-old child died after being given the intravenous dose of the anticancer drug methotrexate intrathecally (into the cerebrospinal fluid in the spinal canal). The doctor was charged with manslaughter, but acquitted.

The use of intrathecal methotrexate together with intravenous methotrexate increases the likelihood of error. The emergency treatment for intrathecal overdose (Poplack 1984) is occasionally successful in preventing death or serious injury (Spiegel *et al.* 1984).

Writing the wrong dose

The prescriber can confuse the dose for one drug and another of similar name or similar action, or write down the wrong dose in aberration. The wrong dose can also be the result of transcription error.

CASE 6.18 (FERNER AND WHITTINGTON 1994)

A man who had suffered from schizophrenia had been able to lead a reasonably normal life on treatment with the major tranquillizer haloperidol which he had received from his general practitioner for many years in the (large) dose of 5 milligrams three times daily. The general practitioner had a computer prescribing system installed, and failed to notice that the dose had been altered in transcription to 0.5 milligrams three times daily. The patient took the newly prescribed dose, became extremely withdrawn and lapsed into a catatonic state. He then developed pneumonia from which he died.

Such an error could arise because the computer held a store of 'usual' dosages for specific drugs, and prescribed this dose automatically unless countermanded, or because a reading or typing error had arisen in copying the handwritten records on to computer.

Writing the dose in such a way that it is wrongly interpreted

The classic error is to write fractional doses without putting a leading zero before the decimal point, so that the dose is wrong by a factor of ten- or 100-fold. For example,

.25 milligrams could be interpreted as 25 milligrams
.5 millilitres as 5 millilitres

Good prescribing practice dictates that:

(1) if it is possible to write the dose as a whole number, then do so;
(2) if it is impossible or more confusing to write the dose as a whole number, then ensure that a zero precedes the decimal point.

Thus:

0.25 milligrams is better written as 250 micrograms
.5-1 gram is better written as 0.5 to 1 gram.

The route can also be interpreted wrongly.

CASE 6.19 (COHEN 1987)

A woman with hypoparathyroidism (underactivity of the parathyroid glands, leading to a low calcium concentration in the blood) was prescribed a vitamin D preparation, 50 000 IU (international units), and this was interpreted to mean IV (intravenously) by a nurse. The pharmacist, however, dispensed the correct dose and form, and the error was discovered when the nurse questioned why the drug had been dispensed in an oral syringe.

The moral of this story is that units should be written as 'units'. This is reinforced by the need to avoid misinterpreting doses such as:

Insulin 4U as Insulin 40 [units].

Prescribing with insufficient knowledge of the prior concentration of the drug in blood

Some drugs have rather low margins of safety, and there is only a small difference between therapeutic and toxic doses. When such drugs have only indirect effects, or poorly measurable effects, then it is often valuable to determine the concentration of the drug in blood.

CASE 6.20 (ANONYMOUS 1986B)

A man was treated with the antimicrobial medicine gentamicin, which is very toxic to the vestibular branch of the eighth cranial nerve (the nerve supplying the organs of balance in the middle ear).

The toxicity of gentamicin is well known, and it is good practice to measure the concentration of the drug in blood just before and about 1 hour after a dose, and to repeat the measurements every few days. The former is the 'trough' or 'pre-' [dose] concentration and the latter the 'peak' or 'post-' [dose] concentration. It is recommended that the trough concentration should be less than 2 milligrams of gentamicin per litre, and the peak concentration be between 4 and 10 milligrams per litre (Data sheet for 'Genticin' (ABPI 1993-4b). The man was treated with the drug for 30 days, but the concentration was measured only twice. The man suffered severe damage to the vestibular nerve.

The monitoring in that case was clearly inadequate, but sometimes the line between unacceptable and acceptable practice is unclear: the mere fact that damage resulted from gentamicin treatment may not be enough to demonstrate that negligence has occurred. It is also necessary to show that no respectable body of medical opinion would have acted in the way that the defendant acted. When a patient became disabled by unsteadiness after gentamicin antibiotic treatment, her action for negligence failed, because the doctors who treated her did so according to an established nomogram (calculation chart) (Brahams 1986b).

Prescribing the wrong dilution or tablet strength

Some drugs are used in much higher doses for one indication (the *indication* is the reason for using them) than another. For example, the drug clonidine, which stimulates the alpha$_2$-adrenergic sympathetic receptors and inhibits the sympathetic nervous system, can be used to prevent the occurrence of attacks of migraine in doses of 25 micrograms twice daily. It can also be used to treat hypertension (high blood pressure), but the doses required are over 10 times higher. Two preparations are marketed in the United Kingdom, 'Dixarit' which contains 25 micrograms of clonidine, and 'Catapres' which contains either 100 or 300 micrograms of clonidine. There is a danger of confusing the various preparations.

The problem also arises with solutions of drugs such as adrenaline for injection. Adrenaline has sometimes to be given intramuscularly, when a small volume is important, and a solution of 1 milligram per millilitre ('1 in 1000') is needed. At other times, a dose has to be given directly into the heart in an attempt to restart it, and a concentrated solution can carry the additional danger of local damage to heart muscle. A solution of 100 micrograms per millilitre ('1 in 10000') is used for this purpose. The potential danger is clear.

Confusion is potentially greater still with the solutions of tuberculin purified protein derivative (PPD), used to test a subject's immunity to tuberculosis. Full-strength solutions contain 100000 units of PPD per millilitre. This strength is required for the test known as the Heaf test. However, test solutions used in another form of the tuberculin test known as the Mantoux test contain 10, 100 or 1000 units per millilitre. Subjects who have strong reactions in the Mantoux test can have unpleasant redness, swelling, and blistering with as little as 100 microlitres (0.1 millilitre) of PPD 10 units per millilitre, and so it is important to use the correct dose of the correct solution. This is made hard by the multiplicity of solutions, and harder still by an alternative, and now outdated, nomenclature of '1 in 1, 1 in 100, 1 in 1000 and one in 10000' which refers to the dilution of the full-strength solution.

For unambiguous prescription, it is perhaps best to write both the dose in units and the volume and concentration of the solution to be used:

> Tuberculin purified protein derivative 1 unit (100 microlitres
> of 10 units per millilitre).

Prescribing the wrong formulation of a drug

Drugs can be made in a variety of special formulations so as to alter their absorption or other properties. For example, it is common to prescribe the calcium-channel-blocking drug nifedipine in a retarded-release form, because the standard capsule contains a solution of the drug which is rapidly absorbed and can cause headache and dizziness initially but which is rather short-lived in its therapeutic action on hypertension or angina.

Such errors appear common (Lesar 1992), and are likely to become more common as the number of available modified-release preparations rises.

Prescribing the duration of treatment incorrectly

Sometimes prolonged prescription of a drug intended for short-term or intermittent use leads to severe damage or death.

CASE 6.21 (ANONYMOUS 1991B)

A consultant wrote in a patient's notes that he should receive 'vindesine days 1+8' for chemotherapy of cancer. The inexperienced junior doctor interpreted this to mean days 1, 2, 3, 4, 5, 6, 7, and 8. It was intended to mean day 1 and day 8. The patient received treatment on all 8 days, developed bone-marrow damage from the drug, and died.

CASE 6.22

A woman with a peptic ulcer was prescribed the preparation 'De-Nol', which contains bismuth, on the advice of a specialist. The general practitioner continued to prescribe the drug for 2 years, although the initial course was intended to be only 6 weeks long. The patient developed an illness, one feature of which was the uncontrolled spasmodic contraction of muscles called myoclonus. Myoclonus has previously been reported as a feature of bismuth intoxication, and no alternative cause was discovered on investigation. However, the patient's illness persisted for over 2 years after the drug was stopped, whereas the cases of myoclonus from bismuth poisoning described in the literature have resolved within a few months.

The issues include: whether the myoclonus was, on the balance of probability, caused by bismuth in this case, whether the long duration of treatment was reason for it, and if so, then whether the general practitioner was negligent in continuing treatment for longer than recommended either in the Data sheet or the *British National Formulary*.

Prescribing wrongly for a given individual

Making an error in the name or identity of the patient

Hospital patients often have gummed paper labels with their name and hospital number printed on them, to ease the burden of form-filling by doctors. When the wrong label is affixed to a prescription or to a laboratory test form, chaos can result, so that the patient is endangered.

Failing to take account of pre-existing disease

Patients suffering from a variety of diseases, including liver, kidney, and lung disease, can be harmed by medicines. An example of this would be asthma, which can be made worse with drugs such as the beta-blockers propranolol and atenolol. Patients with liver disease can be precipitated into coma from hepatic encephalopathy (the brain damage that results from severe liver failure) by sedative drugs such as the benzodiazepine diazepam.

The actions of drugs can also be altered by disease. For example, the heart drug digoxin is excreted from the body mainly by the kidneys, and so can accumulate in kidney failure if the dose is not reduced. Accumulation of digoxin can lead to nausea, vomiting, diarrhoea, abnormalities of the heart rhythm, hyperkalaemia (a raised serum potassium concentration), and death.

Knowledge of pre-existing drug allergy is important before prescribing drugs, as some drug allergies are so severe as to put the patient's life at risk. It is good practice to ask patients whether they have had reactions to any drugs, but in a survey, only about 55 per cent of patients reporting drug reactions had had the reactions recorded in their hospital notes (Cook and Ferner 1993).

Failing to take account of concurrent therapy

The more drugs a patient takes, the greater is the scope for a serious interaction between them, in which one of the drugs causes a severe reaction because of the presence of another. Warfarin, an anticoagulant (a drug used to prevent the blood clotting), is a particularly dangerous drug, because it has a very narrow therapeutic range, its metabolism is variable between one patient and another, and sometimes in the same patient at different times, and its pharmacokinetics and pharmacodynamics can be affected by a wide range of drugs, including common antiarthritic and anti-infective agents.

Case 6.23 (Ferner and Whittington 1994)

A man who was taking the anticoagulant (anticlotting) drug, warfarin, developed gout, and the general practitioner prescribed the anti-inflammatory drug azapropazone. This drug is known to increase the anticoagulant effect of warfarin. The patient had massive gastrointestinal haemorrhage (bleeding from the gut) and died in spite of efforts to save him.

Other drugs with narrow therapeutic ranges can also be affected by adding a new agent to the patient's treatment.

Case 6.24 (Anonymous 1987b)

A 42-year-old woman who had been on lithium treatment (used for manic-depression) for 9 years was prescribed a diuretic ('water tablet') for her high blood pressure. An assay of lithium concentration was made and the concentration was high, but the result was only made available 7 days later, and the woman suffered irreversible damage to the cerebellum (the part of the brain that co-ordinates movement). She was unable to walk unaided, and a substantial settlement was made.

Prescribing with inadequate or incorrect instructions

It is disturbing how frequently patients in the hospital clinic will produce bottles of tablets labelled 'Take as directed', with no further instruction. One of the duties of the prescriber is to make clear the manner in which the product is to be used, and to ask the pharmacist to label it appropriately.

It can be important to specify the frequency, the maximum dose, the relationship to meals, the need for copious fluid, and the possible adverse effects.

Case 6.25 (Gwynne 1986b)

A woman was prescribed the benzodiazepine sedative lorazepam, but was not warned of the potential dangers. The prescriber's error was compounded by the dispenser in his practice, who gave out 2.5 milligram tablets labelled as 1 milligram tablets. The patient drove her car off the road while under the sedative influence of lorazepam, and on expert advice the claim against the prescriber was settled.

Prescribing without the informed consent of the patient

The problem of informed consent before starting treatment is related to the last problem. It could most easily arise in two circumstances: where the patient would need to know of the serious adverse effects which might accompany treatment before making a rational decision as to whether to commence it; and where the treatment is experimental and neither the doctor nor the patient can be sure what adverse effects might tend to occur.

An example of the former case might be epidural anaesthesia, where the anaesthetist should warn the patient of the possible dangers.

The latter problem could be encountered where a patient unknowingly becomes the subject of an experimental clinical trial of a new medicine. If the medicine were for some condition such as rheumatoid arthritis where the patient would generally be conscious and able to decide whether to proceed, then written informed consent would be expected from the patient.

In some circumstances, such as potentially life-saving treatment for unconscious patients, then it might be impossible for the patient or relatives to give consent to the experimental trial. The conditions under which the trial was to be conducted should generally have been specified by an independent ethics committee.

CASE 6.26 (MITCHELL 1995)

A 22-year-old woman had four teeth extracted under general anaesthetic at her dentist's surgery. She had signed a form consenting to the surgery. The anaesthetic was given by a consultant anaesthetist, and while the woman was unconcious he also inserted a diclofenac (pain-killing) suppository. It was inadvertantly placed in the vagina, and the patient, concerned from her subsequent symptoms that she might have been sexually assaulted, informed the police. There was no evidence of any intentional sexual assault, but the matter was referred to the General Medical Council, which in due course found the anaesthetist guilty of serious professional misconduct.

To a senior anaesthetist, 'this case was provocative at first, meddlesome in the middle, and outrageous at the end' (Lunn 1995). A lawyer considered, in the light of this case, that the profession should review the information given to patients before obtaining consent (Jones 1995). This case evoked strong feelings (Graham 1995; Mason and Smith 1995; Rosen 1995).

Prescribing outside or against currently accepted practice

The line between accepted practice and negligence is sometimes thin, and negligence can be so grave as to justify a charge of manslaughter. It is rare, however, for doctors who behave in utmost good faith to be charged with murder. This did happen in a case which was suspected to involve 'euthanasia'.

CASE 6.27 *R* v. *LEONARD ARTHUR* (*THE TIMES*, 15 OCTOBER 1981 *ET SEQ.*)

A baby was born with the features of Down's syndrome (formerly known as mongolism), a condition of the chromosomes in which there is almost invariably some degree of mental retardation. The mother was said to have turned away and said 'I don't want it'.

The consultant paediatrician caring for the baby decided that it should be given no active supporting treatment, but should be allowed a solution of the opioid pain-killing drug dihydrocodeine ('DF118'), and wrote in the hospital records 'Nursing care only'. Dihydrocodeine causes sedation and depresses the breathing.

The baby died 69 hours after birth. A member of the ward staff apparently rang an antiabortion group, Life, with this story, and Life reported the conduct of the paediatrician to the police. The paediatrician was subsequently charged with murder.

A professor of forensic pathology gave evidence for the prosecution, saying that the baby had died from bronchopneumonia, and that 'the administering of the DF118 was the greatest single factor in causing the baby's death'. He also gave the opinion that without the drug the baby would have had an 80 per cent chance of survival.

In a dramatic denouement, the professor was shown a series of slides by the defence, and had to concede that the baby had serious brain and lung damage from birth, so that the prosecution case was misleading. The charge of murder was withdrawn, since the evidence now was that whatever action had been taken by the defendant, the baby's death was likely to have been caused by natural disease. However, the trial continued on the charge of attempted murder.

A well-known paediatrician gave evidence for the defence that it was an accepted viewpoint in paediatrics not to take life, but sometimes to allow a baby to die when it is apparently in the baby's interest.

In his summing up, the judge said: 'It is a prospect one views with some alarm that expert evidence can be given to you in a case of murder which turns out to be incomplete and in that sense inaccurate.'

The paediatrician was acquitted.

There are further stages in the therapeutic process before errors in prescribing can lead to harm, namely dispensing, drawing up, and administration of the medicine prescribed. Each of the processes provides an opportunity for detecting errors made in previous stages, but also for introducing new errors.

6.3 Dispensing errors

Dispensing is the process by which the prescription a doctor writes is translated by a pharmacist into the medicines for the patient involved, and the medicines are delivered to the patient. The pharmacist has to read, and often decipher, the doctor's instructions, then carry them out. It is rare these days for pharmacists to compound medicines out of the raw ingredients, but this is still required sometimes. More commonly, the pharmacist has to decant liquid medicines or count pills from bulk into a smaller container destined for the patient to take away. The pharmacist may have to make up solutions by dissolving powdered ingredients in water or some other diluent.

Dispensing errors are probably common. Many tablets lack identifying marks, and some medicines are available in tablets containing the same dose, but of different forms, depending on the manufacturer. Even very toxic medicines such as the anticancer drugs methotrexate (Klaber 1992) and vincristine (Kosmidis *et al.* 1991) can be marketed in different strengths with very similar physical forms:

CASE 6.28 (KOSMIDIS *ET AL.* 1991)

Three children being treated for leukaemia received accidental overdoses of intravenous vincristine. Vials containing 5 milligrams had been mistaken for vials containing 1 milligram. One of the children died, and the others required several days of hospital treatment.

There is a trend towards prescribing medicines in *original packs* (OPs), that is, in packages that the manufacturer has designed specifically to contain a suitable course for a single patient. Medicines which are prescribed long-term are often available in OPs containing 28 or 30 days' treatment. It is also necessary to transmit the doctor's instructions to the patient and to add prudent warnings to the label. The *British National Formulary* lists warnings suitable for most common medicines. The final task of the dispenser is to ensure that the correct patient receives the medicines.

The role of translating the instructions of the doctor places the pharmacist in a special position of providing a service rather than merely selling a product. This means that the laws regarding strict liability for products do not necessarily apply to medicines supplied by a pharmacist (Dukes and Swartz 1988d).

The Pharmaceutical Society has given guidance on good dispensing practice (Anonymous 1979). It gives details of suitable premises and equipment, the expected standards of cleanliness and hygiene, the adequate control of materials, and certain other matters. For example, 'equipment should include ... a suitable means for counting tablets and capsules. Steps should be taken to avoid cross contamination, particularly when using mechanical counters.'

CASE 6.29

A 42-year-old woman had received the analgesic drug dihydrocodeine as 'DF118' for some time. A pharmacist dispensed tablets labelled as dihydrocodeine, but of different form. When the patient queried this, it was explained that the tablets were the (generic) equivalent of 'DF118'.

Later a further prescription was dispensed, and the tablets were of yet another form. The woman did not question the correctness of the label, which was 'dihydrocodeine'. She subsequently became ill, and it was discovered that the new tablets actually contained aminophylline, an entirely different drug used to treat asthma. The pharmacist had dispensed the wrong tablets.

CASE 6.30 (BOLAN ET AL. 1986)

Nineteen children in a children's day-care centre suddenly developed a 'glowing' red skin and swollen face or eyelids. The children had all received prophylactic treatment with a mixture containing the antibiotic rifampicin. Investigation showed that the pharmacist responsible had made up a solution five times more concentrated than the intended solution, as a result of an arithmetic error.

Pharmacists have a number of duties and functions in addition to their dispensing, such as advising the public on minor remedies, controlling P (pharmacy sale only) licensed medicines, and taking responsibility for quality control of medicines.

Cases in which the wrong drug is prescribed and subsequently dispensed can contain elements of error by the pharmacist as well as the doctor (see Section 6.2).

It sometimes happens that drugs are dispensed against an unsigned or otherwise incomplete prescription.

CASE 6.31 (GUARDIAN, 15 OCTOBER 1994)

A senior nursing sister on a neurosurgical ward realized that there would soon be no more space on a patient's drug chart to record the administration of medicines. She therefore wrote out the names and dosages of the drugs he was to receive on a fresh chart, and telephoned one of the junior doctors to ask him to sign the prescriptions, which included insulin and a morphine derivative. The doctor forgot to do so, and for several days the new, unsigned, chart was used. When the matter was eventually noticed, the sister was suspended, and she was only reinstated after fierce local protest.

6.4 Errors in drawing up and giving medicines

Errors in drawing up (preparing for injection by syringe) and giving medicines can lead to serious harm.

The errors are classified in Table 6.2.

Errors in administration

Giving a drug outside or against currently accepted practice

A practitioner who uses a drug outside or against currently accepted practice and thereby causes harm can be negligent. If a drug is given recklessly and the patient dies, the practitioner can face a charge of manslaughter.

CASE 6.32 (THE TIMES, 27 OCTOBER 1981)

A 52-year-old woman called at a dentist's surgery one evening and complained of severe toothache. The dentist's assistant had already left, but he none the less decided to administer a general anaesthetic and extract the tooth. He performed the operation, and then left the patient with a man who was an unemployed engineer while he went out to tell her husband that the

Table 6.2 Harm from drawing up and giving medicines (Adapted from Ferner 1992)

Errors in drawing up
  drawing up the wrong drug
  drawing up the correct drug in the wrong dose
  drawing up the correct drug in the wrong dilution
  drawing up the correct drug in the wrong formulation
  entraining air, particles or other contaminants with the drug

Errors in administration
  giving a drug outside or against currently accepted practice
  giving the wrong drug by mistake
  giving the wrong dose, dilution or formulation of drug
  giving the drug by the wrong route
  giving the drug in the wrong site
  giving the drug at the wrong rate
  giving the drug to the wrong patient

Mishap that can be due to accident or to error

Extravasation (see p. 110)

---

operation was a success. The patient meanwhile had vomited, and then choked on her own vomit and died.

The dentist was convicted of manslaughter, given a suspended prison sentence, and fined £1000.

CASE 6.33 (*THE TIMES*, 7 JULY 1981)

A Harley Street doctor said that he had agreed to treat the warts on the toes of a 42-year-old antiques dealer, and when the patient became agitated during the procedure, gave him an injection of diazepam ('Valium'). The patient collapsed, and was taken to hospital, where he died after several days of intensive care. Blood samples taken in life showed not diazepam but the short-acting barbiturate anaesthetic methohexitone, at concentrations 10 times higher than expected with standard therapeutic doses.

The doctor was sent for trial on a charge of manslaughter, and the prosecution alleged that he had deliberately misled the hospital staff to protect himself. He had, it was said, intended to administer an anaesthetic dose of methohexitone as a single operator. An expert witness for the prosecution said that 'the use of anaesthetics by a doctor performing surgery on his own was absolutely contraindicated these days'.

In spite of the condemnatory expert evidence, the doctor was acquitted.

Giving the wrong drug

This is especially likely in an emergency.

CASE 6.34 (COLLINS 1991)

An anaesthetist took from the drawer of the anaesthetics trolley an ampoule of what he believed was the respiratory stimulant 'Dopram' (doxapram), and administered it to a patient. The ampoule in fact contained dopamine, a cardiac stimulant, and the patient died. 'There was no evidence that the anaesthetist had checked the drug name on the ampoule before administering its contents.' The doctor was charged with manslaughter under New Zealand law, and convicted, although suffering no other penalty.

Lack of training, time, or care can result in tragic mistakes when drawing up and giving drugs. The most common problem seems to be the confusion of sodium chloride, which is widely used as an innocuous diluent, and potassium chloride, which is available in similar ampoules, but undiluted is a deadly poison when given intravenously.

The *Journal of the Medical Defence Union* has described potassium chloride strong solution as 'The KCl killer'[6] (Hill 1990). The results of erroneous intravenous injection are sufficient to justify this reputation.

CASE 6.35

A house physician made up a solution of an antibiotic for intravenous use by dissolving the powder in what he believed was sodium chloride solution ('saline'). As he injected the solution, his patient collapsed, and he realized that he had used potassium chloride solution and not sodium chloride solution. There was some hesitation in resuscitating the patient, as it had previously been decided that he was 'not for resuscitation'[7]. When in the event resuscitation was attempted, it was unsuccessful.

The Coroner criticized the system whereby house physicians were expected to carry out potentially dangerous tasks such as giving medicines intravenously with inadequate training. This inadequacy is highlighted by a report of house officers' experiences with giving intravenous drugs (Teahon and Bateman 1993).

Potassium chloride and its dangers are considered further in Chapter 10.

Giving the wrong dose, dilution, or formulation of drug

These errors can occur as the final stage in propagating errors made earlier, or can arise *de novo*. Many doctors are incapable of making simple dosage calculations (Rolfe and Harper 1995).

CASE 6.36

A baby weighing approximately 8 kilograms was prescribed 150 milligrams of phenytoin intravenously to control convulsions. The recommended loading dose (the initial dose given to produce therapeutic blood concentrations rapidly, and larger than the maintenance dose) is 15 to 20 milligrams per kilogram, so this was an appropriate dose. A junior doctor gave the contents of six ampoules of phenytoin 250 milligrams, that is, 1.5 grams or 10 times the intended and prescribed dose. The baby suffered severe phenytoin poisoning and was fortunate to survive.

It is very rare for infants to require doses of more than a single ampoule of any drug, and even in adults one might pause before opening six ampoules.

One concern with oral doses of liquid medicines is that the 'teaspoon' measure is incapable of delivering an accurate and repeatable dose. Since 1992, liquid medicines dispensed for children in the United Kingdom have come with a special measure. The 'liquid medicine measure' is a 5 millilitre syringe graduated in 0.5 millilitre (500 microlitre) divisions. Liquid medicine can be drawn up from a bottle through a rubber adaptor, and the correct volume slowly emptied from the measure inside the mouth into the cheek of the infant patient. The device is not intended for injections, and is marked 'for oral use only'[8].

---

[6] KCl is the notation for potassium chloride in chemical symbols.

[7] Patients in hospital who suddenly collapse can sometimes be resuscitated by the efforts of the Cardiac Arrest ('Crash') Team, who rush to the patient and perform external cardiac massage and other treatment. It is an undignified business, and patients with terminal illness can be spared it by an explicit decision that they are 'not for resuscitation'. The emergency telephone number that summons the Cardiac Arrest Team, which varies from hospital to hospital(!), is sometimes used as a short-hand: 'not for 333', for example.

[8] Department of Health Pamphlet COI/HSSH J1606AR 11184/A July 1992.

Giving the drug by the wrong route

It sometimes happens that one drug has to be given intravenously while, at the same time, another is intended for intrathecal use, that is, injection into the space around the spinal cord by lumbar puncture. If the two medicines are drawn up into syringes which are not identified by the doctor giving the drug, tragedy can result.

CASE 6.37[9]

A patient having chemotherapy for leukaemia was to receive intravenous vincristine and intrathecal methotrexate. The lumbar puncture to gain access to the cerebrospinal fluid was performed by one junior hospital doctor under the supervision of another. Inadvertently, the vincristine was given intrathecally in mistake for the methotrexate, and the patient died. The two doctors were found guilty of manslaughter, although they were later acquitted on appeal.

Giving the drug in the wrong site

There is a substantial danger of nerve damage if intramuscular injections are made near to the route of a nerve through the muscle, itself something which varies considerably between one person and another. The safest muscle is generally the anterolateral part of the quadriceps femoris, that is the outer, front aspect of the main muscle of the front of the thigh.

Formerly the practice was to use the deltoid muscle of the outer side of the upper arm, and the upper outer quadrant of the large gluteal muscle of the buttocks. However, the radial nerve runs close to the first site and the sciatic nerve close to the second. Both have been damaged by intramuscular injection.

Sometimes the product licence specifies that an intramuscular preparation has to be given by a particular route. For example, the Data sheet for the intramuscular preparation of 'Voltarol', the non-steroidal anti-inflammatory drug diclofenac, stipulates that it should be given into the upper outer quadrant of the buttock. This is because the drug can damage tissue, and severe necrosis (tissue destruction) of the thigh muscles has sometimes resulted from injection into the quadriceps femoris. For diclofenac, the manufacturers believe that the risk of muscle necrosis outweighs the risk of sciatic nerve damage.

Giving the drug at the wrong rate

The rapid injection of a drug can cause the concentration in the bloodstream to rise very rapidly, and fail to allow time for the drug to be distributed out of the bloodstream into the tissues. The adverse effects of transient very high concentrations can be serious.

CASE 6.38

An anaesthetic registrar gave a patient a bolus injection (a very rapid 'shot') of the antibiotic vancomycin and immediately the patient became scarlet, and his blood pressure became unrecordable. Fortunately, he was resuscitated.

The data sheet for 'Vancocin' (vancomycin) states that the drug must be given over 60 minutes if the hypotension and rash are to be avoided.

It is quite possible for automatic infusion equipment to be set to administer a drug at a rate

[9] *R* v. *Sullman and Prentice* [1993] 4 MedLR 303. See also [1993] 1 MedLRev 373.

which is inappropriate for the patient, or to be set correctly but administer a drug at the wrong rate because of mechanical or electronic faults (Gerber and Apseloff 1993).

Patients can be poisoned when mechanical infusion devices fail.

CASE 6.39 (SOUTHERN AND READ 1994)

A 13-year-old girl was treated with morphine given by a patient-controlled infusion pump. When her bed was moved, the pump was placed about 80 centimetres above her bed, air leaked into the tubing, and she received 40 milligrams of morphine unexpectedly, and developed respiratory depression.

Giving the drug to the wrong patient

This must be a relatively common occurrence where patients are unable to control their own medicines, for example in an old people's home.

CASE 6.40 (KALIMO AND OLSSON 1980)

An 84-year-old man in an old people's home was given the diabetes treatment intended for the patient next to him, lapsed into coma due to hypoglycaemia (a low blood glucose concentration) and died from irreversible brain damage.

Extravasation, a mishap that can be due to accident or to error

Extravasation is the leakage of fluid into the surrounding tissue when it had been intended to enter a blood vessel or other vessel. The most common cause is the displacement of a cannula, that is, a small tube, nowadays usually made of plastic, which is inserted into a vein to allow fluids to pass into the patient's bloodstream. It is sometimes difficult to insert the cannula into a vein, and it may lie in the tissues from the outset. Alternatively, it can become dislodged from the hollow lumen (the cavity or 'bore') of the vein after having been in place for hours or days.

Many solutions are potentially harmful, but can be given into a vein as they are then mixed with the flowing blood and diluted. Common examples include sodium bicarbonate solution, thiopentone sodium solution, and phenytoin solution. Many of the drugs used for cancer chemotherapy are also very toxic to tissues.

CASE 6.41 (HAYES AND CHESNEY 1993)

A 49-year-old woman was given an injection of phenytoin intravenously after a cardiac arrest. The injections were continued for 10 days, via a cannula on the back of the right hand. About a day after an episode of extravasation, the hand became discoloured, and it gradually became gangrenous and had to be amputated.

It is possible that early recognition and prompt treatment might have saved the hand.

6.5 Summary

Doctors, pharmacists, and nurses bear a heavy responsibility for making sure that a patient is prescribed, and correctly receives, the correct medicine in the correct dose. Errors can arise at any stage in the process, and can lead to actions for negligence, and sometimes to trial for unlawful killing.

Part 3

Specific drugs of forensic importance

7

Ethanol

Alcohols are alkyl organic compounds which contain an —OH group. Ethanol (ethyl alcohol), C_2H_5OH, is the chemical name for the alcohol derived from the fermentation of glucose (grape-sugar) and other sugars and starches by the action of yeasts. Since this is economically and socially the most important alcohol, the term 'alcohol' often designates ethanol.

Ethanol is the single most important drug in forensic work, because of its widespread consumption, its undesirable effects, and the law regarding drinking and driving. There are several monographs on the forensic aspects of ethanol (Walls and Brownlie 1985a; Fitzgerald and Hume 1987a; Garriot 1988; Ley 1993a).

There is often a need to make calculations, based on a series of assumptions, when dealing with ethanol cases. To protect the reader from an excess of formulae, these have mostly been placed in Appendix B. The appendix also contains a list of the ethanol contents of some commonly encountered beverages.

7.1 Measurement of ethanol

Ethanol can be measured in blood, breath, or urine by a variety of techniques. Methods that are sufficiently reliable for forensic work include gas chromatography, chemical and enzymic methods, and, for breath, infra-red spectrophotometry; fuel cell potentiometry is also used. The most important methods are discussed.

7.1.1 Sample collection
Blood samples

Blood samples are usually obtained by venesection (literally 'vein cutting'), using a sterile, disposable, hollow needle with a bevelled cutting edge; that is, a 'hypodermic' needle.[1] This is attached to a syringe, also disposable, or an evacuated glass test tube closed by a rubber bung (for example, the 'Vacutainer'). The needle pierces the skin and then the wall of a surface vein such as one in the bend of the elbow. The skin is usually cleaned beforehand. It is common practice in hospital to rub the skin with a small pad impregnated with isopropanol (for

---

[1] The doctor who obtains the sample should be sober, too. A driver who was convicted of failing to provide a blood specimen had the conviction quashed on appeal, where he reported 'the doctor was slurring and I could see that he was drunk. He said "You're not pissing me about" and produced a needle.' The doctor failed to appear at the appeal hearing (*Daily Telegraph*, 2 December 1994).

example, the 'Steret'), or with cotton wool soaked in an antiseptic such as chlorhexidine, which may itself be dissolved in ethanol. This can cause contamination of the blood sample (Dubowski 1986). Care is therefore needed in interpreting results from samples taken from patients in hospital.

Blood samples, once obtained, are kept in or emptied into test-tubes. If analyses are to be made on whole blood or plasma, then it is necessary to stop the blood clotting, and the test-tube will usually contain potassium oxalate or heparin. Bacterial contamination, which is more a theoretical hazard than a proven risk (Dubowski 1986), can result in the formation of ethanol from carbohydrate. To guard against this, sodium fluoride is used to inhibit enzymic oxidation. It has no effect if samples are stored tightly closed, but is helpful if they are repeatedly opened (Somogyi *et al.* 1986). Refrigeration at 4 °C helps to protect against bacterial growth and chemical reaction (Brown *et al.* 1973).

The ethanol concentration in whole blood is lower than that in plasma or serum, because red cells contain fat, and ethanol is insoluble in fat and remains in the watery fluid. It is therefore important to know which fluid was used for analysis.

Urine samples

Urine samples are simply collected, but because the bladder can store urine over several hours, the accuracy of timing is limited. The situation is improved if the subject empties the bladder and then subsequently provides the specimen of 'new' urine. In Britain, an interval of up to 1 hour after the bladder has been emptied is allowed for the subject to produce urine for evidential samples (Walls and Brownlie 1985*e*).

Breath samples

Breath samples for quantitative analysis are produced by blowing into a mouthpiece which is attached to the breath-testing machine in such a way that the first 1.5–2 litres of breath are discarded, and only the last 50–100 millilitres are allowed into the sample chamber. This is important, because the air in the upper part of the airways does not have the opportunity to equilibrate with ethanol in the blood, and cannot provide a reliable measure of blood ethanol concentration.

7.1.2 Measurement of ethanol concentrations by gas chromatography

The general principles are described on pp. 46–7. Breath, whole blood, serum, plasma, urine and alcoholic beverages can all be analysed by the technique. The method is specific, that is, it measures ethanol and not any other substance, and it can be accurate. The accuracy depends on the addition of an accurately measured volume of internal standard, that is a standard which is in the fluid containing an unknown amount of ethanol when it is injected into the chromatograph.

The alcohol *n*-propanol is used as an internal standard, because it is similar to ethanol, but can be easily separated on the chromatography column. The peak due to the accurately measured volume of internal standard can then be compared with the peak due to ethanol. This ratio can in turn be compared with the ratio of peak area from the same volume of internal standard to the peak areas from solutions of ethanol of known concentration. (Walls and Brownlie 1985*h*; Dubowski 1986).

The method is outlined in Appendix B, Section B.1. Lawyers may, on occasion, wish to examine the evidence from gas chromatography in detail (Fitzgerald and Hume 1987c).

7.1.3 Infra-red breath ethanol measurement

The Camic Breath Analyzer (Camic Ltd, North Shields, NE30 1QG, England) and the Lion Intoximeter 3000 (Lion Laboratories Limited, Cardiff CF2 1PP, Wales), which are used as evidential breath-testing equipment by British police forces, work by this method.

Infra-red meters rely on the fact that ethanol can absorb radiation in the infra-red, and there is a characteristic absorption at a wavelength of about 3.4 micrometres, due to stretching of the C—OH bond. The proportion of a beam of infra-red radiation that passes through a gas containing ethanol vapour depends on the concentration of ethanol, because the more there is, the more strongly the infra-red radiation is absorbed. The method is not completely specific for ethanol, and both acetone and toluene can interfere, because they too absorb radiation at 3.4 micrometres. Instruments used for evidential testing take account of acetone (which occurs on the breath of diabetic patients, for example), but not toluene.

The machines only reflect blood ethanol concentration if the breath ethanol concentration is measured in alveolar air (p. 125), and to this end, the machine discards the first 1.5–2 litres of a forced expiration. The final portion of breath fills a sample chamber of fixed length through which the beam shines into a detector. Errors would also occur if the infra-red beam were scattered by droplets or particles. The chamber is heated to prevent droplets condensing, and a fine filter is interposed between the mouthpiece and the chamber to prevent small particles entering the chamber. However, cigarette smoke has particles sufficiently fine that they can affect the reading for some minutes after smoking.

The results of infra-red measurements depend on accurate calibration of the machine using standard ethanol vapour. This is performed with a solution which contains a fixed amount of ethanol, and which is held at a specified temperature, so that there is a known concentration of ethanol vapour above it. The solution is made up to within 1.5 per cent of the desired concentration, and the temperature held constant to within 0.2 °C (Walls and Brownlie 1985c).

The machine is calibrated at zero ethanol concentration and at the known concentration, which is 35 micrograms per 100 millilitres of breath. A specimen from the subject is measured, followed by a further zero ('purge'), another specimen from the subject, one more zero, and a final calibration sample. The two samples for the known concentration should agree if the machine is stable and should be within 3 micrograms per 100 millilitres of the specified value of 35 micrograms per 100 millilitres. Only the lower of the two values from the subject's samples is considered for legal purposes.

7.1.4 Fuel cells

Fuel cells exploit the fact that chemical reactions can generate electricity, as they do in a car battery. The cell consists of platinum or platinum-coated electrodes between which is a solution chosen in such a way that ethanol, but not other substances, will be oxidized by it and generate a voltage (electrical potential difference) which is proportional to the concentration of ethanol. Certain roadside screening meters rely on this method of analysis.

7.2 The pharmacology of ethanol

7.2.1 Exposure to ethanol

Ingestion

Most people who have ethanol in the body have drunk it. As a rough guide, the amount of ethanol in one measure of spirits, one glass of wine, and one half-pint of beer is 10 grams. However, there is a wide variation in the ethanol content among different spirits or wines or beers, and any accurate assessment of intake must consider this. Beverages which contain ethanol are now labelled with the percentage ethanol by volume (per cent v/v, volumes of ethanol per 100 volumes of solution). This is equivalent to the number of millilitres of pure ethanol per hundred millilitres of the drink.

The weight of ethanol contained in a given volume of drink depends both on the percentage ethanol by volume and on the density of absolute ethanol. The density of ethanol varies with the ambient temperature. Its value at 20 °C is 0.791 grams per millilitre, and so for example, a solution which is 10 per cent ethanol by volume at 20 °C contains 7.91 grams of ethanol in each 100 millilitres.

In the days before the European Community, the strength of drinks in Britain was expressed as per cent proof. A spirit which was 100 per cent proof contained just enough ethanol to enable it to sustain the combustion of gunpowder. This was later defined as 57.1 per cent ethanol by volume, although in the United States 100 per cent proof spirit contained 50 per cent ethanol by volume.

Beer is still sold in pubs in England by the imperial pint, which is equal to 568 millilitres. The standard volume ('single') of spirits such as whisky, brandy, and vodka dispensed in an English pub was until recently a sixth of a gill, that is, $\frac{1}{24}^{\text{th}}$ of a pint, or 23.7 millilitres. It is now 25 millilitres.

The concentration of ethanol in blood is usually expressed in mass units, such as milligrams per 100 millilitres of whole blood. Occasionally, laboratories will report blood ethanol results in SI units, such as millimoles per litre. The molecular weight of ethanol is 46.1 grams, so 100 milligrams per 100 millilitres is equal to 21.7 millimoles per litre.

Ethanol can be ingested not only in drinks, but in foodstuffs such as chocolate liqueurs, and in medicines and industrial solvents. The amount of ethanol in liqueurs is said to be up to 12 milligrams per gram (de Gaard 1979)[2]

Methylated spirits

Methylated spirits is ethanol adulterated with methanol (methyl alcohol) or acetone, so as to render it unfit for drinking, and coloured with methyl violet or another dye to make it easily recognizable. It can also be tainted with pyridine or 'Bitrex' to make it unpalatable. Methylated spirits contains 90–95 per cent ethanol, and, except in enormous doses, the effects and toxicity are due to this (Martensson *et al.* 1988; Jones *et al.* 1989).

Inhalation

Ethanol can be absorbed into the systemic circulation through the lungs, but the concentration of ethanol that has to be mixed with inspired air to produce significant concentrations in the

[2] So a kilogram of liqueur chocolates will contain approximately a unit of ethanol, equivalent to a single measure of spirits.

bloodstream is so high that the mixture causes coughing and irritation. However, in experimental studies it has been possible to achieve blood ethanol concentrations of up to 50 milligrams per 100 millilitres (500 milligrams per litre) after breathing ethanol/air mixtures for several hours (Lester *et al.* 1951).

Absorption through the skin

Ethanol is not absorbed through the intact skin in significant amounts (Bowers *et al.* 1942), at any rate, in adults. There are rare cases of new-born babies who have apparently been poisoned as a result of aborbing ethanol through the skin (Autret *et al.* 1982; Dalt *et al.* 1991).

7.2.2 Pharmacokinetics

There are several useful monographs and reviews on the pharmacokinetics of ethanol (Cooper *et al.* 1979*a*; Walls and Brownlie 1985*a*; Fitzgerald and Hume 1987*a*; Holford 1987; Crow and Batt 1988; Pohorecky and Brick 1988).

Rate of absorption

Ethanol undergoes passive diffusion into the body, and is neither actively taken up nor actively excluded. When it has been taken by mouth, ethanol moves across the mucosa, the lining of the inner (luminal) surface of the gut, into the blood which circulates in the capillaries that supply it, until the concentration of ethanol in the blood is the same as the concentration in the lumen of the gut.

The absorption of ethanol from the gut after an oral dose begins on ingestion, but because liquids pass quickly from the mouth via the gullet to the stomach, little absorption takes place until the ethanol enters the stomach. After a time, the stomach empties, its contents flow on into the small intestine, and absorption continues through the much larger surface area of the small intestine.

The mucosal lining of the stomach is thicker than that of the small intestine, and its blood supply is not so rich. The rate of diffusion of ethanol across the mucosa of the stomach is therefore lower than the rate of diffusion across the small intestinal mucosa, and the overall rate of absorption therefore depends on how rapidly the ethanol reaches the small intestine.

Ethanol can be absorbed through the colon and rectum (the large intestine) as well. This might be significant if it is indeed true that some people use red wine as an enema, but is unlikely to be important for those who restrict themselves to oral intake, since absorption will be essentially complete in the small intestine.

Rate of absorption in fasting subjects

Ethanol is rapidly absorbed on an empty stomach. One study (Wilkinson *et al.* 1977) examined the rate and extent of absorption of different doses of ethanol in eight normal subjects. Each subject was studied four times, and each received doses of 11.2 grams (9.4 per cent by volume), 22.4 grams (18.8 per cent), 33.6 grams (28.2 per cent) and 45.0 grams (37.9 per cent) of ethanol made up to 150 millilitres with orange juice.

Numerous blood samples were then taken, and the results interpreted using a mathematical model which described stomach emptying and absorption from the small intestine as first-order processes, and elimination of ethanol from the blood as a saturable process following Michaelis-Menten kinetics (these technical terms are explained in Section 1.2.4).

The average times to reach peak concentrations in blood were 22.5 minutes, 40 minutes, 55 minutes and 60 minutes after drinking 11.2, 22.4, 33.6, and 45 grams of ethanol, respectively.

The mathematical model, which makes several assumptions and approximations, yields a rate constant for the absorption of ethanol from the intestine, k_a, of 25.0 per hour. This is equivalent to a half-life of approximately 1.66 minutes. Put another way, over 98 per cent of ethanol in the small intestine would be absorbed within 10 minutes. Most of the delay in reaching peak absorption in this model is due to the relative slowness of stomach emptying, and this fits what is known about factors that influence ethanol absorption.

In practice, most drinkers will consume ethanol more or less steadily over a period of time, and the rate of ingestion is an important factor in determining how rapidly the peak ethanol concentration is reached.

Factors that influence the absorption of ethanol

Because the rate of absorption of ethanol in the stomach is less than the rate of absorption from the small bowel, the overall rate of absorption is sensitive to the rate of stomach emptying. This in turn depends on the volume and nature of the stomach contents. These influence the activity of the pyloric sphincter, the muscular valve that controls the outflow of contents from the stomach.

Gastric emptying can be slowed by distension of the stomach, as occurs after drinking large volumes of beer, and by muscle spasm of the pyloric sphincter (the muscular valve at the outflow of the stomach) which can result from taking ethanol whose concentration is above 30 per cent by volume, as in neat spirits.

The presence of food in the stomach can reduce the rate of gastric emptying, dilute the ethanol which enters the stomach, and limit the contact between the ethanol and the gastric mucosa. For all these reasons, ethanol absorption is both more rapid and more complete on an empty stomach. One study (Cortot *et al.* 1986) showed that substantial quantities of ethanol can be absorbed through the stomach wall even when the stomach contains food: in this case, homogenized steak, bread and olive oil.

Medicines can also affect the rate of stomach emptying and so alter the rate of ethanol absorption. The most important of those drugs that slow gastric emptying are shown in Table 7.1.

The operation of partial gastrectomy, in which part of the stomach was removed as a treatment for peptic ulcer disease, was commonly performed up to about 1980. It accelerates gastric emptying.

All these factors are expected to change the rate of absorption of ethanol after oral ingestion.

Bioavailability

The oral bioavailability, that is the proportion of an oral dose which reaches the systemic circulation, is less than 1, because some ethanol is broken down by the enzyme alcohol dehydrogenase in the walls of the stomach and intestine before it can reach the bloodstream. This effect may be important. Jones (1984) showed that the overall elimination rate was much higher than the terminal elimination rate usually measured, and this is likely to be because a

Table 7.1 Drugs that affect, or would be expected to affect, the rate of stomach emptying, and so influence the rate of ethanol absorption.

Drugs that slow gastric emptying
    Drugs which have an anticholinergic action, and so inhibit the effects of the parasympathetic nervous system, such as:
        atropine
        chlorpromazine and promazine
        disopyramide
        procyclidine
        propantheline
        tricyclic antidepressant drugs (e.g. amitriptyline)

    Drugs which have an adrenergic action, and so stimulate the effects of the sympathetic nervous system, such as:
        amphetamines
        dexfenfluramine
        phenylpropanolamine (in cough mixtures)

    Drugs which have an opioid action, such as:
        antidiarrhoeal medicines (including loperamide and 'Lomotil')
        buprenorphine
        codeine
        diamorphine (heroin)
        dextropropoxyphene (in co-proxamol)
        methadone
        morphine
        pethidine

Drugs that hasten stomach emptying, notably:
    the antiemetics metoclopramide and cisapride, and the antibiotic erythromycin

---

substantial proportion is broken down before it enters the systemic circulation (von Wartburg 1989). This is called *pre-systemic elimination* or *first-pass metabolism*.

Women may have less alcohol dehydrogenase in the gut wall, and so absorb a greater proportion of ethanol into the systemic circulation. There was no significant difference between the oral and intravenous bioavailability in women, whereas there was in men (Frezza *et al.* 1990). The matter is contentious (Seitz *et al.* 1990; Sweeney 1990; Zedeck 1990; Gentry *et al.* 1994; Levitt 1994), and direct measurements in rats have failed to find any role for the stomach in breaking down ethanol before it is absorbed into the circulation (Smith *et al.* 1992). Brown *et al.* (1995) showed that, although inflammation or atrophy of the stomach lining can reduce local alcohol dehydrogenase activity, they do not influence the extent to which ethanol is absorbed.

The antiulcer drugs cimetidine and ranitidine inhibit alcohol dehydrogenase, and are said to increase the bioavailability of ethanol (Di Padova *et al.* 1992). This is contentious, too, and several negative studies have been reported (Kendall *et al.* 1994; Toon *et al.* 1994).

Distribution

Once ethanol has entered the systemic circulation, it is distributed throughout total body water. Total body water accounts for about 60–70 per cent of body weight, but is different in males and females, and depends on size as well as weight. In men, it decreases with age.

Useful equations based on over 700 people aged 17–86 were derived (Watson *et al.* 1980), and are given in Appendix B. The amount of ethanol in the body at a time when the blood ethanol concentration is known can be calculated from a knowledge of the subject's total body water.

Only a proportion of the blood is water, and only the watery part contains ethanol. The fatty part contains none. It is therefore necessary to correct the blood ethanol concentration to allow for this. The correction can be determined by drying a sample of blood, but it is usual to assume that blood is 80 per cent water (Watson 1988). The concentration of ethanol in the watery component of blood is therefore 1.25 times the concentration in whole blood:

$$\text{concentration in water} = \frac{\text{concentration in blood}}{\text{fraction of blood that is water}}$$

The amount of ethanol in the body is therefore given by:

$$\text{ethanol (mg)} = \frac{\text{TBW (dl) x blood ethanol concentration (mg/dl)}}{\text{fraction of blood that is water}}$$

where TBW = total body water, mg = milligrams, and dl = decilitres.

The volume of distribution as usually defined is the ratio of the amount of a substance in one unit volume of blood to the total amount in the body, and here is equivalent to TBW/fraction of blood that is water.

Much of the forensic understanding of ethanol comes from the classical treatise by Widmark, published in 1932, in which he defined the amount of alcohol in the body, A, in terms of the concentration in blood, C_0, the body weight in kilograms, p, and a factor 'r', which represented the volume of distribution per kilogram body weight.

Widmark's equation,

$$A = r \times p \times C_0$$

is analogous to the equation above. He found experimental average values of 0.68 for r in men, and 0.55 in women. These values are equivalent to a body composition of 54 per cent water in men, and 44 per cent in women, values which are lower than those found by direct experiment.

There are advantages in calculating the total body water from the subject's height and weight (and age in men), and correcting the blood ethanol concentration to the amount in the aqueous portion of blood, since this approach uses more (readily available) information than Widmark's approach based on weight and sex alone. This is especially true for individuals of unusual shape. An example is given in Appendix B, Section B.3

Fitzgerald and Hume (1987*e*) have argued that the use of total body water is unnecessarily complicated, and that it still ignores differences between individuals of the same height and weight but different shape. The 95 per cent confidence intervals for the estimates of total body water are ± 4 litres of the mean value, that is, about ± 10 per cent (Watson 1988). In a group of subjects, 95 per cent of true values for total body water would be expected to lie within this range. The corresponding 99 per cent confidence interval about the mean would be approximately ± 15 per cent. This compares with the 'low', 'average' and 'high' r factors which Fitzgerald and Hume (1987*d*) suggest, of 0.52, 0.68, and 0.86, a spread of ± 25 per cent. Calculations of total body water, using more information about the individual, are therefore more precise than calculations based on Widmark's r.

Elimination of ethanol

Ethanol is broken down by the enzyme alcohol dehydrogenase to form acetaldehyde, and this is further metabolized to acetate. It may also be broken down by a microsomal oxidase enzyme (Lieber 1977; 1994). Alcohol dehydrogenase can be saturated, that is, it can reach its maximum working rate, at relatively low ethanol concentrations, so that ethanol elimination then proceeds at this maximum, constant, rate. A small amount of ethanol is eliminated unchanged in the urine, the breath, and the sweat. These routes are significant because they allow blood ethanol concentration to be estimated from urine or breath.

The quantitative analysis of ethanol elimination has used two approaches. Either a simple zero-order model is used, in which it is assumed that the rate of removal of ethanol is constant throughout the relevant range of concentrations; or a concentration-dependent, capacity-limited (Michaelis-Menten) model is employed. This describes the disappearance of ethanol in terms of the maximum velocity, V_{max} and the concentration at which the enzyme is half-saturated, K_m (see p. 124).

Widmark's equation for the elimination of ethanol

Widmark calculated the weight of absolute ethanol metabolized in some time-interval, t, from the equation:

$$C_t = C_0 - \beta \cdot t$$

where C_t is the blood ethanol concentration at some time, t, C_0 the ethanol concentration at some initial time, 0, and β a constant which represents the average amount of ethanol removed in unit time. β was expressed as milligrams ethanol per gram of blood per minute, or (β_{60}), per hour. Some later workers have expressed β as milligrams ethanol per 100 millilitres of blood per hour.[3]

The elimination rate has also been expressed as the total weight of ethanol eliminated per hour and as the total weight of ethanol eliminated per kilogram body-weight per hour. These can be converted to an elimination rate in milligrams per 100 millilitres per hour by assuming either the weight and Widmark's r or the volume of distribution, which anyway are needed in the first place to calculate the total amount of ethanol eliminated.

Holford (1987) summarized the results of 11 studies of oral ethanol in which the disappearance rate was calculated using a form of Widmark's analysis. Several studies have looked at the elimination rate after different doses of ethanol. Average values ranged from 12.6 milligrams per 100 millilitres per hour to 26.8 milligrams per 100 millilitres per hour. The scatter of elimination rates with dose is shown in Fig 7.1.

It should be possible to determine the disappearance rate for ethanol from just two measurements of blood ethanol concentration provided the interval between the first and the second sample is known. In practice, the determination cannot be made very accurately, because of ignorance of the state of absorption of ethanol and because of intrinsic variability in the measurements which can introduce errors. There is no way of knowing in an individual case what these errors might be. None the less, expert judgment often has to rely on only one concentration measurement, and two may seem luxurious.

Neuteboom and Jones (1990) examined the apparent ethanol disappearance rate in over

[3] The conversion factors are: milligrams per 100 millilitre per hour = (milligram per gram per hour) × 105.6 milligrams per 100 millilitre per hour = (milligram per gram per minute) × 6336 [1.056 is the relative density of blood in normal people].

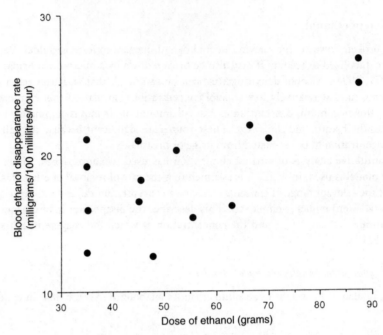

Fig. 7.1 The measured elimination rate of ethanol from the blood (milligrams of ethanol per 100 millilitres of blood per hour) plotted against the dose of absolute ethanol (grams) for 11 separate studies, assuming that the elimination rate is constant for any one study (after Holford 1987).

1300 drivers arrested for drinking, in whom blood ethanol concentration was measured twice. The second concentration was higher than the first, suggesting continued absorption, in 2 per cent of drivers. Rates below 10 milligrams per 100 millilitres per hour were not studied, and of those drivers who were studied, some 80 per cent had ethanol concentrations above 100 milligrams per 100 millilitres. Estimated ethanol disappearance rate was between 12 milligrams per 100 millilitres per hour and 38 milligrams per 100 millilitres per hour in 95 per cent of drivers, though 0.4 per cent had apparent rates above 48 milligrams per 100 millilitres per hour.

An interesting finding was that the mean ethanol elimination rate increased as the blood ethanol concentration increased. This may be the result of concentration-dependent pharmacokinetics, or of enzyme induction in habitual heavy drinkers; but it could also be due to ongoing redistribution of ethanol; and apparently low rates of elimination at low concentrations could be due to continued absorption.

Back-extrapolation

A common problem in medicolegal work is to calculate what the ethanol concentration would have been when some event occurred, knowing the blood (or breath) ethanol concentration at some later time. One approach is to accept the imperfections in Widmark's formula, and to make explicit the assumptions which have been used, including:

(1) that the subject had already absorbed all the ethanol into the system at the time of the event. (This assumption is likely to be true if more than 2 hours elapsed from the end of drinking until the event);

(2) that the subject has not drunk since the event occurred; and

(3) that the subject eliminates ethanol in the average way expected according to Widmark's equation.

Since there is wide variation in the rate of ethanol metabolism between individuals, this may cause difficulty. There is also the problem that, particularly at low ethanol concentrations, Widmark's equation can be in error.

The last assumption can be replaced by using the upper and lower bounds for the ranges of variables which are used. In particular, instead of using an average value for the rate at which ethanol disappears from the blood, the highest and lowest rates observed in a group of subjects would be used.

Reasonable values to assume are:

(1) lowest likely rate = 12.5 milligrams per 100 millilitres per hour;

(2) average rate   = 18.7 milligrams per 100 millilitres per hour; and

(3) highest likely rate = 25 milligrams per 100 millilitres per hour.

The average value, based on the data in Holford's review, is 25 per cent faster than the rate that has been suggested by Walls and Brownlie (1986e). Both values fall within the range suggested; and the rate of 18.7 milligrams per 100 millilitres per hour has the additional advantage of being midway between the upper and lower bounds of the range.

Detailed calculations are illustrated in Appendix B, Section B.4.

Reliability of back-extrapolation

There are good theoretical reasons why back-calculation might give erroneous results, and there is also experimental evidence. Al-Lanqawi *et al.* (1992) studied 24 men given approximately 50 grams of ethanol (roughly equivalent to two thirds of a bottle of wine, or 2-3 pints of beer), measuring their blood ethanol concentrations over the next 9 hours.

The mean rate of elimination was 18.6 milligrams per 100 millilitres per hour, with 95 per cent confidence intervals of 13.4 and 23.8 milligrams per 100 millilitres per hour. This is equivalent to saying that there is a 95 per cent chance that the true mean rate lies between 13.4 and 23.8 milligrams per 100 millilitres per hour. These limits are very close to those established above from Holford's earlier review.

Three different rates of elimination were then used to back-extrapolate from the observed values at 4 and 6 hours to the values 1 to 5 hours earlier. The calculated results were compared with the previously measured results. Errors in back-extrapolation were fairly small when the experimentally determined average rate of 18.6 milligrams per 100 millilitres per hour was used, with mean errors less than 3 milligrams per 100 millilitres. Much larger errors were seen in some individuals, and these were greater at earlier times. The worst errors in back-extrapolation over times as long as 4 hours were around ± 20 milligrams per 100 millilitres.

When an elimination rate of 15 milligrams per 100 millilitres per hour, commonly assumed in such calculations, was used, the average difference between the true and calculated results rose from 4 milligrams per 100 millilitres 5 hours after drinking to 21 milligrams per 100 millilitres 1 hour after drinking, and the worst errors were up to 40 milligrams per 100 millilitres when extrapolating for 4 hours. Errors of similar magnitude were apparent if the highest observed rate was used.

The study confirms the wide margin for error when an average value for ethanol elimination rate is applied to an individual. Since it was conducted under controlled conditions, it is likely that the study underestimates the errors that occur in practice, when the precise time that the ethanol was drunk is uncertain, and the subject may have taken food with it, for example.

The assumption that the subject has already absorbed all the ethanol into his system at the time of the incident is critical. This is clearly illustrated in an important theoretical paper on the Gumbley case[4] (Jackson et al. 1991). The delay between the end of drinking and the accident was only 30 minutes. Assuming that absorption was complete in 30 minutes, then only 0.2 per cent of drinkers would have had a blood ethanol concentration below 80 milligrams per 100 millilitres; but with slow absorption after large amounts of alcohol, over half of all drinkers might have had concentrations below the legal limit at the time of the accident.

The effect of blood ethanol concentration on ethanol elimination

Ethanol elimination proceeds at an approximately steady rate over a fairly wide range, but not the whole range, of ethanol concentrations likely to be encountered. Lundquist and Wolthers (1958) examined ethanol elimination in 10 healthy young subjects with this in mind. They found that the rate of ethanol disappearance was lower at low concentrations, but approached a maximum at concentrations higher than about 100 milligrams per 100 millilitre, that is that ethanol showed saturable (Michaelis-Menten) kinetics. Saturable kinetic processes are described by V_{max}, the maximum rate of the reaction, and K_m, the concentration at which the reaction rate is half of the maximum rate (see p. 21). The mean values for the two parameters that define the Michaelis-Menten equation were found to be a K_m of 9.2 milligrams per 100 millilitres, and a V_{max} of 22 milligrams per 100 millilitres per hour. This means that the disappearance rate approaches more and more closely to a maximum of 22 milligrams per 100 millilitres per hour as the concentration of ethanol in the blood increases above 9.2 milligrams per 100 millilitres (Fig. 7.2).

Other studies, reviewed by Holford (1987) gave a range of K_m between 8.2 and 12.8 milligrams per 100 millilitres, and a range of V_{max} between 18 and 31 milligrams per 100 millilitres per hour.

Figure 7.3 illustrates the way in which the rate of ethanol elimination is determined both by the concentration of ethanol and by the K_m.

Lewis (1986) has calculated theoretical ethanol concentration-time curves based on a V_{max} of 22.8 milligrams per 100 millilitres per hour, a K_m of 9.5 milligrams per 100 millilitres, and an absorption half-life of quarter of an hour, and shown that the blood ethanol disappearance rate is 12 milligrams per 100 millilitres per hour after a dose of 20 grams taken over 6 minutes by a man of 70 kilograms, and 18 milligrams per 100 millilitres per hour after a dose of 50 grams.

At very high concentrations of ethanol, processes such as excretion through the lungs and in the urine may become more important, and these processes are not saturable. Lundquist and Wolthers (1958) estimated that these non-metabolic routes accounted for 3 per cent of ethanol elimination at 50 milligrams per 100 millilitres, but 15 per cent at 300 milligrams per 100 millilitres.

Practical importance of concentration-dependent kinetics

There has been very little formal analysis of the relative merits of these two methods of describing ethanol elimination. Any description that involves two parameters (for example K_m

[4] Also reported at [1989] AC 281.

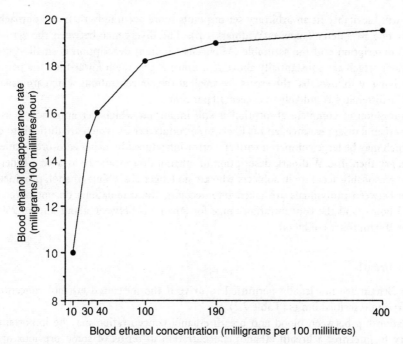

Fig. 7.2 The elimination rate of ethanol from the blood (milligrams of ethanol per 100 millilitres of blood per hour) plotted against the dose of absolute ethanol (grams), assuming that the process is saturable, with a maximum velocity (V_{max}) of 20 milligrams per 100 millilitres per hour, and a concentration at half-maximum reaction rate (K_m) of 10 milligrams per 100 millilitres

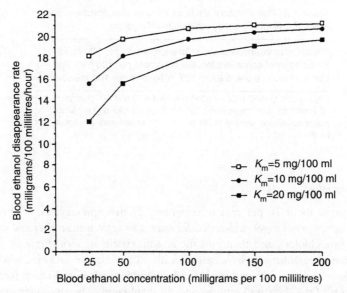

Fig. 7.3 The elimination rate of ethanol from the blood (milligrams of ethanol per 100 millilitres of blood per hour) plotted against the dose of absolute ethanol (grams), assuming that the process is saturable, with a maximum velocity (V_{max}) of 21.8 milligrams per 100 millilitres per hour, and three different values of concentration at half-maximum reaction rate (K_m): 5, 10, and 20 milligrams per 100 millilitres.

and V_{max}) will inevitably fit an arbitrary set of points more accurately than an approach that allows only one parameter (such as Widmark's β). The divergence between the zero–order (Widmark) description and the saturable (Michaelis–Menten) description is small at ethanol concentrations which are substantially above K_m. Since K_m is much lower than the permitted limit for driving, it follows that the errors are small at the concentrations which are usually of interest. The difference is unlikely to exceed 10 per cent.

The assumption of complete absorption is still important whichever approach is used in examining ethanol disappearance, and is likely to introduce errors which are difficult to quantify but which may be large compared with any error introduced by using zero–order kinetics.

In summary then, the Widmark description of ethanol disappearance as a zero–order process will be reasonably accurate in subjects who are no longer absorbing ethanol, provided that differences between individuals are taken into account, the calculations do not cover more than 2 or 3 hours; and the concentration range for ethanol is between about 25 and 250 milligrams per 100 millilitres of blood.

Ethanol in breath

Drivers in Britain are not legally permitted to drive if the measured ethanol concentration exceeds certain prescribed limits (Table 7.2).

The relationship between blood and breath ethanol concentration may be important if it is necessary to interpret a breath ethanol concentration in terms of some previous or subsequent concentration, or to estimate the amount of ethanol consumed from the breath concentration.

Table 7.2. The statutory limits of ethanol concentration above which it is illegal to drive in the United Kingdom

Breath ethanol concentration: 35 micrograms per 100 millilitres
Blood ethanol concentration: 80 milligrams per 100 millilitres
Urine ethanol concentration: 107 milligrams per 100 millilitres

If the breath ethanol concentration is between 35 and 50 micrograms per 100 millilitres, then the motorist can opt to give a separate specimen; the police can decide whether blood or urine should be taken, and usually opt for the former.

Relevant lung physiology

Air, which contains about 78 per cent nitrogen and 21 per cent oxygen, is drawn into the lungs, via the trachea (wind pipe), which divides again and again into smaller and smaller tubes (bronchi, then bronchioles), and then into the alveoli, elastic air sacs (Fig.7.4). The alveoli, about 300 million in each lung, behave mechanically like miniature balloons, whose walls are pulled outwards in inspiration (breathing in) and pushed inwards in expiration (breathing out) by the movements of the chest wall muscles and the diaphragm. The alveoli are made of membranes which allow gases to pass through. On one side is air, and on the other side is a network of capillaries carrying blood drained from the veins of the body.

As it passes through the upper air passages, the air is made warmer and moister. In the

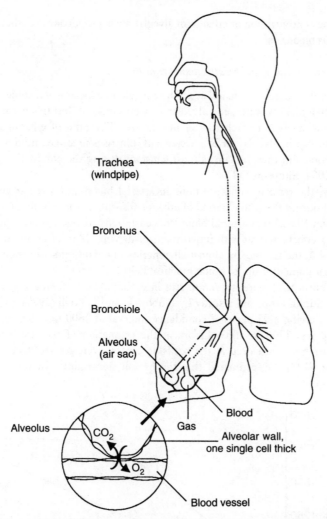

Fig. 7.4 The respiratory system. Air passes through the mouth and nose to the trachea (windpipe), bronchi (the larger tubes in the lungs), and bronchioles (the smaller tubes in the lungs), to the alveoli (the air sacs). Each alveolus has a wall one cell thick that is in contact with a blood vessel. Gases, including oxygen (O_2), carbon dioxide (CO_2), and ethanol vapour, can cross to and from the bloodstream in this way.

alveoli, oxygen in the inspired air is exchanged across the thin alveolar membrane for carbon dioxide in the blood which flows through alveolar capillaries. Other gases, such as the anaesthetic agent halothane, can also pass across the alveolar membrane. Any air not reaching the alveoli does not take part in the exchange of gases.

Ethanol is volatile, and so ethanol in the blood can pass across the alveolar membrane into the alveolar air, and be exhaled in expired air. The *vapour pressure* of a substance is a measure of its volatility, that is, its readiness to evaporate from a liquid to a gas. The vapour pressure of a substance above a solution is proportional to its concentration in the solution, and so the ethanol concentration in alveolar blood influences the ethanol concentration in alveolar air. At equilibrium, the concentration of ethanol in alveolar air is proportional to the concentration in systemic venous blood.

Changes in the ratio of blood and breath ethanol with time

It would be possible to infuse ethanol at a constant rate in experimental subjects until the concentrations in blood, body water, and alveolar air were constant, but this has not been done. In practice, equilibrium is not reached after oral intake. The ratio of ethanol concentration in venous blood to that in alveolar air is not constant, but rises to a maximum over the period of ethanol absorption and then remains almost constant during the elimination phase (Fig. 7.5) (Martin *et al.* 1984; Simpson 1987*a*).

Interestingly, the ratio of concentrations in arterial blood and alveolar air is much more nearly constant during the whole period of ethanol absorption and elimination, and it could be argued (Simpson 1987*a*) that arterial blood concentrations correlate more closely with central nervous system effects and so with impairment of driving. It is, after all, arterial blood that delivers ethanol to the tissues. As almost all experimental data refer to venous concentrations of ethanol, this argument is not of much practical help.

In the post-absorptive state, there are still interindividual differences in the blood:breath ethanol concentration ratio, and a study by Dubowski and O'Neill (1979) estimated the value as 2280 ± 241 , giving a 95 per cent confidence interval of 1800 to 2760; the experimentally observed range was 1706 to 3063. Errors in the estimation of blood ethanol from breath ethanol concentrations measured at the roadside can be even greater than this (Jones 1985, 1987). Simpson (1987*b*, *c*) estimated that the overall uncertainty for the whole procedure,

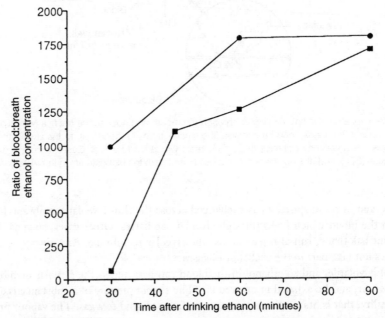

Fig. 7.5 The ratio of venous blood:breath ethanol concentration plotted against time from drinking (minutes) for two different studies (Martin *et al.* 1984; Simpson 1987*a*).

including potential errors in the machines and their calibration, was slightly higher, but more than 90 per cent of the uncertainty was due to differences between individuals. In Britain, a ratio of 80 000/35 (nearly 2300 : 1) is assumed (Walls and Brownlie 1985*f*).

The readings by an infra-red breath ethanol measuring machine were compared with corresponding blood ethanol concentrations measured by different methods and in different laboratories. Repeat readings of breath samples within one laboratory varied, with a coefficient of variation of ± 4 per cent (that is, 95 per cent of results were within ± 8 per cent of the mean value). The relationship with blood concentrations was much more variable, and the breath instrument read zero when there was still detectable ethanol in blood (Jones *et al.* 1992).

Difficulties in measurement of alveolar breath ethanol concentration

Exhaled air is a mixture of alveolar air and air from the bronchi and bronchioles which has not taken part in gas exchange, so-called 'dead-space air'. The first part of the expired air contains most of the dead-space air, and the proportion of alveolar air increases as expiration continues. The dead space in normal lungs has a volume of 100-200 millilitres, and the forced vital capacity, which is the greatest volume of gas that can be exhaled in a single breath, is around 3 litres in men and 2.5 litres in women. It has been recommended that only the last 30 per cent of the breath be used to represent alveolar ethanol concentration (Walls and Brownlie 1985*f*).

The vapour pressure above a solution increases as the temperature of the solution increases. This means that the blood:breath ethanol concentration ratio will increase as blood temperature increases, and the assumed ratio will be in error if the subject has a fever or hypothermia.

It is assumed that end-expired air represents alveolar air, and that most subjects will breathe out most of their forced vital capacity in a few seconds; indeed, it is normal to breathe out over 70 per cent of the forced vital capacity in one second. Patients with asthma or chronic bronchitis, diseases in which the rate of expiration is decreased, will not be able to breathe out as fast as normal. Patients with emphysema, a disease in which the alveolar airspaces are damaged, may have considerably increased dead space, and so may not give samples containing wholly alveolar air.

The concentration of ethanol in beer is usually below 5 grams per 100 millilitres in round numbers, and the concentration in the blood of conscious subjects is usually less than 0.5 grams per 100 millilitres. This tenfold difference in concentration is reflected by a tenfold difference in the concentration of ethanol vapour above the two liquids. Great care must therefore be taken to avoid measuring vapour from ethanol-containing drinks which are still in the mouth, as might happen if drink were trapped behind a dental plate; belching will also increase the figure if the stomach still contains ethanol.

In the United States, law enforcement agencies set the time between the last consumption of ethanol and breath-testing as at least 20 minutes in some states, and at least 30 minutes in others (Caddy *et al.* 1978).

In one experiment (Caddy *et al.* 1978), subjects were asked to swill a volume of drink round the mouth for 15 seconds and then spit it out; breath ethanol concentrations were subsequently measured at frequent intervals until two consecutive ethanol concentrations were zero. Beverages contained 4 per cent, 12 per cent, 43 per cent, 45 per cent and at least 95 per cent of ethanol (presumably by volume). The breath ethanol concentration returned to zero within 20 minutes of swilling at least 95 per cent ethanol, and the time taken to do so was substantially shorter when drinks contained lower concentrations of ethanol. Vigorous mouth-rinsing with warm distilled water reduced the time taken for ethanol to disappear from the breath.

In summary, it is unlikely that there will be a direct effect of mouth ethanol on breath readings after 20 minutes, but the breath:blood ethanol concentration will still be changing at that time.

Factors influencing the kinetics of ethanol

Sex

The differences in body composition and the difference in activity of alcohol dehydrogenase in the stomach wall of men and women have already been referred to. The ethanol elimination rate appears to be the same in healthy men and women, but the removal of acetaldehyde, formed by the breakdown of ethanol, is faster in women (Arthur *et al.* 1984). In one study of the disappearance rate at different times during the menstrual cycle, women were shown to have higher rates during the mid-luteal phase than the follicular or ovulatory phase, although the differences were small compared with interindividual differences (Sutker *et al.* 1987).

The question of pre-systemic elimination in men and women is discussed on p. 119.

Age

Age is an important determinant of total body water in men, and it therefore influences the volume of distribution of ethanol and the peak ethanol concentration after a standard dose per kilogram body weight; apparently ethanol elimination is not influenced by age between 20 and 60 years (Vestal *et al.* 1977; Jones and Neri 1985).

Genetics

Monozygotic (identical) twins have more similar ethanol kinetics than dizygotic (non-identical, or fraternal) twins (Kopun and Propping 1977).

Choice

When alcoholic subjects were allowed to drink freely, their mean blood ethanol concentrations were higher than when they followed a programme for treatment: they drank more ethanol (Mello and Mendelson 1970). This result was less surprising than the mean blood ethanol concentrations during free-choice drinking, which were as high as 240 milligrams per 100 millilitres.

Food

Blood ethanol concentrations after a drink are lower if there is food in the stomach while drinking. Early theories included the degradation of ethanol by food in the stomach and the stimulation of ethanol metabolism, but it now seems likely that food primarily slows the absorption of ethanol (Schultz *et al.* 1980). High-energy meals, and meals with high protein contents, cause a greater reduction in C_{max} (the maximum concentration reached) and the area under the ethanol concentration-time curve than low-energy or low-protein meals (Pikaar *et al.* 1988).

Exercise

Exercise does not alter the kinetics of ethanol significantly in healthy volunteers (Pikaar *et al.* 1988).

Race

Intravenous ethanol disposition was measured in Inuit (Eskimo), Native Americans (American Indians), and White subjects. Both the metabolic rate, calculated from the infusion rate required to keep blood ethanol at approximately 125 milligrams per 100 millilitres for 60 minutes, and the disappearance rate, calculated from the decline in blood ethanol concentrations after the infusion finished, were greatest in White subjects and least in Inuit subjects (Fenna *et al.* 1971). However, a later and larger study (Bennion and Li 1976) failed to find any difference in ethanol disposition between White and Native American subjects.

7.3 Specific medicolegal problems with ethanol

Experts and lawyers are recurrently faced with the same problems in prosecuting or defending those accused of driving with excess ethanol in the blood or breath. Jones (1991) has listed the top 10 defence challenges used by drinking drivers in Sweden as:

(1) 'the hip-flask ploy';[5]
(2) laced drinks;
(3) inhalation of ethanol vapour at work;
(4) trauma or disease;
(5) use of skin antiseptics containing ethanol;
(6) alleged mix-up of blood specimens;
(7) formation of alcohols in the sample after sampling;
(8) drug-ethanol interaction;
(9) consumption of medicines or tonics containing ethanol;
(10) resuscitation by infusion of fluids (including blood) that contain ethanol.

This useful list, and Jones's subsequent discussion, include some defences I have not met, and exclude others. Some important specific problems are dealt with here.

Hip-flask defence

The 'hip-flask' defence depends on the subject drinking after an alleged offence of driving with excess alcohol in the blood, but before he or she undergoes a test to determine the concentration of ethanol in breath or blood: 'I was so shocked by what happened, officer, that I took a swig of brandy from my hip-flask'.

The expert can be asked to calculate whether the amount drunk after the incident would account for the result, or alternatively, what the reading would have been if the subject had only consumed some stated, and usually small, amount before the incident.

The calculation can show that there is reasonable doubt that the defendant's blood ethanol concentration exceeded the legal limit at the time of an offence, which is helpful for the

[5] Jones's description. The term 'hip-flask defence' may be more neutral in tone.

defence; or that the defendant's ethanol concentration was still, in all probability, above the legal limit, even when the post-offence consumption is taken into account. It can also show a discrepancy between the account given of the total ethanol consumption and the measured ethanol concentration. Details of such calculations are given in Appendix B.

Lacing defence

The essence of the lacing defence is the accused's assertion that he or she was only drinking dilute ethanol, in the form of beer or wine, for example, but that a 'friend' had covertly added more concentrated ethanol, usually in the form of spirits such as vodka or whisky. Though no longer a defence in the United Kingdom to the charge of driving with excess alcohol in the blood, lawyers may present evidence of lacing to the court to show special reasons why their client should not be disqualified from driving.

It is often possible to show that the defendant would have needed to drink, unawares, very large volumes of spirits to produce the observed ethanol concentration. Detailed calculations are again described in Appendix B.

One related matter, namely whether a defendant could be expected to realize that a drink was laced, has not been formally tested. A small pilot experiment with colleagues suggests that most are unable to detect significant quantities of vodka in beer. A related experiment has shown that even determined, experienced, subjects can be unable to distinguish brandy from whisky (Campbell *et al.* 1994).

Level so high that defendant would have been in coma

Solicitors are sometimes asked to defend clients with extremely high blood ethanol concentrations. On one occasion, it was sought to argue that the client's ethanol concentration was so high that he would have been unable to drive with so much ethanol in his system.

CASE 7.1

'We act for Mr… who is charged that he drove a motor vehicle after consuming so much alcohol that the proportion of it in his breath exceeded the prescribed limit…The Lion Intoximeter Breath Analyser produced figures of 189 and 191 micrograms [per 100 millilitres of breath]…[This is equivalent to 432 milligrams per 100 millilitres of blood]. We are led to believe that a blood alcohol reading of 400 and more is likely to produce death or at least deep coma…'

Table 7.3 Sequence of central nervous system depression due to ethanol

	Target	Result
First	Higher centres	Feeling 'relaxed'
		Errors of judgement
		Loss of social inhibition
Second	Coordination	Dysarthria (slurred speech)
		Fumbling movement
		Loss of balance
		Nystagmus (oscillation of eyeballs)
Third	Sensation	Reduced pain perception
Fourth	Consciousness	Coma
Fifth	Brain stem functions	Respiratory depression, death

Standard textbooks (Cooper *et al.* 1979*b*; Ellenhorn and Barceloux 1988; Garriot 1988; Ley 1993*b*) carry tables of the relationship between blood ethanol concentration and the clinical effects. There is general agreement on the approximate sequence of changes in behaviour and physiology (Table 7.3). However, the concentrations at which these changes occur are very different in different subjects. There is a particularly marked difference between unhabituated and habituated drinkers, but tolerance is very variable within these broad categories.

There is scientific evidence that some people can 'take their drink' with fewer outward signs than others. The standard works regard concentrations of over 500 milligrams ethanol per 100 millilitres of blood as 'probably fatal'. This view is derived from studies such as those by Kaye and Haag (1957) on patients with 'uncomplicated fatal acute alcoholism', which concluded that 'patients with alcohol levels about 500 milligrams [ethanol] per 100 millilitres [of blood] or above are foredoomed, in the absence of effective therapy, although at death the blood alcohol value may be only a fraction of that figure'.

Survival at much higher concentrations is now well-documented.

CASE 7.2 (JOHNSON *ET AL.* 1982)

A 24-year-old woman came to hospital with abdominal pain. She was conscious and talking, but slightly confused, and her blood ethanol concentration was 1510 milligrams per 100 millilitre. Her pain settled, the blood ethanol concentration fell, and she left hospital after 2 days.

Although it must be exceptional for patients to tolerate concentrations three times the 'lethal' concentration and still be talking, less extreme tolerance seems common. In one survey, patients seen in a Pennsylvanian emergency department who admitted to drinking had blood ethanol concentration measured. In 76 patients, none of whom was clinically 'intoxicated', the median concentration was 265 (range 120–540) milligrams per 100 millilitres (Urso *et al.* 1981). Eighteen alcohol abusers attending for detoxification at an Australian clinic had ethanol concentrations in the range 300–450 milligrams per 100 millilitres of blood with 'very little clinical evidence of intoxication' (Davis and Lipson 1986).

Habituated drinkers can clearly tolerate extremely high blood ethanol concentrations with very little outward sign that they are drunk.

Breath and blood concentrations inconsistent

Subjects can sometimes provide specimens of two kinds, such as blood and breath or blood and urine. This happens in the United Kingdom when the police breath test shows a value of less than 50 micrograms of ethanol per 100 millilitres. The defendant can then opt to replace the breath test result with the result of a blood or urine test (the police decide whether to use blood or urine).

In some circumstances, the difficulty may arise that two sorts of test are apparently discrepant.

CASE 7.3

'Our client was breathalyzed, and because of his Camic reading, i.e., 42, he was given the opportunity of providing a specimen of blood for analysis...it was...found to contain 81 milligrams of alcohol per 100 millilitres of blood.'

The Camic reading is a breath ethanol concentration. The solicitor was concerned that the alcohol content of the blood might have increased during storage. This was a misunderstanding of the different units used to express concentration of ethanol in blood and breath. The breath value was in fact 42 micrograms per 100 millilitres, compared with a legal limit of 35 micrograms per 100 millilitres; whereas the blood reading was 81 milligrams per 100 millilitres, compared with a limit of 80 milligrams per 100 millilitres.

Using the standard conversion factor of 80 000/35, the breath ethanol concentration of 42 micrograms per 100 millilitres is equivalent to 96 000 micrograms per 100 millilitres of blood, that is, 96 milligrams per 100 millilitres. There is a discrepancy, but it can be accounted for in several ways:

1. A delay between the Camic reading and the blood sampling. This is the most obvious explanation, since a police officer would have obtained the breath reading, but a police surgeon would have to be called to take the blood sample. A delay of about 1 hour would probably have been long enough for the blood ethanol concentration to fall by 15 milligrams per 100 millilitres.
2. The subject did not have an average blood:breath ratio. If the samples had in fact been taken simultaneously, then the concentration ratio is 81 000/42, that is, 1929:1. This is below average, but within the range of normal for blood:breath concentration ratios in the post-absorptive state.
3. The subject did have an average blood:breath ratio, but was not in the post-absorptive state. The blood:breath ratio increases gradually over more than 90 minutes after drinking, so a lower ratio than usual might simply reflect sampling within this 90 minute period.
4. A less likely possibility is that a small quantity of drink was trapped behind a dental plate or in a tooth cavity and may therefore have affected the reading.
5. There always remains the possibility of experimental error. The difference between the actual and expected blood readings was 19 per cent, and might be due to some technical error. This is rather unlikely if the specimen was analysed in the proper way by an approved laboratory, but not impossible. Nor is it impossible for samples from two subjects to be switched.

Concentration enhanced by interaction with drugs

The interactions between ethanol and drugs are potentially important, since a substantial proportion of the population is taking medicines obtained on prescription or over the counter, and some may take illicit drugs such as cannabis, Ecstasy, and opioids.

There are two possible sources of interaction. The drug may alter the concentration of ethanol in the blood, for example, by reducing the amount absorbed or decreasing the rate of metabolic breakdown. It can also alter the way in which a subject responds to a given concentration of ethanol in the blood, for example, because the drug has sedative or respiratory depressant effects which add to those of ethanol. Three cases illustrate the questions asked of experts in this area.

Phenytoin

Phenytoin is an anticonvulsant drug which can affect the way in which the liver breaks down other drugs.

CASE 7.4 PART 1

'We act on behalf of ... who has been charged with driving with excess alcohol as the result of an accident...[he] informs us that he is an epileptic and he takes the anti-convulsant drug phenytoin (1×100 mg) three times daily. We understand that a side-effect of the taking of these drugs is a quantity of the drug is excreted through the saliva in the mouth, and would therefore be expelled when blowing into a breath testing machine.' The solicitors ask whether this is in fact the case. If so, would it have affected the reading?

There are three separate points to consider.

1. Does phenytoin get into saliva?   Saliva is a protein-free 'ultrafiltrate' of the watery plasma component of blood. Phenytoin does get into saliva, but because most phenytoin in plasma is bound to protein, the concentration of the drug is much smaller in saliva than in plasma, and in most subjects is only about 100 micrograms per 100 millilitres (1 milligram per litre) of saliva, when the blood concentration is in the therapeutic range.

2. Does the phenytoin in the saliva get into the breath testing machine?   There are two possible ways that this might happen. Phenytoin vapour, like ethanol vapour, might be breathed into the machine in the gaseous state. However, the vapour pressure of phenytoin at 37 °C is negligible, so the amount breathed in will be negligible. The other way is in droplets of saliva. However, breath testing machines have filters which exclude all but the smallest particles from the sample analysis chamber. The amount entering the machine by this route is therefore negligible, too.

3. If phenytoin entered the breath testing sample chamber, would it have given a reading?   The Intoximeter detects ethanol using a catalytic fuel cell. The manufacturers claim that it has a high specificity for ethanol and does not respond to carbon monoxide or most drugs. Phenytoin does not contain a hydroxyl (−OH) group, and is unlikely to give a reading on this system.

Taken together, these factors make it most unlikely that the phenytoin made any contribution to the breath ethanol reading.

CASE 7.4 PART 2

The solicitors were not entirely deterred by the expert evidence, and wrote that 'we now understand that one of the side-effects of taking the anti-convulsant drug phenytoin can result in liver damage. Results of tests carried out on our client by his General Practitioner reveal that his liver is not functioning properly and this is a result of the medication which he is taking... We wonder whether the malfunction in our client's liver could affect the ability of his body to "break up" its alcohol content...'

Phenytoin is an inducer of hepatic enzymes, that is, it increases their activity. Conventional biochemical tests of liver function measure the serum concentration of the pigment bilirubin, formed by the breakdown of haemoglobin and excreted by the liver; and the activity in serum of several 'liver enzymes'. Abnormalities of liver enzyme tests are common in patients who take phenytoin, but they do not mean, in general, that the function of the liver is impaired. In particular, gamma-glutamyl transpeptidase can be induced; and alkaline phosphatase (which also reflects bone turnover) can be increased because there is increased metabolism of vitamin D, and hence relative deficiency. Because it induces enzymes, phenytoin is more likely to increase the rate of ethanol metabolism than reduce it. Rare cases of hepatic necrosis from phenytoin do occur, but this causes a severe clinical injury and one-third of such patients die.

In summary, abnormal liver function tests in a patient taking phenytoin do not, by themselves, suggest that the patient's ability to metabolize ethanol is impaired.

Glyceryl trinitrate (GTN)

Glyceryl trinitrate is a drug used to treat angina (heart pain brought on when the heart is working hard, for example during exercise).

CASE 7.5

'Our client has a heart condition and he has informed us that before he left home on the evening in question, he had taken two glyceryl trinitrate tablets and he states he took two further tablets before he left the public house…he believes that glyceryl trinitrate tablets could have affected the disposition or metabolism of alcohol in his body…'

The usual dose of glyceryl trinitrate is 500–1000 micrograms, sucked under the tongue. The drug dilates both arteries and veins, and it might therefore act to increase blood flow through the liver. This would increase the rate at which ethanol passed through the liver, but because the capacity of the liver to metabolize ethanol is limited, is unlikely to materially alter the disappearance rate. Glyceryl trinitrate has a half-life in the body of about 3 minutes, so any effect on ethanol metabolism will be transient.

'Lomotil' + propranolol ('Half-Inderal LA')

Sometimes subjects are taking more than one medicine in addition to the ethanol that they have consumed.

CASE 7.6

'Our client was in fact suffering from an upset stomach, and was taking paracetamol, kaolin morph [sic] and Indurella [sic] and Lomotol [sic] painkiller tablets…We would be grateful for your expert opinion on the question of the possible effect of the medication…on the level of alcohol recorded in Mr…'s blood.'
The Camic breath test reading was 56 micrograms ethanol per 100 millilitres of breath.

On further enquiry, the medicines he had taken were confirmed to be four tablets of the antidiarrhoeal agent 'Lomotil', a mixture of the opioid drug diphenoxylate (10 milligrams total) and the anticholinergic agent atropine (100 micrograms total); 180 millilitres kaolin and morphine mixture, equivalent to 12.6 milligrams total of morphine; 8 tablets of paracetamol (4 grams total) and six tablets of propranolol as 'Half-Inderal LA' (240 milligrams total).

Morphine, atropine, and diphenoxylate can all slow stomach emptying, and so might reduce the rate of absorption of ethanol. Propranolol speeds gastric emptying by about 30 per cent. The net effect of all the drugs is most likely to have been some reduction in gastric motility, prolonged absorption, and a correspondingly reduced peak ethanol concentration.

Concentration would have been lower at the time of the offence

It sometimes happens that the defence wish to argue that the ethanol concentration would have been lower at the time of the offence than it was subsequently found to be by the police, even though no further ethanol had been consumed after the offence. This contrasts with the 'hip-flask' defence discussed above.

This is only likely if two conditions are satisfied:

1. the subject has not absorbed all the ethanol in the stomach and intestines at the time of the offence; and
2. there is a material interval between the time of the offence and the time of the test for ethanol being taken.

The rate and extent of absorption depend on the factors mentioned on pp. 117–18. Such factors may persuade the expert one way or another, though the only certain indication that the ethanol concentration would have been lower at the time of the offence is the existence of a second sample (of the same nature) showing that the ethanol concentration continued to increase after the first sample had been obtained. This would imply that the subject had been on the rising part of the ethanol curve, always provided that no further ethanol had been taken. If the concentration in a second sample were lower than the concentration in the first sample, then either the subject was in the post-absorptive state at the time of the offence, and continued to break down ethanol, or was absorbing at the time of the offence, but had ceased to absorb further ethanol by the time of the second sample.

Defendant unable to blow

The breath analysis requires that the subject blow sufficiently hard and sufficiently long to produce a sample of alveolar air. The machine used may have pressure and volume sensors to ensure that this happens. If the subject fails to perform as the instrument requires, then he or she may be liable to a charge of failing to provide a specimen of breath for analysis.

CASE 7.7

A solicitor represented a client who had been dieting because he had hypercholesterolaemia (a high concentration of cholesterol in the blood). When he 'tried to provide a roadside breath test he instructs us that he did so to the best of his ability so much so that after his attempts to blow up the bag he felt dizzy almost to the point of blackout'. The sample was inadequate. He again failed to give an adequate sample at the police station. Although he offered to give a blood specimen, the station officer decided that he was deliberately withholding a specimen of breath, and he was charged with that offence.

When examined some months after the alleged offence, the man had a raised blood pressure of 170/108. The tendon reflexes (such as the knee-jerk) were all brisk.

His peak flow rate[6] was measured on three occasions by asking him to breathe out as fast as possible into a Wright peak flow meter, and the results were 300, 450, and 350 litres per minute. These results are more variable than is usual, and suggest either an inability to understand what was required, a degree of nervousness, or voluntary restriction of the peak flow rate. He was also asked to blow through a mouthpiece with sufficient force to maintain a column of mercury 30

---

[6] The 'peak expiratory flow rate', 'peak flow rate' or simply 'peak flow' are almost self-explanatory terms. They refer to the rate at which a subject can blow air out of the lungs in a big breath, as when blowing out the candles on a birthday cake. Patients with asthma or another cause of airways obstruction cannot blow out as fast as normal: the peak flow rate is reduced. Normal values depend on age, height, and sex.

millimetres high for 30 seconds, while his heart rate was monitored. His heart rate rose from 75 to 120 beats per minute before he started to blow, and rose still further during the 30 seconds of blowing.

The brisk reflexes, variable peak flow rate, and marked rise in pulse rate in anticipation of the blowing test all pointed to an abnormal degree of anxiety, but there was no neurological, muscular, skeletal, or respiratory disease which could have explained the apparent inability to blow.

Dizziness did not occur on prolonged blowing against a resistance, so it was difficult to argue that there was a physical illness behind the man's inability to give a breath specimen. He was subsequently convicted.

Chest disease can be so bad that the patient is indeed unable to blow. Spirometry (measurement of respiratory volumes and rates of flow) can be helpful. A forced expiratory volume in the first second (FEV_1) above 2.3 litres, a forced vital capacity (FVC, the volume of air expelled from the lungs when a subject takes the biggest breath in that he or she can manage, and then breathes out as long and as hard as possible) exceeding 2.6 litres and a peak expiratory flow rate greater than 330 litres per minute should be sufficient (Gomm *et al.* 1991). However, the FEV_1 can vary from hour to hour, so the values at the time of sampling cannot necessarily be deduced from spirometry performed some time later.

Solvent inhalation

Workers exposed to organic solvents sometimes claim that the solvent has affected a subsequent breath ethanol measurement. For example:

CASE 7.8 (DENNEY 1990)

A 26-year-old man spent 4½ hours spraying a car in an unventilated workshop, drank 2 pints (1136 millilitres) of lager (5 per cent ethanol by volume) and was then arrested; samples of breath contained 73 and 68 micrograms ethanol per 100 millilitres. The solvents inhaled were methanol, toluene, and xylene.

In an experiment, Denney (1990) exposed this man, and another involved in a similar case, to solvent fumes, and measured apparent 'breath ethanol' concentrations with two instruments, the Lion Alcolmeter S-D2, which contains a fuel cell, and the Lion Intoximeter 3000, which uses infra-red absorption. Both subjects found breathing solvent unpleasant, but tolerated 165 minutes of exposure. Breath ethanol readings remained zero in one subject, but a maximum reading of 9 micrograms per 100 millilitres of breath was obtained under slightly different conditions with the second subject, by Intoximeter. 'Recovery from the inhalation of solvents is normally rapid and could only be expected to lead to very slightly inflated breath alcohol levels on evidential tests carried out less than 30 minutes after exposure to the solvents has ceased.'

However, Edwards *et al.* (1986) studied a 52-year-old man who had been exposed to lacquers and paint thinners for many years, and had mildly abnormal liver function tests. An infra-red device, the Intoxylizer 5000, showed a breath 'ethanol' equivalent to a blood concentration of 310 milligrams per 100 millilitres, but gas chromatography failed to detect any ethanol in blood. However, the blood contained 1.1 milligrams of toluene per 100 millilitres. Since the blood:breath concentration ratio for toluene is only about 15:1, the corresponding breath toluene concentration would have been 73 micrograms toluene per 100 millilitres, and toluene absorbs infra-red radiation at the wavelength used by the Intoxilyzer 5000 (3.5

micrometres). Toluene was the likely cause of machine interference in this case.

In summary, there is some evidence that toluene, and perhaps other solvents, could affect the breath ethanol reading on some machines, but it might well be necessary to investigate every individual case to be sure whether any effect was significant.

One final point on this subject: Walls and Brownlie (1985d) refer to a number of cases in which those who intentionally abuse solvents have been convicted of driving while under the influence of drugs.

7.4 Summary

Ethanol (ethyl alcohol) is the single most important drug in forensic work, because of its widespread consumption, its undesirable effects, and the law regarding drinking and driving. Measurements of ethanol concentrations in breath, blood, and urine are subject to error, and require careful interpretation. When concentrations are measured some time after the event, then many factors need to be taken into account in estimating the likely concentration at the time of the event. Differences within and between subjects in the rate of absorption, the distribution, and the rate of elimination of ethanol all contribute to uncertainties in the calculations, as do interactions with food and drugs. The effects of increasing concentrations of ethanol on the central nervous system become increasingly severe, but differences in individual tolerance make it difficult to predict the effects of any given concentration in a particular subject.

8

Benzodiazepines

The benzodiazepines are anxiolytic (they reduce anxiety) and hypnotic (they induce sleep).

8.1 History

Chlordiazepoxide ('Librium') was the first benzodiazepine to be marketed, and has been available since 1960. By the mid-1970s, benzodiazepines were prescribed to around 3 per cent of the population in several European countries (Marks 1985). The remarkably widespread use of the drugs was due in part to their perceived safety in acute overdosage, especially when compared with barbiturate sleeping tablets. It was also in part the result of their wide promotion. Benzodiazepines could be used to calm any anxiety and to soothe any insomniac to sleep. One advertisement from 1967 shows a series of seven scenes linked by text which reads: 'Anxiety is in every ward and every clinic, preceding birth, anticipating death, complicating treatment. But where there is anxiety, in hospital or general practice, there is *Librium*'. Another advertisement of the same period is for the benzodiazepine nitrazepam ('Mogadon'). 'Of course, *Mogadon* means sleep for almost everybody, but often it means more than that'. The headline is above a series of vignettes showing a student, a businessman, a young mother and baby, and an older woman.

The image of benzodiazepines as harmless drugs which could help to relieve the everyday anxieties and ensure a good night's sleep has gradually faded into an image of overprescribing by doctors who tried to treat the social problems of their patients with medicines. The medicines were safe in overdosage, at least in normal people, but they were able to induce dependence.

8.2 The drugs

There are several useful monographs on the benzodiazepines (Trimble 1983; Smith and Wesson 1985; Hindmarch *et al.* 1990).

Over 35 benzodiazepines have been marketed somewhere in the world, and about 20 are available in the United Kingdom. All the drugs have anxiolytic, hypnotic, muscle relaxant, and anticonvulsant effects. There are differences in the degree to which these effects are manifest with any specific member of the group, and some drugs, such as clobazam, are used for one indication (as an anticonvulsant) rather than another. Midazolam and diazepam are available intravenously, and can be used to sedate patients undergoing minor surgical procedures such as endoscopy (a general term for 'looking inside a patient', usually used to mean the examination of the gullet, stomach and upper small bowel through a flexible fibre-optic tele-scope[1], unless it is further qualified). Effects last longer if a drug has a long half life or is broken down to an active metabolite which itself is long lasting. The compound desmethyl-diazepam is the active metabolite of chlordiazepoxide, chlorazepate ('Tranxene'), diazepam ('Valium'), flurazepam ('Dalmane'), ketazolam ('Anxon'), medazepam ('Nobrium') and prazepam ('Centrax'). These compounds therefore all have long-lasting effects owing to the long half-life of desmethyldiazepam which is around 80 hours. By contrast, triazolam ('Hal-cion') has a half-life of 3 hours, and its active hydroxy metabolites may also be short lived, so that its effect does not persist.

The benzodiazepines all act at specific receptors in the brain which are closely linked to certain receptors for the endogenous neurotransmitter GABA (gamma-aminobutyric acid), the $GABA_A$ receptors. When $GABA_A$ receptors, or the related benzodiazepine receptors, are activated, they affect chloride channels in the outer membranes of nerve cells, increasing the flow of chloride ions out of the cell, and this inhibits the discharge of the nerve cell.

8.3 Acute effects

The benzodiazepines have a number of effects in addition to their primary therapeutic actions of inducing sleep and relieving anxiety.

Termination of seizures

The significance of the benzodiazepine-induced inhibition of neuronal discharge is most obvi-ous when the drugs are used to terminate epileptic convulsions. In this situation the drug is usually given intravenously, and the convulsions often cease after a minute or so.

Respiratory depression

A second inhibitory effect can become manifest in this circumstance, namely respiratory depression. This is most likely to occur in patients who are already suffering from other forms of respiratory depression, such as those due to chronic obstructive airways disease (a form of lung damage which is usually brought about by cigarette smoking). It is also more likely in patients who have already taken a drug with depressant properties on respiration, the most common being ethanol.

The respiratory depression can be so severe that the patient would die without further treatment, in the form of either artificial ventilation or flumazenil ('Anexate')—an antidote to benzodiazepines.

Intravenous benzodiazepines are sufficiently dangerous that they should only be given when adequate facilities exist to deal with respiratory depression if it occurs, or where the dan-ger of withholding them outweighs the risk of respiratory depression.

Amnesia

Benzodiazepines are able to inhibit the formation of memories, and this is a distinct clinical advantage for patients undergoing unpleasant procedures such as endoscopy or electrical car-

[1] This procedure is more properly called fibre-optic oesophago–gastro–duodenoscopy, or 'OGD'.

dioversion (correcting abnormal heart rhythm by delivering a direct current shock to the heart). There is no retrograde amnesia, so that events prior to the administration of the benzodiazepine should be remembered. The drugs inhibit memory for a longer period than they suppress consciousness, and many doctors have had the experience of holding a conversation with a patient about the results of a recent endoscopy, only to be asked by the patient the next day if the results were yet available.

CASE 8.1 (LURIE *ET AL.* 1990)

A 30-year-old 'gentle, calm' man was given 10 milligrams diazepam intravenously and then underwent upper gastrointestinal endoscopy (the gullet, stomach, and first part of the small bowel were examined through a flexible telescope). While still lying on the endoscopy table after the examination, the patient asked when his endoscopy was to be. Told he had already had it, he said he would not be lied to, became enraged, struck his physician, and had to be forcibly restrained. The staff performed a second endoscopy.

The amnesia is not confined to intravenous benzodiazepines, and there are anecdotes of doctors who have taken short-acting benzodiazepines to help them snatch a few hours of sleep on international flights, and later have been completely amnesic for their arrival, passage through customs, and first few hours abroad (Morris and Estes 1987). Benzodiazepines can also impair memory because of the sedation and loss of concentration that they cause.

A study of the effects of the short-acting benzodiazepine triazolam examined whether memory was impaired for events the morning after a night-time dose of the drug (Bixler *et al.* 1991). Eighteen patients with insomnia were divided into three groups. One group received triazolam 500 micrograms or placebo; one, temazepam 30 milligrams or placebo; and one placebo only, on 12 successive nights. Memory in the morning, daytime, and evening was assessed.

Only temazepam improved sleep significantly more than placebo in this small study. Immediate memory the morning after a dose of drug was the same whether placebo or a benzodiazepine had been taken. However, daytime amnesia occurred in five of six patients (during 12 of 40 days) following triazolam, but not following temazepam, and in only one patient (out of 18) after placebo. 'Examples of memory impairment included a subject who began to leave a grocery store without paying for her purchases until reminded by the clerk'. Evening recall of word lists learnt during the morning was impaired by triazolam and also by temazepam.

This interesting small study suggests that amnesia is common after triazolam, that the amnestic effect is present after the sedation has worn off, and that triazolam and temazepam interfere with learning the morning after a night-time dose.

Amnesia is of forensic importance, because it can happen that patients who are taking a benzodiazepine are arrested for a crime and then argue that it was the result of absentmindedness, or that they are unable to recall any of the relevant facts (McClelland 1990). The paradigm is of patients who are caught shoplifting, and then plead that they had forgotten to pay for the goods in question because they were taking a benzodiazepine.

Todd (1976) had called attention to 'pharmacogenic shoplifting' as a result of seeing five previously honest people who had allegedly taken goods from supermarkets without paying, and who all put goods into their own shopping bags as well as a supermarket basket or trolley, but did not present the goods in the shopping bags for payment. There was no obvious attempt to conceal what was done, and the goods in the shopping bags often included items that the accused seldom or never used. The drugs involved are not discussed, other than to say that they were legitimately taken for a therapeutic purpose.

Laurence and Bennett (1992*b*) comment that, 'whilst it is natural to regard such claims with suspicion, those of us (not taking a benzodiazepine) who have nearly walked out of a self-service shop carrying goods we have neglected to present for payment will not be over ready to dismiss the possibility (though amnesia selective for payment must arouse scepticism).' They suggest that it is useful to examine whether the drug might have contributed to absent-mindedness, so that there is reasonable doubt that the accused had formed the necessary intent to steal.

Stofer (1984) quotes four typical Swiss cases of shop-lifting associated with benzodiazepine consumption. These led to a *'diminution de la responsibilité'* for the crime as adjudged by the court.

Mortimer (1991) has classified shoplifting into three groups according to whether an intention (*mens rea*) was present, dubious, or absent. The first group includes people who are aware that stealing is wrong, but who are unconcerned by this and set out to steal. Such people, whom she characterizes as 'blunted conscience thieves' include patients rendered disinhibited by drugs or alcohol. The benzodiazepines might cause such behavioural disinhibition by pharmacological inhibition of those higher centres that control behaviour, in the same way that ethanol can cause disinhibition of behaviour.

'Mentally disordered individuals who describe an alteration in consciousness at the time of the offence, suggesting depersonalization, derealization, dissociation or twilight state' form a group in whom it is dubious whether the intention was present to commit a crime at the relevant time. Persons who absent-mindedly fail to pay for goods fall into the third group, those in whom the intention was absent. The classification helps the expert to lay out the possible explanations of events, but the analysis will not necessarily convince the court.

Amnesia for an alleged crime is no defence to having committed it, but the genesis of the amnesia can be important. A man who failed to remember if he had committed a crime while befuddled and drowsy from the non-specific sedation caused by a benzodiazepine would be in a rather different position from a man who acted in a perfectly clear-headed and reasonable way but could subsequently remember nothing of events because of the specific antegrade amnesia induced by the same drug. McClelland (1990) makes the point that hysterical amnesia is more likely if strong emotion at the time of the crime combines with drugs to suppress the memory of events as a psychological defence mechanism. In the case of such hysterical amnesia, the failure to recall events says nothing about the state of mind of the accused during them.

Impairment of mental and motor skills

Benzodiazepines, like other sedative drugs, can impair the motor (movement) skills required for operating machinery, especially for driving motor-vehicles. There is epidemiological as well as laboratory evidence for this.

Skegg *et al.* (1979) examined the prescriptions for 57 people injured or killed while driving or cycling, and compared them with the prescriptions in 1425 similar (control) subjects who had not been injured or killed. Those who had been involved in a serious driving accident were five times more likely to have been prescribed a minor tranquillizer in the 3 months before the accident.

The effect of single doses of placebo, temazepam, and flurazepam on driving performance the next morning were examined in 12 healthy women (Betts and Birtle 1982). Both drugs significantly impaired driving ability 12 hours after a dose.

Older subjects do not break down the benzodiazepine triazolam as rapidly as younger subjects, so that the same dose of drug causes higher plasma concentrations in older subjects than in younger subjects (Greenblatt *et al.* 1991). The higher concentrations cause greater sedation, more interference with the 'digit symbol substitution' test of mental alertness, and more prolonged effects.

Paradoxical reactions to benzodiazepines

Some people become sleepy when drunk, while others become aggressive. It is argued that the depressant effects of ethanol are first manifest in those higher parts of the brain that control our behaviour and so allow uncontrolled and unconsidered actions. Benzodiazepines have very similar depressant effects to those of ethanol, and it is not surprising that they occasionally lead to paradoxical reactions of hostility, rage, or aggression when they would be expected to cause relaxation and drowsiness (McClelland 1990). As Oliver (1990) puts it: 'However, cortical restraint is also damped down, releasing or aggravating whatever aggressive propensities remain'.

Hall and Zisook (1981) have reviewed reactions that occur in individuals who would not otherwise be thought predisposed to such behaviour. The reactions 'are, in general, uncharacteristic [of the individual], rare, most often idiosyncratic, and consequently extremely difficult to predict on the basis of past behaviour'.

Paradoxical reactions are most likely to occur within 1 or 2 weeks of starting treatment or increasing the dosage (Lader 1987). Aggression and loss of control are the most well-known reactions, though depression can also occur. The loss of control can lead to criminal behaviour, and it is not always clear whether the dyscontrol is due to therapeutic doses of the benzodiazepine or to ethanol consumed during treatment:

CASE 8.2 (TERRELL 1988)

A 40-year-old woman who was treated with alprazolam drank a quantity of whisky and then broke into her neighbour's house and laid waste to it. She caused $50 000 worth of damage and also cut both forearms on broken glass. She then returned home, fell asleep, and woke up with only dim memories of breaking glass. She went to the police, was admitted to a psychiatric hospital, and subsequently recovered completely.

The likelihood of paradoxical aggression seems higher in patients with personality disorder, and the data sheet for 'Valium' (diazepam) takes this into account:

'Abnormal psychological reactions to benzodiazepines have been reported. Rare behavioural effects include paradoxical aggressive outbursts, excitement, confusion, and the uncovering of depression with suicidal tendencies. Extreme caution should therefore be used in prescribing benzodiazepines to patients with personality disorders.'

This warning is important for prescribers, but it is precisely patients with personality disorders who can be the most persistent in demanding treatment for psychosomatic ills.

Benzodiazepine-induced fantasies

There are several reports of women who believe that they have been molested during sedation with intravenous benzodiazepines. This has been discussed in Section 5.4.2. The problem is not confined to women.

CASE 8.3 (PLAYFORD 1992)

A 70-year-old man was sedated with midazolam before endoscopy. Shortly after the procedure, he complained that he had been sexually assaulted by two female nurses. One hour later he remembered neither the event nor his accusation.

8.4 Longer-term effects

Addiction

The addictive properties of benzodiazepines were recognized only rather tardily. One major reason for this is the similarity between the symptoms that occur on withdrawal of benzodiazepines after chronic usage and the symptoms of anxiety for which the drugs are initially prescribed. Another reason is that patients rather rarely resort to increasing the dose of a benzodiazepine to obtain the therapeutic effect. Such 'dose-escalation' is an important feature of addiction to other drugs, where the subjects become 'tolerant' to the effects of normal doses and so require increasing doses to give the same effect.

However, important work in the early 1980s (Petursson and Lader 1981; Tyrer *et al.* 1983; Ashton 1984) drew attention to a syndrome of withdrawal that could occur in up to one-third of patients treated with benzodiazepines for 6 months or more. The difficulty remains of identifying those patients who have suffered true withdrawal symptoms and those who have felt a recurrence of their initial symptoms of insomnia or anxiety, made worse now by the *fear* of a withdrawal syndrome.

Some features are sufficiently specific to be useful in diagnosing the withdrawal syndrome, and even relative sceptics accept that this is so (Edwards 1992). These features include:

(1) seizures, especially tonic-clonic (grand mal) seizures, characterized by episodes in which at first the patient's body goes stiff and then the limbs jerk rhythmically;
(2) acute toxic confusional state (delirium), in which the patient becomes confused as to the time, the place, and the people about, and can suffer from hallucinations in which sights or sounds are imagined, or can misinterpret sights or sounds as threatening or unusual;
(3) perceptual disturbances, especially:
    (a) oscillopsia, that is, jerking of the field of view with movements of the eyes or head;
    (b) hyperacusis, that is, painful awareness of sounds;
    (c) tinnitus, that is, an unpleasant continuous sound heard in the absence of any external stimulus;
    (d) dysguesia, that is, an unpleasant perversion of taste, especially a metallic taste in the mouth; and
    (e) dysaesthesia or hyperaesthesia, disturbances of feeling that impart an unusual and unpleasant quality or an abnormal and disturbing sensitivity.

Other important but less specific symptoms include: feelings of anxiety or fear, insomnia, weakness, tremor, muscle cramp or pain, abdominal discomfort, anorexia and nausea, urinary frequency, and palpitation.

The reliability of the diagnosis of benzodiazepine withdrawal is increased if the time-course of the symptoms is consistent with it. The symptoms would not be expected to occur until the drug has been given for a long enough time to induce dependence. This time is now thought to be around 4 to 6 weeks for some patients (Power *et al.* 1985). Nor would they occur until the dose of benzodiazepine was reduced. They would be expected within a few hours of significant reduction in dosage or complete cessation of treatment with a drug having a short half-life, and within a day or two of the cessation of a drug with a long effective half-life. The symptoms certainly continue for several weeks. Some (Ashton 1984; Higgitt *et al.* 1985) have argued that they can persist for up to a year.

The prescriber would do well to keep in mind guidance issued on the prescribing of benzodiazepines (Committee on Safety of Medicines 1988):

(1) the drugs should only be used to relieve anxiety for two to four weeks, and then only if it is severe, disabling, or causing the sufferer unacceptable distress;
(2) they should only be used to treat insomnia that is severe, disabling, or causing the sufferer unacceptable distress;
(3) the lowest dose effective in relieving symptoms should be used;
(4) the treatment should not continue for more than 4 weeks;
(5) the treatment should be 'tapered off' gradually, that is, the dosage should be reduced in stages over several days.

Current data sheets for benzodiazepines reflect this view of the Committee on Safety of Medicines, and contain additional warnings which the prescriber would be expected to heed.

The medicolegal question of whether a particular patient has been harmed in a particular way by a particular drug is complex. The complexities are increased when the expert has to consider whether a reasonably responsible medical practitioner would have acted as the plaintiff's practitioner did, given the state of the art at the time, usually several years in the past. These difficulties have led to the abandonment of large scale actions against the prescribers or manufacturers of benzodiazepines by those who may have become addicted to them.

8.5 Abuse

The benign image of the benzodiazepines has been further tarnished by the increasing degree to which certain members of the class, particularly temazepam, have been abused. This phenomenon has only been apparent in the past decade, and at first was confined to the northwest of England and to western Scotland.

Addicts find some special 'gain' in benzodiazepines. Nine men with a history of drug abuse took part in a behavioural study (Troisi *et al.* 1992). They positively liked oral doses of the benzodiazepine lorazepam, but rather disliked the non-benzodiazepine anxiolytic buspirone: when offered the choice, eight out of nine preferred lorazepam (see also Sellers *et al.* 1992).

The favourite method of abuse was to draw up the liquid content of gelatine capsules of temazepam ('soft eggs') and inject it intravenously. In an effort to prevent this, the manufacturers reformulated temazepam capsules as a solid gel, and tablets containing temazepam also became available. The result has been less a reduction in abuse than an increase in the enterprise of abusers (Strang *et al.* 1992), coupled with a higher toll in complications related to injection.

Nearly half of a group of 208 patients attending one of several drug addiction clinics in Britain in 1992 had injected benzodiazepines at some time. Most had used either temazepam capsules or diazepam tablets; though many had used temazepam tablets or other preparations (Strang *et al.* 1994).

Methods of dissolving the solid gel include shaking it with boiling water, heating with water in a spoon, or attempting to dissolve it in isopropanol, vinegar or citric acid (Ruben and Morrison 1992). Devastating problems arise when temazepam is injected not into a vein but into an adjacent artery (Nott *et al.* 1993) or elsewhere. Five of eleven abusers who received intra-arterial temazepam injections and were seen subsequently in hospital required amputations (Nott *et al.* 1993). The tablets are sometimes crushed and extracted with hot water, then filtered. The filter material, such as a cigarette filter, can itself result in serious injury or death (Vella and Edwards 1993).

Benzodiazepine abuse is linked to criminal activity, both to finance the abuse and because apparently injection of temazepam prior to committing a crime reduces fear and diminishes inhibitions, while the abuser may believe it possible to invoke amnesia or the effects of the drug in mitigation should he or she be caught. The amnesia can, of course, be genuine:

CASE 8.4

A 29-year-old man who had been addicted to intravenous heroin (diamorphine) for 8 years was arrested after four rather ineffectual attempts at robbery of a garage, a fish and chip shop, a general stores and another garage, all in the space of an hour or so. He claimed to have taken about 250 milligrams of heroin intravenously and 20–30 20 milligram temazepam capsules, either intravenously (one account) or orally (another account).

He was taken into custody at midnight and interviewed the next morning. The police officers interviewing him asked a number of specific questions about the events of the previous night. The suspect maintained that he was 'out of his head on temazepam' and could not recall clearly what happened. At one point, one of the police says 'I accept that I am not familiar with the effects of drugs, but you had obviously hadn't had that much that you couldn't walk about and visit different places and talk to people.'

The expert view was that the temazepam taken by the defendant could have resulted in exactly that: an apparent ability to walk about and talk normally to people, coupled with an inability to remember the events subsequently.

8.6 Summary

The benzodiazepines are important for their acute and chronic effects on patients who can be harmed, on those who may perpetrate crimes under their influence knowingly or unknowingly, and on those who abuse them. Their importance is the greater because of their widespread use.

9

Insulin

Insulin is a hormone, that is, a 'chemical messenger', secreted by specialized cells called the B cells (formerly the β cells) in the pancreas of vertebrate animals. The pancreas synthesizes a large molecule called preproinsulin, which is broken down to proinsulin and then to insulin and C-peptide. When a molecule of insulin is released from the pancreas, a molecule of C-peptide is released with it. The rate at which the normal pancreas secretes insulin (with C-peptide) varies, and is mainly determined by the concentration of glucose in the bloodstream. The insulin secretion rate is high when the blood glucose concentration is raised above normal, and falls to zero when the blood glucose concentration is below normal. Insulin itself affects cells in the liver, the muscles, and the fatty tissue, and increases the rate at which these cells take up glucose. It also prevents glucose being formed from the storage compound glycogen. These two effects combine to reduce the blood glucose concentration.

9.1 Control of blood glucose concentration

Glucose concentration in the blood is maintained within a fairly narrow range in healthy people, and usually will stay between 3 and 7 millimoles per litre, though after a large meal of sugary food, it may rise as high as 10 millimoles per litre. If the glucose concentration is too high, the rate of insulin secretion increases, cells take up the glucose more avidly, and the level falls. If the concentration of glucose falls, then insulin secretion diminishes, the cells take up less glucose and release glucose from glycogen stores, and so the blood concentration rises again.

9.2 Hypoglycaemia

The brain relies entirely on glucose as a fuel, and without glucose its function ceases. After about 60 minutes of glucose deprivation, cells in the brain are irreversibly damaged. Before this stage is reached, there are progressive and well-documented alterations in brain function. The condition of an abnormally low blood glucose concentration is called *hypoglycaemia*.

Hypoglycaemia can very occasionally be due to a tumour of the pancreatic islet B cells, an insulinoma, which secretes insulin in an uncontrolled way. It is more often due to inappropriate doses of insulin or other drugs intended to lower the blood glucose concentration, particularly the sulphonylurea drugs such as glibenclamide and chlorpropamide. About 10 per cent of insulin-treated diabetic patients will have an episode of hypoglycaemia sufficiently severe to warrant medical treatment within any 1 year, and, in one study, about 30 per cent of patients taking glibenclamide had experienced symptoms suggesting hypoglycaemia in a period of 6 months (Jennings *et al.* 1989).

The symptoms of hypoglycaemia can be rather non-specific, and the cardinal feature is that the symptoms are present when the blood glucose concentration is measured to be low and regress when enough glucose is given to restore the concentration to normal. Since prolonged hypoglycaemia can cause irreversible brain damage, there are cases in which the symptoms of hypoglycaemia will not regress even if the blood glucose concentration is restored to normal. Sweating and tremor are common, because adrenaline is released in response to hypo-glycaemia. Disturbance of vision ('spots before the eyes'), slurred speech, odd behaviour, aggression, and confusion occur because the nerve cells in the brain are failing.

There has been considerable legal debate on the state of mind of persons who were hypo-glycaemic when they committed criminal acts. This is discussed in Section 3.4.3. The diffi-culties of assessing the state of mind of the accused can be compounded by a complete amnesia for events occurring during these episodes of hyperglycaemia (Tattersall 1995).

Experiments in normal people show that the body starts to respond when the blood glucose concentration falls below about 3 millimoles per litre (Herold *et al.* 1985). Below 2.5 milli-moles per litre, there is a measurable fall in mental concentration and in vision (Pramming *et al.* 1986; Hoffman *et al.* 1989), though the subject is not aware that anything is amiss until the glucose concentration is lower still, and convulsions and coma are only likely if the blood glucose concentration falls below 1 millimole per litre.

In elderly patients, the effects of hypoglycaemia can mimic those of stroke (Gutsche *et al.* 1969; Axelgaard *et al.* 1986), and the correct diagnosis could easily be overlooked.

CASE 9.1

An 81-year-old man was admitted to hospital because he had suddenly become very agitated. He was given an injection of the sedative haloperidol, and 1 hour later he collapsed unconscious with signs of a stroke. His blood glucose was measured and found to be less than 1 millimole per litre, so he was given an injection of glucose and recovered consciousness almost at once. It subse-quently transpired that he had taken one of his wife's tablets of the antidiabetic drug gliben-clamide.

In other circumstances, he could have suffered irreversible brain damage, and this would have been attributed to a stroke.

9.3 Diabetes mellitus ('sugar diabetes')

Diabetes mellitus is the disease that results when the B cells are unable to provide sufficient insulin to control the blood glucose concentration, and is characterized by a higher concentra-tion of glucose in the blood than normal, particularly after a sugary meal. When there is a very severe lack of insulin, then cells cannot adequately use glucose and in its place fats are broken down. One by-product of the breakdown of fats is the production of organic acids, such as β-hydroxybutyric acid and acetoacetic acid, which are themselves injurious. This severe lack of insulin leads to the condition of diabetic ketoacidosis. Sufferers die if they are not treated promptly with insulin.

The average amount of insulin needed by a normal adult is about 24 units per day, although diabetic patients can become resistant to the effects of insulin, and may need several times this amount.

9.4 Types of insulin

Until the 1980s insulin for pharmaceutical use was purified from beef or pig pancreas, but a greater part of the insulin now available is 'human insulin', manufactured by biosynthesis in yeasts ('pyr') or bacteria ('crb' and 'prb') or by enzymic modification of porcine insulin ('emp'). The 'human insulins' contain exactly the same sequence of amino-acids as native human insulin. The amino-acid sequences in porcine and bovine insulin differ from those in native human insulin by 2 per cent and 6 per cent respectively. There are only very minor differences in the action of the three insulins, but the biochemical differences are sufficient to allow them to be distinguished by immunological assays. This sometimes makes it possible to detect homicidally administered insulin.

Insulins of bovine, human, or porcine sequence are available in different forms. Soluble insulin (known as 'regular insulin' in the United States) is the preparation most rapidly absorbed from injections given subcutaneously (under the skin). It can be given intravenously. Insulin can be complexed with the protein protamine, obtained from the testes of male salmon, to make it less soluble, and so slow the rate at which it is absorbed. Such insulin is called isophane insulin, sometimes known as NPH insulin. It can also be crystallized with zinc salts, which produces insulin zinc suspension (IZS), another relatively insoluble and slow-acting preparation. Neither isophane nor IZS insulins should be given intravenously. The longest-acting insulin, protamine zinc insulin, is the least soluble, and can act for over 24 hours after a subcutaneous injection (see Appendix C, Section C.15).

9.5 Insulin poisoning

Insulin injected into people who are not diabetic can cause hypoglycaemia. It does not cause hypoglycaemia if it is given by mouth, because the acid in the stomach and the enzymes in the gut effectively destroy it.

> CASE 9.2
>
> A woman told a friend that she was frightened to go home because her husband might be dead. Their daughter was diabetic and the woman had put 500 Units of her insulin in the husband's tea. The husband drank some of the tea, which anyway tasted unpleasant, but suffered no ill effects. The woman was charged with attempted murder, but the husband did not give evidence and the woman was bound over to keep the peace.

If the insulin is of porcine or bovine origin, then it can be possible to detect its presence in the bloodstream by radioimmunoassay, a technique which uses the differences in immune response caused by the different insulin structures. However, if the insulin is of human sequence, then there is no assay technique that will distinguish the victim's own insulin from the injected insulin. The demonstration that insulin was injected then becomes more difficult.

It has sometimes proved possible to demonstrate high concentrations of insulin in the tissues at skin injection sites, and this can be done even after death.

> CASE 9.3 (BIRKINSHAW ET AL. 1958)
>
> The classical case was described by Birkinshaw et al. (1958) The previously healthy wife of a male nurse was found dead in the bath. A post-mortem examination suggested that she had drowned,

but there was no sign of violence. The glucose concentration in mixed heart blood obtained 7 hours after death was 12 millimoles per litre, which is rather higher than would normally be expected in life. When the police searched the house, they found her sweat-soaked pyjamas and also hypodermic syringes and needles. When the body was reexamined, four needle marks were found over the buttocks. 'The tissues underlying these marks were therefore excised...'. There was no direct method for assaying insulin concentrations at that time, so the authors made crude extracts from the tissues and injected them into mice. The effects were equivalent to those of over 500 milliUnits of insulin per gram of tissue, and to a total insulin content of 84 Units. The biological properties of the extracts were also shown to be those of insulin. Experiments with injection of known amounts of insulin into cadaveric tissue showed that only two-thirds of the injected amount could be extracted, and that after a time, only half would be found. The total dose was therefore likely to have exceeded 164 Units of insulin.

The woman had been injected with a lethal dose of insulin. The sweat-soaked pyjamas were consistent with the profuse sweating which occurs in hypoglycaemia; and it is now well known that heart blood, especially right heart blood, obtained some time after death, is a wholly unreliable indicator of the blood glucose concentration before death.

Immunoassay, which can demonstrate the presence of insulin in the subcutaneous tissue, makes the detection of injected insulin more straightforward now (Phillips *et al.* 1972; Dickson *et al.* 1977; Fletcher *et al.* 1979; Fletcher 1983). It requires that antibodies against insulin are allowed to bind to insulin in thin tissue slices ('sections'). There are then several ways of showing where the antibodies have bound.

CASE 9.4 (HOOD *ET AL.* 1986)

A five-month-old girl was found dead, and the only abnormality at post-mortem was a group of needle marks on the left thigh. Her uncle had insulin-treated diabetes.

Tissue was taken and stored frozen. Measurements were made of the concentrations of insulin in blood and of glucose in the vitreous fluid of the eye. Antibodies to insulin were localized along the needle tracks in the thigh tissue, and in the pancreas, but could not be demonstrated in other tissues. Insulin concentration in the blood was 1400 milliUnits per litre, which is about 50 times the level that would have been expected in life. The glucose concentration in the vitreous humour was low, suggesting that the baby had been hypoglycaemic at the time of death.

As the authors comment, 'high insulin levels alone are not proof of exogenous insulin administration, and the interpretation of postmortem insulin levels can be problematic'. However, the localization of insulin along the needle tracks was excellent evidence of homicidal insulin administration.

If remains are examined several months after death, the difficulties of extraction are considerable and quantitative results should be treated with caution (Heyndrickx *et al.* 1980).

If the injection site is not known or the insulin was given into a vein, then careful quantitative analysis can be used. This relies on the fact that the pancreas releases one molecule of C-peptide for every molecule of insulin. The disappearance of C-peptide is about five times slower than the disappearance of insulin, but the ratio of insulin to C-peptide is known in normal subjects. If a normal subject becomes hypoglycaemic as a result of an insulin injection, then his own (endogenous) insulin secretion is inhibited, and so C-peptide secretion is also inhibited, and the C-peptide concentration in blood falls to low levels. The insulin concentration, however, will be high, because of the injection. The combination of low blood concentrations of glucose and C-peptide with a high concentration of insulin is the characteristic pattern of hypoglycaemia due to injection of insulin. Normally, the concentration of insulin in picomoles per litre should be less than the concentration of C-peptide in picomoles per litre

(Grunberger *et al.* 1988; Missliwetz 1994). Care is necessary, because concentrations of both insulin and C-peptide are often expressed in other units.

Patients who have hypoglycaemia which is not easily explained have sometimes been injecting themselves with insulin, and several studies have reported insulin and C-peptide concentrations in the venous blood in such patients and in the victims of crime (Couropmitree *et al.* 1975; Hasche *et al.* 1982; Mayefsky *et al.* 1982; Guillausseau *et al.* 1983; Bidot-Lopez *et al.* 1987; Haibach *et al.* 1987; Johnson *et al.* 1987; Grunberger *et al.* 1988)

CASE 9.5

A non-diabetic baby boy of five months had several unexplained episodes of pallor, sweating, and collapse while in hospital with a chest infection. On the fourth occasion, blood samples were taken, and showed a glucose concentration of 1.8 millimoles per litre (normal fasting concentration 3–7 millimoles per litre), a potassium concentration of 2.3 millimoles per litre (normal 3.5–5.2 millimoles per litre), an insulin concentration of 43 000 milliUnits per litre (or 43 Units per litre; normal fasting level less than 12 milliUnits per litre) and a C-peptide concentration of 0.16 nanomoles per litre (normal fasting level 0.2–0.63 nanomoles per litre).

Seven hours later, the insulin concentration was 125 milliUnits per litre and the C-peptide concentration 0.08 nanomoles per litre.

The baby had classical symptoms of hypoglycaemia, which was confirmed by the low blood glucose concentration. The blood insulin concentration was extremely high, but the C-peptide concentration was low. The low blood potassium concentration is consistent with an overdose of insulin, since a subsidiary action of this hormone is to cause potassium in the blood to enter cells.

9.6 Summary

Insulin is no longer 'the perfect murder weapon'. Porcine and bovine insulin can be distinguished from native human insulin at sites of subcutaneous injection and in the bloodstream. Injected human insulin does not contain C-peptide, and so blood tests can show that insulin has been administered to victims who survive attacks. Even if the victim dies, subcutaneous or intramuscular insulin can be demonstrated by antibody staining. There is, though, no evidence as to the relationship between insulin and C-peptide in blood after death, so it might still be difficult to demonstrate that someone had been murdered with intravenous human insulin.

10

Potassium chloride and other potassium salts

Potassium is the most important cation (positively charged chemical species) within cells, whereas sodium is the most important cation in the extracellular fluids including plasma (the fluid component of blood). The potassium concentration in the plasma during life is approximately 4 millimoles per litre and inside the red blood cells the concentration is approximately 140 millimoles per litre. This difference is maintained by an enzyme system in the membrane envelope of cells. The enzyme system, the Na^+K^+ ATPase, uses chemical energy to pump sodium out of the cell and potassium into the cell.

10.1 Potassium concentration in plasma

The potassium concentration in plasma is usually maintained between about 3.5 and 5.0 millimoles per litre. However, it can fall if there is abnormal potassium loss from the gut in diarrhoea or vomit, or in the urine as a result of drugs such as thiazide or loop diuretics (types of 'water tablet'), or for other reasons. The condition of an abnormally low plasma potassium concentration is called *hypokalaemia*. The concentration can rise excessively high when the kidney is unable to excrete potassium efficiently, either as a result of disease, or because of the action of drugs such as the potassium-sparing diuretics or the angiotensin converting enzyme inhibitors. The condition of an abnormally high plasma potassium concentration is called *hyperkalaemia*.

In nerve cells and heart muscle cells, the chemical energy used to establish a difference in the concentrations of the cations potassium and sodium inside and outside the cell can be converted into electrical energy. This is the basis for electrical conduction in the heart and nervous system. If the plasma potassium concentration falls lower than about 2.5 millimoles per litre, then heart tissue can become abnormally easy to excite, and as the concentration rises above 6.5 millimoles per litre there is a risk that normal excitation will be prevented.

Three important forensic consequences follow from these facts. First, the concentration of potassium in plasma depends on the continued supply of chemical energy to the enzyme in the cell membrane, and the continued integrity of the membrane. Therefore, plasma concentrations of potassium which would have been dangerous in life can be found after death as a matter of course.

Secondly, certain drugs can dangerously increase or reduce the potassium concentration in plasma. The intravenous administration of a strong solution of potassium chloride can have this effect instantaneously.

Thirdly, changes in the concentration of potassium in the plasma can have a dramatic effect on the behaviour of heart muscle and also nerve transmission, and therefore can have serious or fatal effects.

10.2 Potassium concentration after death

After death, the energy supply is not renewed, and potassium leaks out of the cells into the plasma. Since the concentration in red cells is approximately 45 times the concentration in plasma, and blood is 40 to 50 per cent red blood cells by volume, the plasma concentration alters dramatically even if the leakage is relatively slight.

Coe (1974a, b) reviewed post-mortem biochemical measurements in blood, and stated that 'the release of potassium from cells occurs so rapidly after death as to make evaluation of potassium metabolism impossible by any known method'. Jetter (1959) had shown that within 1 hour of death the potassium concentration in human heart blood plasma had risen to 18 millimoles per litre, and that it had risen to about 25 millimoles per litre by 24 hours after death. The rise varied from subject to subject, and appeared to depend on the temperature at which the body was kept. Some knowledge of changes in blood potassium concentration around the time of death in children comes from a study made in India (Walia et al. 1963).

Leakage of potassium out of cells can occur if the enzyme in red blood cell membranes is rendered inactive by cold. This happens, for example, if blood is taken from the patient and then stored in a refrigerator at about 4°C. The cell membranes are not ruptured, but potassium leaks out because the activity of the enzyme pump is greatly reduced. There is nothing to show during subsequent analysis that the increase in plasma potassium concentration occurred in the refrigerator and not in the patient.

The heart drug digoxin can inactivate the Na^+K^+ ATPase and an increase in the plasma potassium concentration above normal can be a sign that the patient is suffering from severe digoxin poisoning.

Membrane damage can cause leakage of potassium, whether the damage occurs before or after the blood sample used to measure potassium is taken. Haemolysis (the breakdown of red cells) can occur when blood is taken from the patient, especially if it is necessary to pull hard on the syringe to draw blood off. Haemolysis that occurred when the blood was taken is the most likely cause of a spuriously elevated plasma potassium concentration. Because haemoglobin leaks out of the damaged red cell as well, haemolysis can usually be detected by a pink discolouration of the plasma.

Breakdown of cells in disease can also cause an increased concentration of potassium in the blood. Red cell, white cell, and muscle cell breakdown can all, in certain circumstances, lead to a significant, and sometimes a dangerous, rise in potassium concentration.

The clinical causes of hyperkalaemia have been reviewed (DeFronzo et al. 1982; Paice et al. 1983), as has drug-induced hyperkalaemia (Ponce et al. 1985).

10.3 Spuriously high plasma potassium concentration

Two causes of spuriously high plasma potassium concentrations are sampling blood from a vein which is close to the site of an intravenous infusion ('drip') of fluid that contains potassium, and placing a correctly obtained sample into a container which itself contains potassium.

This latter error can occur if a sample is placed into a bottle containing potassium edetate for haematological specimens (a 'pink tube') or potassium oxalate and sodium fluoride for glucose analysis (a 'yellow tube'). If the person obtaining the sample realizes that the wrong tube has been used, and transfers the blood to the correct tube, the laboratory is unable to tell directly whether contamination has occurred.

CASE 10.1

The clinical biochemist in charge of a hospital laboratory gave evidence during a murder trial. He stated that a specimen of blood from a girl who died had a plasma potassium concentration of over 10 millimoles per litre. This concentration is almost invariably fatal. Counsel for the defence produced for him a report from his own laboratory on a blood sample from a boy who was well and who left hospital shortly afterwards. The report gave the plasma potassium concentration as 27 millimoles per litre without any further comment.

The biochemist was asked to explain the result. 'I would suggest that it had been contaminated. Well, yes, it is difficult to think of any explanation [except] that it is contaminated, because it was so high.' This was what the defence wanted, since the explanation might also apply to the blood sample from the alleged murder victim.

The difficulties in interpreting post-mortem plasma potassium concentrations have led forensic pathologists to examine other body fluids, notably the vitreous humour (the transparent thick fluid in the rear part of the eyeball). Coe (1974*b*), reviewing his own work and that of others, pointed out that the rise in vitreous humour potassium concentration with time is of the order of 0.17 millimoles per litre per hour after death, but that the difference between individuals is so great that even within the first 24 hours after death, the calculated time of death, based on the measured vitreous humour potassium concentration and the assumed rate of rise in concentration could be in error by 10 hours either way, and the errors were worse still after the first 24 hours had passed.

10.4 The effects of an increase in plasma potassium concentration

A sudden increase of potassium concentration in the plasma can stop the heart beating. This effect is put to use to stop the heart when a surgeon is performing open-heart surgery. The technique was introduced by Melrose in the 1950s (Melrose 1978). The patient is attached to a heart-lung machine, and then the heart is filled with a solution containing high concentrations of potassium. Initially, very high concentrations of potassium and of other ions were used. Melrose's solution contained 25 millimoles of potassium ions per litre. Later such extremely concentrated solutions were found to damage the heart (Gay and Ebert 1973) and were replaced by more modest ones which have a potassium concentration of about 8 millimoles per litre, and a similar osmolality (osmotic strength, which is determined by the number of osmotically active particles–molecules and ions–in the solution) to plasma.

The volume of plasma is about 2.5 litres in an adult, so that it contains about 10 millimoles of potassium. An injection into the bloodstream of a further 10 millimoles will double the concentration for a brief period, and this can be enough to stop the heart. The standard 10 millilitre ampoule of potassium chloride strong solution BP contains 20 millimoles (1.5 grams) of potassium chloride, and therefore 20 millimoles of potassium. This is more than enough to kill a patient if injected in error. The lethal dose by rapid intravenous injection was estimated to be 30 to 35 milligrams per kilogram body weight on the basis of one human and two rabbit deaths (Bhatkhande and Joglekar 1977).

Oral potassium salts have occasionally been reported to cause serious poisoning, both in children (Welti and Davis 1978; Illingworth and Proudfoot 1980;) and in adults (Bedford 1954; Yap *et al.* 1976; Welti and Davis 1978; Saxena 1988) The following case serves as an illustration.

CASE 10.2 (WELTI AND DAVIS 1978)

The mother of a 2-month-old baby boy added 3 grams of potassium chloride to her breast milk, in accordance with the advice in 'a popular health book'[1] for treating infant colic. The baby was calmed, but the next morning showed symptoms of colic again,and was again given potassium chloride with his feed. A few hours later he collapsed and was rushed to hospital, where the serum potassium concentration was found to be 10.1 millimoles per litre. The baby died 28 hours after admission.

10.5 Negligence

General considerations are outlined in Chapter 6, and Case 6.35 provides a specific example of the dangers of potassium chloride.

Hill (1990) reviewed 10 cases reported to the Medical Defence Union over a period of 5 years in which inadvertent injection of potassium chloride led to claims of medical negligence. Six patients died, one suffered permanent neurological damage after cardiac arrest, one lost a big toe, and one suffered a cardiac arrest but was resuscitated and recovered completely.

CASE 10.3 (HILL 1990)

In a typical incident, a nursing sister was asked for a solution of calcium gluconate, and presented the doctor with a 'syringe filled with 10 millilitres of clear colourless fluid' which was then injected. 'After about 2 to 3 millilitres the patient called out in pain that his body was burning and so [the doctor] pulled out the needle and then watched as he started to gasp and then arrested' The fluid was potassium chloride.

The doctor was found guilty of disgraceful conduct for failing or neglecting to take necessary precautions that the medication injected was calcium gluconate.

CASE 10.4 (HILL 1990)

A surgeon wished to anaesthetize a man's big toe prior to removing an ingrowing toe-nail. He injected what he thought was a solution of the local anaesthetic lignocaine, but it was in fact potassium chloride strong solution, and the toe became gangrenous and had to be amputated. The man had previously injured his foot and was seriously disabled as a result of the further injury. His claim was settled for £16 000 (about $30 000).

Eight of these incidents were the result of confusion between ampoules of sodium chloride, which is innocuous, and potassium chloride, which is potentially lethal. Hill pointed out that manufacturers were not legally obliged to make the ampoules of the two solutions easy to distinguish, and they did not as a routine do so. One manufacturer would supply, at extra cost, otherwise plain ampoules of potassium chloride distinguished by a black plastic cap. One Regional Health Authority used only those ampoules, but Hill asked 'why does not every

---

[1] David, A. *Let's have healthy children.* (3rd ed). New York.

health authority and every hospital insist that its KCl [potassium chloride] ampoules should be readily identifiable?' The next year, the incident described in Case 6.35 took place.

Other dangers have also been described. Intravenous fluids are usually given from sealed sterile plastic bags containing 500 or 1000 millilitres of solution. The standard solutions include 0.9 per cent sodium chloride, also known as 'physiological' or 'normal' saline and 5 per cent D-glucose (dextrose) in water. Drugs are often added to infusion fluids, and the plastic fluid bags contain outlets for the fluid, and inlets for the needle of a syringe so that drugs can be added. One such drug is potassium chloride strong solution, given to patients who are receiving intravenous fluids and have low plasma potassium concentrations.

Two cases were reported (Williams 1973) in which patients collapsed soon after potassium chloride had been injected into a non-rigid plastic fluid container. The collapses were ascribed to potassium poisoning, and experiments showed that potassium could pool in the bag, and very high potassium concentrations could be infused for a short while. The problems could be overcome by adequate mixing, achieved by inverting the plastic fluid bag.

10.6 Murder

Potassium chloride has sometimes been used for murder. Because the amount of potassium needed to stop the heart of an adult is contained in one ampoule of the standard potassium chloride solution found on hospital wards, and because post-mortem changes in the plasma potassium concentration effectively obscure any hyperkalaemia present before death, such murder is difficult to demonstrate. Argument over post-mortem potassium concentrations arose in *R* v. *Beverley Allitt*.

CASE 10.5

A 15-month-old baby girl was admitted to hospital with a recurrence of wheezing, diagnosed as asthma. She was very ill, and treatment was given both by mask and intravenously. She had an episode of collapse when she went very blue, but was resuscitated. While the consultant paediatrician caring for her was explaining the recovery to the girl's mother, the girl again collapsed, and could not be resuscitated, despite prolonged efforts. The heart tracing had initially shown asystole (no electrical activity), but sinus rhythm (a normal rhythm) was restored for a few seconds. The rhythm then degenerated to ventricular tachycardia (a fast, regular and inefficient rhythm of the ventricles) and ventricular fibrillation (a chaotic and completely ineffective rhythm of the ventricles). The trace during sinus rhythm was said to show abnormally broad complexes[2]. A blood sample was taken about 45 minutes after the second collapse, and a post-mortem sample was also taken. They both contained in excess of 10 millimoles of potassium per litre of plasma. The samples were not haemolysed.

A potassium concentration of that order was explanation enough for a fatal collapse.

Subsequently, the blood was found to contain a subtherapeutic concentration of lignocaine, the local anaesthetic drug which is also used to treat certain heart rhythm abnormalities, including ventricular tachycardia and ventricular fibrillation. None of those present at the resuscitation recalled lignocaine having been given.

Argument centred around the nature and meaning of the hyperkalaemia. The characteristic abnormality of the electrocardiograph trace in hyperkalaemia is tall, peaked T-waves, but these were not recorded. The broad complexes which were seen can occur in hyperkalaemia, but are non-specific (see, for example, Ettinger *et al.* 1974). The cardiac arrest itself could have elevated

---

[2] The electrocardiogram is a recording of the electrical activity of the heart. The tracing has a vertical scale in millivolts and a horizontal scale in milliseconds. Each normal heart beat is accompanied by a series of complexes (groups of deflections or 'waves'), designated P, QRS, and T; there is sometimes a U-wave.

the potassium concentration, because metabolism may have been impaired, the blood was likely to have become acidic, and cells may have been damaged by lack of oxygen.

The prosecution called expert evidence to the effect that the potassium concentration would not have risen above 10 millimoles per litre during resuscitation, and that the concentration found after death would not have increased so rapidly as to vitiate the result, and that taken with the observation of widened electrical complexes observed by others, the only possible conclusion was that a dose of potassium had been given intravenously to cause the second cardiac arrest.

We do not know whether the jury were convinced by this or by other evidence (for example, the evidence that the nurse stood by while the baby went blue, and did nothing, or the mother's statement that as the baby was dying in her arms, the defendant was present: 'I will never ever forget. She was just staring'). In any event, the nurse, Beverly Allitt was convicted of this and three other murders.

The difficulties in interpreting potassium concentrations are illustrated by another murder case[3].

CASE 10.6 (BRAHAMS 1990c; GRAY 1992 AT THE BIRMINGHAM MEDICO-LEGAL SOCIETY)

A patient with terminal cancer of the pancreas was delirious and in pain uncontrolled by large doses of diamorphine (heroin). His relatives begged the senior house officer (resident doctor) to do anything to help. He asked a nurse for potassium chloride and lignocaine, and when asked what for is said to have drawn his finger across his throat and said 'I'm going to send somebody out there'. Gilbert Gray QC described this in a memorable phrase as 'a scatological aside intended to lighten the atmosphere'. The doctor injected a mixture of lignocaine and potassium chloride, and the patient died peacefully a few minutes later. The nurses told the administrators, who called the police.

The doctor was committed for trial on a charge of murder, and a pathologist's expert report gave the cause of death as acute potassium poisoning. It is likely that this view was at first supported by a forensic toxicologist, but in court the prosecution admitted that the expert was no longer wholly convinced that death was due to potassium overdose. Brahams cites three other possible causes of death: opiate poisoning from the very large doses of diamorphine which had been given; the cancer itself; and pre-existent coronary artery disease. There was also, less helpfully, the possibility that death was due to lignocaine poisoning.

The defence were in a position to call two professors who taught at the London hospital where the senior house officer had recently trained, and who had conducted experiments showing that potassium could improve the pain relief afforded by other drugs. Their evidence suggested that he might reasonably have believed potassium to enhance the effect of lignocaine, and that its use was supported by other responsible practitioners.

The prosecution decided in the circumstances to offer no evidence, and the judge directed the jury to return a verdict of 'not guilty'.

The case was reminiscent of that of Dr Leonard Arthur (Case 6.7), except for the 'scatological aside'. In that case, too, a doctor acting in what he perceived to be the interests of his patient, and with the support of the family, gave treatment which was construed by the nursing staff as murderous. In both cases the prosecution foundered on unreliable expert evidence.

10.7 Suicide

Hospital staff occasionally commit suicide by injecting themselves with potassium (Bhatkhande and Joglekar 1977; Chaturvedi et al. 1986).

[3] R v. Thomas Stephen Lodwig

CASE 10.7 (FARMER *ET AL.* 1985)

A 30-year-old woman was found dead with an intravenous needle connected by tubing to a syringe containing clear fluid. The fluid from the syringe contained nearly 1500 millimoles of potassium per litre.

Right ventricular heart blood, and vitreous humour from both eyes were assayed in samples taken at post-mortem 48 hours after death, and contained 54, 8.9, and 9.5 millimoles per litre of potassium. The authors concluded that these values were not useful in determining the cause of death: estimates of the change in vitreous humour potassium concentration after death from natural causes suggested that a concentration of up to 12 millimoles per litre would be expected 48 hours after death.

10.8 Summary

Potassium chloride is available in hospitals in ampoules containing undiluted potassium chloride strong solution. These can be confused with innocuous solutions, particularly sodium chloride solution. The intravenous administration of concentrated solutions of potassium usually kills the patient.

Changes occur in the plasma potassium concentration after death that make any post-mortem measurement difficult to interpret.

11

The antipsychotic drugs: phenothiazines, butyrophenones, and other agents

Psychological illnesses can be divided into neurotic and psychotic illnesses. Neurotic illnesses, such as anxiety and depression, are exaggerations of the normal emotions, but (generally) leave the thought processes intact. Psychotic illnesses are marked by a break from normal thought processes. The abnormal thoughts can take the form of hallucinations or delusions, for example. A patient who is miserable because he has no power to influence the wrongs of the world is neurotic; a patient who believes that the Martians are trying to destroy him, or that he himself is a Martian, is psychotic[1].

The two most important psychotic illnesses are schizophrenia and manic-depressive psychosis. Depression, which is generally not accompanied by thought disorder, can sometimes bring with it delusions of unworthiness or worthlessness.

The drugs used to treat psychotic disease, especially schizophrenia, are called antipsychotic drugs, major tranquillizers or neuroleptic drugs. Several are listed in Table 11.1.

The paradigm antipsychotic drug is chlorpromazine ('Largactil' in the United Kingdom, 'Thorazine' in the United States), whose sedative properties were said to have been discovered when it was examined for its efficacy in treating worm infestations. An injection of chlorpromazine can quieten patients who are acutely disturbed or violent, but does not cause depression of respiration in therapeutic doses. It can make normal subjects 'sleepy, apathetic and indifferent to the environment' (Laurence and Bennett 1992c).

Since psychotic patients do not always adhere to oral therapeutic regimes, it is common for depot preparations to be given by intramuscular injection every few weeks in hospital clinics. The drugs most often used for this are fluphenazine decanoate ('Modecate'), flupenthixol decanoate ('Depixol Injection') and haloperidol decanoate ('Haldol Decanoate'). Patients can then manage in the community[2] whereas before the introduction of these drugs they would have required long-term psychiatric in-patient care. The adverse effects can be correspondingly long-lasting.

CASE 11.1 (GWYNNE 1986A)

A man went to his general practitioner for an injection of cholera vaccine before he went on a trip to Africa. The doctor in error drew up and gave an injection of flupenthixol decanoate. The businessman was so sleepy that he had to postpone his trip for a week, and a claim for damages was settled.

Forensic problems with antipsychotic drugs come from their adverse effects, from the interaction between the mental disorder for which the drugs are given and the drugs them-

---

[1] I was taught that a psychotic patient believes 2+2=5; a neurotic one knows that 2+2=4, but worries about it.
[2] In theory, at least.

Table 11.1 Major tranquillizers (neuroleptic drugs) and other drugs used to treat psychoses

Butyrophenones
    benperidol ('Anquil')
    droperidol ('Droleptan')
    haloperidol (e.g. 'Haldol', 'Serenace')
    haloperidol decanoate ('Haldol Decanoate') a depot preparation

Phenothiazines
    chlorpromazine (e.g. 'Largactil')
    fluphenazine hydrochloride ('Moditen')
    fluphenazine decanoate ('Modecate') a depot preparation
    methotrimeprazine ('Nozinan')
    pericyazine ('Neulactil')
    perphenazine ('Fentazin')
    pipothiazine palmitate ('Piportil depot') a depot preparation
    prochlorperazine ('Stemetil')
    promazine ('Sparine')
    thioridazine ('Melleril')
    trifluoperazine ('Stelazine')

Other antipsychotic drugs
    clozapine ('Clozaril')
    flupenthixol hydrochloride ('Depixol')
    flupenthixol decanoate ('Depixol Injection') a depot preparation
    fluspirilene ('Redeptin')
    loxapine ('Loxapac')
    pimozide ('Orap')
    remoxipride ('Roxiam')

selves, and from interactions between the antipsychotic drug and other drugs. There is, in addition, the difficulty that the drugs are sometimes given to subdue patients who do not give consent but who are not yet, or at all, the subject of compulsory treatment under an order of the Mental Health Act 1983.

11.1 Problems with adverse effects of antipsychotic agents

The antipsychotic action of phenothiazines and other compounds such as haloperidol ('Haldol', 'Serenace'), which is a butyrophenone, is related to their ability to antagonize the effects of the nerve transmitter substance dopamine in the central nervous system. The ability to antagonize the effects of dopamine confers on these drugs the ability to cause movement disorders. These are principally dystonic reactions, parkinsonism and tardive dyskinesia. A comprehensive review of the legal aspects of these movement disorders has recently been published (Wettstein 1985).

Dystonic reactions usually occur in young people, and are manifest by an abnormal increase in the tone (the tautness or tension at rest) in some muscles and not others. Particularly characteristic are contraction of the muscles which arch the back, curve the neck backwards, and clench the jaw. There can also be *oculogyric crises* in which the patient's head is involuntarily twisted upwards and the eyes turn up in their sockets, much in the manner of an actor feigning a seizure. The dystonic reaction is acute (of rapid onset) and can occur after a single dose of treatment. It produces a picture which is sufficiently bizarre to be mistaken sometimes for hysteria.

Akathisia is an incessant restlessness which is manifest as 'fidgeting'. The patient crosses and uncrosses his arms or legs, shifts from one side of the chair to the other, or sits, then stands, then sits again. This is a central effect of dopamine antagonists, and experiments in normal volunteers given these drugs confirms that akathisia occurs acutely. It is also seen as a part of the tardive dyskinesia discussed below.

Parkinsonism is a movement disorder of tremor, difficulty in initiating movement, and an increase in muscle tone. It occurs especially with treatment continued for months or years. It is usually reversible after treatment stops, though the symptoms can take months to disappear. It responds to treatment with drugs used in the naturally occurring form of Parkinson's disease. The anticholinergic drugs are usually used, since they are perhaps less prone than dopamine to precipitate the psychiatric symptoms for which the antipsychotic drug was initially given.

Tardive dyskinesia is a movement disorder that occurs after continued treatment with antipsychotic medicines, and is therefore common in those schizophrenic patients who have spent long periods in psychiatric hospitals. The characteristic form is *orofacial dyskinesia* in which the patient has incessant and involuntary movements of the mouth, lips and tongue, with chewing, twisting movements of the lips, protrusion of the tongue, and facial restlessness and grimacing. It most often occurs after years of exposure, but the briefest recorded interval between exposure to antipsychotic treatment and development of tardive dyskinesia is 1 month (Chouinard and Jones 1979) The disorder is more likely if high doses of antipsychotic drugs are given, is made worse by the drugs used to treat parkinsonism, and remits only slowly or not at all after treatment is stopped (Barnes 1988). It can become manifest for the first time after treatment is stopped, and pre-existing tardive dyskinesia can become worse after stopping treatment, before it subsequently improves. The dopamine receptors, blocked by the antipsychotic drug, eventually become supersensitive to even small amounts of dopamine, as an adaptive response. Then the supersensitivity persists for some time after treatment is stopped before the receptors again respond normally to dopamine.

11.2 Cause and effect

Acute dystonic reactions occur soon after a dose of drug, are distinctive in clinical features, and subside within hours to days. It is not usually difficult to demonstrate that the drug was responsible, though doubt might arise if exposure to another drug capable of causing muscle spasm were suspected. The most pertinent example is 'Ecstasy', which can cause disturbed behaviour and also trismus (clenching of the jaw) and opisthotonos (tightening of the muscles of the back to make the spine arch backwards) (Henry 1992). A patient who had taken 'Ecstasy' might be given a major tranquillizer and then manifest these symptoms, and it would be difficult to know whether it was the 'Ecstasy' or the antipsychotic drug that provoked them.

Clenching of the jaw can also occur as a manifestation of tetanus, a serious bacterial infection. In at least one instance, a hospital was sued for negligence in failing to deal effectively with an outbreak of tetanus involving four patients. It transpired that, although one patient did indeed have tetanus, there was no outbreak: the other three patients had all received the antiemetic drug metoclopramide ('Maxolon') and developed trismus (C. Ellis, personal communication).

Parkinsonism can be due to natural Parkinson's disease or to a number of other causes, including antipsychotic drugs, but also the viral infection of encephalitis lethargica, and as a sequel to poisoning with carbon monoxide, *inter alia*. Parkinson's disease usually affects middle-aged or elderly people, and is rare below the age of 50 years. The likelihood is that drugs rather than natural disease will have caused parkinsonism in younger patients, but the uncertainty increases with the patient's age. The most obvious distinguishing feature is remission of the disease after cessation of treatment, but, as explained above, even this is not completely certain.

Orofacial dyskinesia is not invariably drug-induced, either. Several studies have shown that such movements can be seen in psychiatric patients who have never been treated with antipsychotic agents, and can be a manifestation of old age. The association is perhaps strengthened by the increased incidence of orofacial dyskinesia in patients with no teeth or ill-fitting dentures. The crucial question of whether orofacial dyskinesia in an individual patient is likely to be an adverse effect of antipsychotic medicines has been touched on in Wettstein's review (Wettstein 1985), but is unlikely to be resolved easily, since patients with severe schizophrenia who have not been treated with drugs are rare, and the opportunity to observe the natural history of their disease without drugs correspondingly uncommon.

11.3 Neuroleptic malignant syndrome

A serious and sometimes fatal complication of antipsychotic drugs is *neuroleptic malignant syndrome*, a syndrome of mental confusion, swings in blood pressure, and muscle rigidity with a high fever and fast heart rate. The condition is sufficiently rare that many practitioners have not seen it, so they can take the features of fever and increased heart rate to indicate infection and treatment can be delayed.

11.4 Sudden deaths with phenothiazines

Patients treated with high doses of phenothiazines, and occasionally other antipsychotic drugs, can die suddenly and unexpectedly (Wakasugi *et al.* 1986). This usually happens after continued treatment with high doses, but occasionally occurs after a single large dose, given intramuscularly to calm particularly disturbed or violent patients. Since blood concentrations are substantially higher after intramuscular dosing than after oral dosing, failure to adjust the dosage when altering the route of administration is a particular hazard (Thompson 1994).

Because of the circumstances in which they are used, it is usually unclear whether the drugs caused sudden death, or whether sudden death was part of, or the sequel to, the disturbed behaviour for which the drugs were given.

There is also a feeling, as yet unsubstantiated, that sudden death in these circumstances may be more common in Afro-Caribbean (Black) patients than in other groups. The problems of deciding whether the drugs are causative are compounded by controversy over the incidence of psychotic illness in this group.

The putative mechanism by which phenothiazines, particularly, can cause sudden death involves a change in the electrical activity of the heart, manifest in the electrocardiogram as prolongation of the Q–T interval[3]. This is known to occur with thioridazine, and perhaps other phenothiazines, in overdosage, and is known to predispose to serious heart rhythm disturbance, notably a disturbance of ventricular rhythm called *torsade de pointes*. Ventricular rhythm disturbance can be fatal.

The Royal College of Psychiatrists' Committee on Psychopharmacology has commented on the problem (Hirsch and Barnes 1994): 'The use of very high dose is a last resort and such treatment should be regarded as an individual trial in each patient, to be carried out advisedly, under specialist guidance, and with caution. It is not for routine use.' The Royal College has also issued guidelines in the form of a consensus statement on the use of high-dose antipsychotic medication (Thompson 1994).

11.5 Clozapine-induced disorders of the white blood cells

Clozapine is an important antipsychotic drug which has become available in the 1990s. It differs from the phenothiazines and butyrophenones in showing only weak activity as a dopamine antagonist, and in being effective in psychotic patients who have failed to respond to those agents.

A high incidence of bone marrow damage, with agranulocytosis (failure to produce granulocytes, an important subtype of white cells), diminishes the therapeutic value of clozapine. The estimated incidence of *fatal* agranulocytosis was 1 in 300 patients before the problem was recognized (ABPI 1993–4*d*). Its use is therefore restricted to patients who have a normal white blood cell count and who can have blood samples taken and the white cell count measured every week for 18 weeks from the start of treatment, then every 2 weeks for as long as the treatment continues. These limitations place severe organizational obstacles in the path of a prescriber wishing to start clozapine treatment.

11.6 Remoxipride-induced disorders of the blood

Remoxipride is another antipsychotic drug introduced in the 1990s which is chemically distinct from clozapine. It has recently been reported to cause aplastic anaemia (a shortage of red blood cells due to reduced or absent production). The manufacturers have written to doctors warning them not to prescribe the drug to patients with abnormal blood counts, nor to continue it if the blood count becomes abnormal. Patients should be told of the possible significance of abnormal bleeding or signs of infection (Barker 1993). The message has been reiterated by the Committee on Safety of Medicines (1993), who suggest in addition that the blood count should be monitored every week for 6 months, and every month thereafter.

These provisions will limit the value of remoxipride as initial or maintenance therapy for schizophrenia.

11.7 Psychiatric effects of antipsychotic drugs

Shaw *et al.* (1986) and others have suggested that there is a link between dopamine antagonists, akathisia, and suicide or violence against others. Either the dopamine antagonists such as

---

[3] The horizontal distance on the tracing from the start of the Q-wave to the end of the T-wave is the *Q–T interval*. The normal distance depends on heart rate, but should not be more than about 420 milliseconds..

chlorpromazine and haloperidol can cause akathisia and suicidal or homicidal thoughts independently, or the akathisia is so unpleasant that the patient contemplates suicide.

Psychotropic drugs can apparently cause somnambulism (sleepwalking) (Luchins *et al.* 1978; Charney *et al.* 1979; Scott 1988), though the story of Lady Macbeth suggests that psychiatric disturbance may itself cause somnambulism. Two cases illustrate the forensic significance.

CASE 11.2 (SCOTT 1988)

A 44-year-old ambulance driver was treated with thioridazine ('Melleril') for 'stress-related psychosis'. He would talk in his sleep, lash out, and wander out of bed. [It is uncertain from the report whether the treatment began before the nocturnal disorder]. One night his wife awoke to find her husband with his hands around her throat. He was admitted to hospital, where he was observed to be restless and to wander every night. The episodes stopped when he stopped taking thioridazine and lost weight.

The authors believed that the somnambulism and violent behaviour were caused by the phenothiazine. It is also possible that they were related to hypoxia (a low oxygen tension in the blood) due to obstructive sleep apnoea (obstruction of the respiratory passages and prolonged pauses in breathing due to obesity), perhaps made worse by the thioridazine.

CASE 11.3 (LUCHINS *ET AL.* 1978)

A 39-year-old woman developed schizophrenia, was treated with thioridazine and improved enough that she left hospital and ceased treatment. One year later the symptoms reappeared, and she was treated with thioridazine together with trichloroethanol, a hypnotic (sleeping draught). One night, after 3 months of treatment, she rose at 3 a.m. and stabbed her daughter to death. A psychiatrist who examined her the next morning found her to be schizophrenic and 'dissociated'.

She was tried for murder, acquitted by reason of insanity, and consigned to a psychiatric hospital.

While an in-patient taking phenothiazines again, she sleepwalked several nights each week. She was studied with sleep electroencephalograms (recordings of brain electrical activity). She only sleepwalked during stage 4 sleep (a stage of sleep with characteristic brain-wave activity), and thioridazine increased the duration in phase 4. She stopped sleepwalking if phenothiazines were stopped.

The authors do not consider whether the killing would have occurred if the woman had not been taking thioridazine.

Both cases suggest that there would be reasonable doubt of intent in a case where an act of violence was committed by a patient who was sleepwalking while on phenothiazines.

11.8 Summary

The major tranquillizers, used to treat schizophrenia and other psychotic illnesses, can have serious adverse effects on the central nervous system that lead to a variety of movement disorders. Fatal complications from using these drugs include neuroleptic malignant syndrome, and sudden death that is probably due to cardiac arrhythmia. The newer agents clozapine and remoxipride are particularly liable to cause blood disorders. Case reports link sleepwalking and other behavourial disturbance to major tranquillizers.

12

Opiates and related drugs

Opiates are those drugs derived from the sap of the opium poppy, especially morphine and codeine. Several derivatives and related drugs have been synthesized, and these are collectively referred to as *opioids*. Important members of the class include:

buprenorphine ('Temgesic')
codeine
dextropropoxyphene (propoxyphene, 'Darvon', in the United States; and a component of co-proxamol, 'Distalgesic')
diamorphine (heroin)
dihydrocodeine ('DF118')
dipipanone
fentanyl
methadone
morphine
pethidine (meperidine, 'Demerol', in the United States)
tramadol

The drugs are used principally to treat moderate (codeine, dextropropoxyphene) or severe pain. They also depress respiration, cause vomiting and constipation, and have psychological effects including euphoria (an elevation of mood) and dysphoria (the induction of an unusual and unpleasant state).

An important sign of opioid ingestion is marked bilateral constriction of the pupils ('pin-point' pupils in English, '*en tête d'épingle* [pin-head]' in French). The sign can occur with other conditions including pontine haemorrhage (a form of brain haemorrhage) and organophosphorus poisoning, but opioid poisoning is an important and potentially treatable cause.

Opioids are important for several reasons:

(1) They are potent drugs that can inadvertently cause death in therapeutic use, or in combination with other drugs, or in overdosage;
(2) They are liable to abuse by drug addicts;
(3) They can be used for murder.

12.1 Opioids in therapeutic doses

Death in therapeutic doses is most likely to occur in patients with increased susceptibility to the drugs, and such susceptibility is in part predictable. The drugs cause respiratory depression, and that is a particular danger for people with the chest diseases chronic bronchitis or emphysema. The opioids are also liable to precipitate the form of acute brain failure known as hepatic encephalopathy in patients who have severely deranged liver function. It is now clear that whereas morphine itself is metabolized by the liver, the metabolites (breakdown products) are excreted by the kidney. Since at least one breakdown product is active, patients with kidney failure risk developing opioid toxicity with morphine.

Opioids are also relatively contraindicated in cases of head injury and other causes of an increase of the intracranial pressure, both because they raise intracranial pressure and because they cause changes in the pupils that can mask the effects of an uncontrolled increase in the pressure. It is traditional to use codeine, which has a rather weaker effect on the pupils.

12.2 Negligence

Opioids are powerful drugs, and in overdosage can cause respiratory depression and death. Practitioners therefore have to take care in prescibing them.

CASE 12.1

A general practitioner performed a circumcision on a 9-year-old boy in his surgery. Because the operation and its sequel were potentially painful, the doctor gave an intramuscular injection of analgesic (pain killer) and the boy left the surgery with his father. He collapsed at home 2 hours later, and died in spite of efforts at resuscitation.

Initially, the general practitioner claimed to have given dihydrocodeine ('DF118'), which is available as a solution containing 50 milligrams of drug in 1 millilitre. Subsequent to laboratory tests on the blood, the doctor admitted that he had actually administered 10 milligrams of diamorphine, which is available as a powder that has to be dissolved before injection. Ten milligrams is an adult dose. The effects were delayed because the injection was given into the muscle, so that absorption was slowed.

The doctor was recklessly negligent. He was charged with manslaughter and pleaded guilty.

CASE 12.2

A boy of 9 months developed diarrhoea and vomiting, as several sibs had done. His father took him to the general practitioner, who wrote a prescription for oral rehydration solution (a mixture of sugar and salts that is dissolved in water, and is used to replace losses of fluid due to diarrhoea).

Afterwards, the doctor apparently administered to the child some drops from a bottle of medicine. The father went with the boy to a pharmacy and then took him home. By the time they reached home, the baby was drowsy. He then became blue and stopped breathing. Fortunately, he was resuscitated, and survived after several days of intensive care.

At hospital, it had been noted that his pupils were very constricted, and this clue led to examination of the blood. The blood contained somewhere between 10 and 100 times the therapeutic concentration of morphine.

A preparation of morphine, 'Oramorph concentrated oral solution' is dispensed with a calibrated dropper, and contains 100 milligrams of morphine in 5 millilitres. A reasonable explanation of events is that the general practitioner administered some of this solution, 'for diarrhoea', the baby received an iatrogenic overdose, and the disastrous consequences were due to respiratory depression. 'Oramorph' is not licensed for the treatment of diarrhoea.

12.3 Deliberate overdosage

The effect of opioids on respiration can be enhanced by ethanol, and this can be extremely rapid. It has particularly proved to be the case for dextropropoxyphene, which is one of the weakest opioid analgesics, and widely used as co-proxamol (formerly 'Distalgesic') in Britain, and as a single analgesic ('Darvon') for use in moderate pain in the United States. Overdoses taken with ethanol can cause death within a matter of minutes, so that there is a tendency for people to die who would in other circumstances have reconsidered their decision to take tablets (Sturner and Garriott 1973; Tennant 1973; Whittington 1977). One case referred to a soldier who swallowed 20 65 milligram propoxyphene capsules and died within about 35 minutes (Tennant 1973).

The rapidity with which death ensues after overdosage was crucial in a case of alleged manslaughter:

CASE 12.3

A 47-year-old man, who was known to abuse both alcohol and his wife, returned home to her one night, and demanded that she count out tablets for him to take, as he was 'no use to anyone'. She complied by counting out 70 co-proxamol tablets, which he took with a half-bottle of gin. Co-proxamol ('Distalgesic') tablets contain 325 milligrams of paracetamol and 32.5 milligrams of dextropropoxyphene.

The man's wife called an ambulance, and the crew who arrived a few minutes later found that the man was dead, with tablet wrappers beside him. The wife did not say at that stage that she had helped her husband kill himself, but rang the Coroner's Officer the next morning. The wife's story was that after he had taken the tablets, she gave her husband a cup of coffee in an attempt to revive him then dialled the emergency services. She was charged with aiding and abetting a suicide and with manslaughter because she had apparently delayed calling for an ambulance until her husband was near death or already dead.

At trial, the expert for the prosecution admitted that death after overdose of dextropropoxyphene-paracetamol and ethanol could occur 'within a few minutes'. The widow was acquitted.

12.4 Addiction to opioids

Opioids are classical drugs of addiction, and are most often injected intravenously. The image of Lascar seamen smoking opium in seedy dens in the East End of London has given way to the image of the junkie 'shooting up' in a public lavatory or seedy bed-sit. The favoured opioid for intravenous injection by addicts is diamorphine (heroin), but market forces and personal preference ensure that other drugs are also widely abused.

Addicts are tolerant to very much higher doses of opioids than previously unexposed subjects, but when the tolerance is exceeded, they too can succumb to respiratory depression and sudden death. This occurs especially when addicts have been through a period of relative or absolute abstinence, and then take the dose of opioid to which they were previously accustomed. The drug sold on the street is usually 'cut' (diluted) with another powder such as chalk, talcum powder, glucose, or powdered milk (Clouston 1994) so that it is only about 15-30 per cent pure when sold. If an unusually pure batch of the drug is sold, then addicts may take more of the drug than they estimated, and suffer dose-dependent adverse effects as a result. There have been sporadic outbreaks of deaths from this cause in British cities. The diluent itself can cause serious damage to the lungs and blood vessels. Addicts can also die as a result of abusing two or several drugs simultaneously.

Death from drug addiction is often linked not directly to the drugs that are abused but to the circumstances of their abuse. The intense desire for a 'hit', an injection of drug, overwhelms any desire for self-preservation and the addict is prepared to risk injury and infection to secure a 'high'.

12.5 Body-packers

The transport and distribution of drugs of abuse is a major industry. One common method of concealment of drugs of abuse is in body cavities. The drugs are wrapped in impermeable material, usually condoms, and then swallowed, or 'stuffed' into the rectum ('back passage', the lowermost part of the large intestine) or vagina ('front passage', the lowermost part of the female genital tract). Those who smuggle drugs in this way are called 'body-packers', 'stuffers', or 'mules'. Very large numbers of packets can be swallowed. In one French case, 173 packets were recovered (Gherardi *et al.* 1988).

There are several methods of detection of concealed packages in people who are suspected by the customs or police of smuggling drugs. Physical examination, including digital examination of the rectum and vagina, identified over half the 35 positive cases amongst 197 suspected cases seen at Helsinki Airport (Karhunen *et al.* 1987). Plain radiographs of the abdomen showed concealed packages in nine smugglers of 158 suspects detained at Manchester Airport (Horrocks 1992). In an unusual case, a would-be body-packer presented with abdominal pain, and was shown to have an oval opacity on plain abdominal radiography. This proved to be a honey-filled condom, which he had swallowed in a trial run of the method, and which he subsequently passed *per rectum* (Bayliss 1993). Radiography is also of use in checking that no further packages remain.

The smuggled drug can sometimes be detected in the urine of the smuggler, either because there is some leakage from the packets of drug or because the smuggler is also an abuser. Gherardi *et al.* (1988) were able to detect diamorphine (heroin) in 9 of 10 smugglers, and cocaine or its breakdown products in 49 of 50. Unfortunately, the drug is often not detected in urine for several days, and so the urine test is not a reliable way of finding whom to detain (Shah 1988).

Even if no drug of abuse is found in the urine, it occasionally happens that other drugs are: the breakdown products of hyoscine butylbromide ('Buscopam') were detected in the urine of a body-packer who had taken that drug to prevent him excreting his consignment while in transit (Wehr and Alzen 1989).

While many body-packers who come to medical attention are detected by customs officers, some present as a result of complications of the trade:

CASE 12.4 (STEVENSON AND HUME 1991)

A 28-year-old man was arrested after drugs had been stolen from a chemist's shop. He became drowsy and was taken to hospital where he was noted to have pin-point pupils, and treated with naloxone (a short-acting antidote to opioids). He woke up, explained that he had injected two crushed tablets of the opioid pentazocine before his arrest, and demanded to be discharged from hospital. He returned to police custody, where he later collapsed. On re-admission to hospital he had a respiratory arrest from which he was resuscitated. Examination showed that he had concealed in his rectum a polythene bag containing tablets of morphine, buprenorphine, and pentazocine, all opioids stolen from the chemist's shop.

The symptoms of drug intoxication after leakage of the contents of a package will depend on the nature of the concealed drug. Packers can also present with intestinal obstruction from the packages, and there is a case recorded of a packer suffocating after attempting to swallow an over-large package.

12.6 Murder with opioids

Morphine (and in Britain, diamorphine) are the prime agents used in the relief of severe pain in patients who are in the later stages of incurable disease. In this use, the risks of respiratory depression are acceptable. However, the law in Britain and the United States does not permit euthanasia, so that using the opioid primarily to hasten a patient's end would be illegal. The problem is morally complex, and if the patient has told her medical attendant that she will leave him a substantial legacy, there can be important forensic problems, as illustrated by the case of Dr John Bodkin Adams. This was remarkable in many ways, not least that it formed the subject of a book written by the man who was judge at his trial (Devlin 1985).

CASE 12.5 (DEVLIN 1985 '*EASING THE PASSING*')

John Bodkin Adams was a successful general practitioner in the English south coast town of East-bourne. He had amongst his patients several well-to-do retired people. One was a Mrs Edith Morrell, a woman aged about 79 years who had a disabling stroke in 1948 and died in 1950. Seven years later the doctor was tried for murdering her, allegedly with morphine (morphia) and diamorphine (heroin). In the last 10½ months of her life, Dr Bodkin Adams prescribed Mrs Morrell 165 grains (approximately 10.5 grams) of morphine, and 139½ grains (approximately 8.9 grams) of diamorphine. When arrested, he had said 'Easing the passing of a dying person is not all that wicked. She wanted to die. That cannot be murder. It is impossible to accuse a doctor.'

The Crown argued both that the dosage of opioids in the months before Mrs Morrell's death was excessive and that the last one or two injections of opioid prescribed by the doctor were given expressly to kill Mrs Morrell and so secure a legacy. The defence were able to find complete nursing records for the patient's illness, and so confront the fading memories of the nurses and others involved.

Experts for the prosecution argued that the maximum permissible daily dose of morphine was ½ grain (approximately 30 milligrams) and the maximum daily dose of heroin ¼ grain (16 milligrams). As the judge points out in his account, tolerance to opioids varies considerably, and can be acquired. Mrs Morrell had been alert and even cheerful for most of the time that she was receiving the drugs, so that it was difficult to argue convincingly that she was chronically poisoned.

Dr Douthwaite, a clinical pharmacologist from Guy's Hospital, initially put forward the view that the doctor had forced opioid addiction on to his patient so as to bring her under his control. There was little evidence for that, and indeed it seemed that she exercised considerable control over her doctor.

In the few days before Mrs Morrell died, Dr Bodkin Adams had given her diamorphine, but at first had stopped giving morphine and then re-instituted it. Douthwaite reformulated his argument, and maintained that the only possible explanation for the doctor withdrawing the morphine and then re-introducing it was that he intended to murder his patient.

Douthwaite's view was difficult to sustain, since the alternative explanation offered by the defence, that Dr Bodkin Adams was experimenting to alleviate his patient's restlessness at night, was at least plausible. In retrospect, Douthwaite would have known that there is cross-tolerance between morphine and diamorphine, so that whatever the defendant's object, he was unlikely to kill the patient by his change in the treatment schedule. He faced the additional difficulty that it contradicted his previously expressed view that Dr Bodkin Adams had schemed to murder his victim, or at least to render her addicted and subjugate to his will, by chronic administration.

The crucial question put to Douthwaite by the defence was whether he would accept that while he was forced to the view that the actions of the defendant could only mean an intent to murder, another doctor might not reach the same conclusion. Douthwaite answered: 'It is clear, is it not? There could always be a difference of opinion.' This left open a reasonable doubt as to the intent behind the change in treatment.

The judge pressed Douthwaite to confirm that he was not merely saying that the treatment had caused death, but that it had done so only because it was intended to kill, and not because of error, ignorance, or incompetence. Douthwaite agreed that this was his view. Douthwaite would have advised the prosecution over whether to bring the case to trial, and might then have felt obliged to support it. 'He was too staunch'; his evidence was 'disastrous'.

The jury brought in a verdict of not guilty after deliberating for under an hour. Dr Bodkin Adams was later convicted of misconduct in his prescribing, fined £2400, and struck off the Medical Register.

One unsatisfactory part of the story was that Bodkin Adams was rumoured to be a bounty hunter who had dispatched several patients so as to benefit from their legacies. The Crown had at one time entertained the possibility of showing *system*, that is, a method of operation which was sufficiently similar in several different cases as to show that they formed part of a common plan, even though the evidence of murder might not be strong enough to support a conviction on just one of the crimes. There remains the possibility that, had the prosecution relied on 'system', Bodkin Adams would have been convicted, whether rightly or wrongly.

Euthanasia was the alleged motive for the administration of dihydrocodeine ('DF118') to a new-born infant with Down's syndrome in the case of the paediatrician Leonard Arthur (Case 6.27). Dr Arthur had prescribed the drug to ease the suffering of the baby, but had withheld feeding. It was argued that his prescription had sedated the baby and caused respiratory depression and death. He was charged with murder, but the charge was later modified to attempted murder when it became clear that the baby was suffering from severe lung damage at the time of birth, and likely to die in any event. He was acquitted.

12.7 Summary

Opioids are potentially dangerous drugs in therapeutic use, particularly because they can cause respiratory depression. They are important drugs of abuse, and they can also be used for criminal ends, including murder.

13

Vaccines

Vaccines (from *Vaccinia*, cowpox) were introduced in the eighteenth century by Edward Jenner who discovered that inoculation of a previously unaffected subject with cowpox, a mild skin affection, could protect from subsequent infection with smallpox, a potentially lethal viral disease. It is now recognized as a form of *active immunization*: the immune system is primed to respond effectively to subsequent infections with the same or similar immunological properties.

The principle of protecting individuals from infections by boosting immunity has now been extended to the protection of populations. The chances of acquiring an infection such as polio depend on its prevalence in the community, and provided the prevalence is low, the risk for an individual remains small. The ethical problem is that for any individual in a community where the prevalence of infection is low, the benefits of preventive treatment are correspondingly low, but it is necessary to give preventive treatment to ensure that the prevalence of infection remains low. The instability of the system was illustrated when fears of brain damage due to pertussis (whooping cough) vaccine caused many parents to leave their children unimmunized against whooping cough, with the result that there were epidemic outbreaks of pertussis in England in the late 1970s and early 1980s, when the 'attack rate' rose from about 4 per 100 000 in 1974 to 175 per 100 000 in 1982 (Cherry 1984).

Damage as a result of preventive treatment in a previously fit member of the community who individually gains little from it is a serious matter. It is also a matter which has led to considerable litigation.

13.1 Recommended immunization

Parents are advised in the United Kingdom that healthy children who have no contraindications to immunization should have diphtheria, tetanus, pertussis (whooping cough), measles, mumps, rubella (German measles), poliomyelitis ('polio') and *Haemophilus influenzae b* immunization. General practitioners have a responsibility to see that immunization rates are maintained, and are offered a financial incentive to see that they are.

One interesting problem has arisen in connection with a campaign aimed at boosting immunity to measles in advance of an epidemic threatened for the winter of 1994–95. The vaccine used (MMR vaccine) was a combined mumps, measles, and rubella vaccine, and the rubella (German measles) component was first grown in cells from a fetus aborted because the mother had contracted rubella in pregnancy. Religious groups strongly opposed to abortion have in consequence opposed immunization with the vaccine.

13.2 Vaccine-damaged children

13.2.1 Pertussis vaccine

Pertussis (whooping cough) was an important cause of death and serious illness before the Second World War. There were, for example, over a quarter of a million cases and over 7 500 deaths from pertussis in the United States in 1934 (David and Jalilian-Marian 1986). Children between about 3 and 6 months of life are particularly susceptible. The disease is now rare. It is characterized by weeks of cruelly-prolonged bouts of coughing, each paroxysm ending in a lengthy inspiration that caused a stridulous 'whoop'. The complications of the illness include long-term lung damage, with bronchiectasis (distortion of the air-passages that consequently become chronically infected), and seizures due to hypoxic brain damage or to intracerebral haemorrhage (bleeding within the brain) related to coughing.

The disease is known to be due to the bacterium *Bordetella pertussis* (first described by Bordet in 1906). A vaccine prepared from killed bacteria is used to immunize against the disease, and it is commonly given as one component of 'DTP', 'DPT', or 'triple' vaccine, against diptheria, tetanus, and pertussis. DTP is available in the United Kingdom as 'Trivax' and 'Trivax-AD'.

Immunization aims to stimulate an immune response, and to this end vaccines should be given after the baby's immune system has matured sufficiently to mount an immune response, and this is only so after 2 or 3 months of age. It also aims to protect the child during its period of greatest vulnerability, and for pertussis this is between about 3 and 6 months of age. The recommendations on immunization are therefore a compromise, and in the United States it is recommended that an infant receive the first dose of triple vaccine at 2 months, whereas in the United Kingdom the first dose is traditionally given at 3 months of age.

Whether pertussis vaccine causes neurological damage is debatable. David and Jalilian-Marian (1986) have reviewed the incidence of convulsion after pertussis vaccine. Reported rates range from 1 case in 1750 doses of DTP to 1 in 800 000 doses (Griffith 1978; Cherry 1984).

13.2.2 Legal actions over pertussis-induced brain damage

The lawyer is faced with the specific problem of demonstrating causation in a particular case, not the general proposition that a vaccine can, on rare occasions, cause a particular sort of injury. In the 1980s the Kinnear case, one of over 200 cases, was selected as a test case, but doubts about the facts caused the case to collapse part-way through (Anonymous 1986c). In that case, the action was against the health authority, the general practitioner who had administered the vaccine, and Boroughs Wellcome who manufactured it.

A second test case, the Loveday case, was then heard. The defendant was the general practitioner, but Boroughs Wellcome became co-defendants at their own request, even though there was no evidence that they had manufactured the vaccine in question. This curious circumstance meant that the defence were fighting over well-prepared ground. Nineteen medical experts, including paediatricians, paediatric neurologists, and epidemiologists, were called. Lord Justice Stuart-Smith delivered a written judgement that ran to 300 pages, in which he concluded that pertussis vaccine was not proved on the balance of probabilities to cause irreversible brain damage. As Professor Gordon Stewart, one of the experts in the case, agreed in cross-examination, there was no distinct clinical syndrome in pertussis-vaccine-associated cases [of neurological disease] that distinguished them from cases not associated with the vaccine (Anonymous 1986c; Meade 1986; Brahams 1988a; Dyer 1988a; Scheifele 1988).

The questions of whether pertussis vaccine did in fact cause Susan Loveday's brain damage, and whether her general practitioner was negligent in immunizing her with it, were never decided.

A Scottish case, the Bonthorne case (Brahams 1985c, 1986a) and a Canadian case, the Rothwell case (Goldman 1988), were also dismissed. In the United States, pertussis vaccine may have contained an epidemic of whooping cough, but it has led to an epidemic of legal claims against vaccine manufacturers, with an estimated 11 lawsuits filed for every million doses of vaccine distributed in 1985 (Hinman 1986). It is not known how many such suits have been settled, though a substantial number were presumably settled out of court: vaccine manufacturers spent $16.2 million in settling 52 cases (Iglehart 1987).

The Irish Supreme Court decided the appeal of a recent Irish case in favour of the plaintiff, Kenneth Best, against the Wellcome Foundation in an action that also involved the general practitioner and the health board.

CASE 13.1 (JUDGEMENT OF CHIEF JUSTICE FINLAY, 3 JUNE 1992; LAURANCE 1993)

A baby boy was vaccinated with DTP and, according to his mother at trial (19 years later), had seizures the same evening and repeatedly over the next several weeks. When eventually seen by a specialist some 4½ months later, the boy was diagnosed as having infantile spasms, a manifestation of serious neurological disease, and he remained gravely mentally retarded.

The pertussis component of the DTP vaccine was manufactured by Boroughs Wellcome in 1968 and the batch, number BA3741, was submitted to a series of tests, including some laid down by British statute and other additional tests. The British version of the standard potency test pre-scribed only the minimum potency, whereas the American version current at that time also pre-scribed a maximum potency, which this particular vaccine batch exceeded by 2½ times. In a non-statutory test, the mouse weight gain test, the batch gave wholly unsatisfactory results, for no reason that was documented at the time. None the less, the company released the vaccine for use, and a dose from this batch was administered to the plaintiff by the general practitioner's nurse.

The trial judge accepted:
(1) that the infant had received Wellcome DTP vaccine;
(2) that a very rare effect of that vaccine is to cause neurological damage;
(3) that the likelihood of toxicity from the vaccine was probably linked to its potency;
(4) that Wellcome were negligent in allowing a vaccine to be released which failed to pass the tests that it had elected to perform, even though they were not required by statute; and
(5) that if the vaccine had been the cause of the neurological disease, the signs would have been manifest within hours.

The mother stated that it was her clear recollection that the child had had a seizure in the evening after immunization, and that she had telephoned the doctor that evening and on several occasions over the succeeding weeks, until she had eventually prevailed on him to refer her son to a specialist.

At the original trial, the judge preferred the evidence of the general practitioner that he had made no note of any fits in the 2 months after the immunization, and that therefore there had been none. The appeal judges, in overturning this judgement and favouring the evidence of the mother, allowed the connection to be made between the vaccination and the infantile spasm, and so completed the chain of causation from Wellcome's negligence to the boy's brain damage.

13.3 Vaccines other than pertussis

The threat of an epidemic of influenza in the United States and Puerto Rico encouraged the immunization of over 40 000 000 people with a vaccine (A/New Jersey) based on a strain of swine influenza virus. Several hundred cases of Guillain-Barré syndrome (an ascending paralysis that can involve the muscles necessary for breathing) were seen in the weeks after immunization, which was likely to have accounted for up to 90 per cent of all the cases of the syndrome seen in vaccinated patients in the 2 or 3 weeks after immunization, and to have been the most likely cause in the first 5 weeks after immunization (Greenstreet 1984).

CASE 13.2 (BRAHAMS 1985*A*)

A 22-year-old man, who was immunized when he was unwell and probably feverish, had a stroke from cerebral infarction within hours of a second dose of cholera–typhoid–paratyphoid A–paratyphoid B vaccine, and the general practitioner was found guilty of negligence.

In the United States, manufacturers have been held liable when insufficient warning has been given of possible adverse effects, and they have occurred. For example, the manufacturer was liable when a man who received oral poliomyelitis vaccine subsequently developed poliomyelitis and was paralysed from the waist down. The manufacturers had known of the potential for harm, but had not advertised the risk in such a way that the plaintiff could decide for himself whether it was a risk he was prepared to accept. In another case, the manufacturer was held liable when the mother of an infant who had been immunized contracted paralytic poliomyelitis (David and Jalilian-Marian 1986).

13.4 Compensation for vaccine-induced damage

Several countries, including the United Kingdom, Germany, France, Denmark, Japan, the United States, and Canada, have introduced compensation schemes so that those who have, on the balance of probabilities, sustained damage from vaccines, can be compensated without any need to show negligence on the part of the manufacturer or the prescriber (Dukes and Swartz 1988*f*). Ironically, the British scheme has been in operation since 1979, and was granting substantial sums in compensation at a time when the courts held in the Loveday case that there was no scientific demonstration on the balance of probabilities that pertussis vaccine did in fact cause brain damage.

13.5 Summary

Mass immunization benefits the community, but sometimes causes damage to perfectly healthy individuals. This causes social and legal problems. It is often extremely difficult or impossible to be reasonably certain that immunization with a particular vaccine led to harm in an individual, so there are problems for medical experts, too. Compensation schemes have gone some way towards reconciling protection of the community and protection of the individual.

14

Paracetamol (acetaminophen in the United States)

Paracetamol is a widely available analgesic (pain-killer) which is remarkably safe in therapeutic dosage. Its forensic importance lies in the problems associated with paracetamol overdosage.

Tablets usually contain 500 milligrams (0.5 grams) of drug; combination tablets such as co-codamol and co-dydramol also contain 500 milligrams of paracetamol, but co-proxamol ('Distalgesic', 'D–G') only contains 325 milligrams per tablet.

14.1 Therapeutic dosages of paracetamol

The standard single dose of paracetamol in an adult is 0.5–1 gram. The dosage may be repeated after 4–6 hours, but the maximum daily dose must not exceed 4 grams.

Paracetamol is now the preferred analgesic and antipyretic (temperature-lowering drug) in children below the age of 12 years. Smaller doses of paracetamol are appropriate in childhood, and depend on the age and size of the infant or child: these are given in the *British National Formulary*.

14.2 Overdosage of paracetamol
(Ferner 1993; Thomas 1993)

Deliberate paracetamol overdosage is common in the United Kingdom (though not elsewhere).

Accidental overdosage can also occur. There is a danger that patients may take several medicines, all with different names, and all containing paracetamol. The *British National Formulary* lists about 40 such preparations. Some brand names, previously applied to preparations containing aspirin, are now also applied to products that include paracetamol. Examples are 'Anadin Extra' (compare with 'Anadin'), 'Aspro Paraclear' (compare with 'Aspro'), 'Beecham's Powders Capsules with Decongestant' (compare with 'Beecham's Powders Tablets') and 'Disprin Extra' (compare with 'Disprin'). The situation is made worse by the inclusion of paracetamol in remedies such as 'Boots Cold Relief Tablets', 'Feminax' and 'Night Nurse' (Aronson 1994).

The danger in overdosage is the development of damage to the liver and kidneys. The damage is due to the production of an active metabolite (breakdown product) called N-acetyl-para-benzoquinoneimine (NABQI) that can bind to tissue proteins, including enzymes, and stop cells from functioning.

NABQI is not produced in significant amounts after therapeutic doses. When NABQI is produced after overdosage, it binds preferentially to sulphur-containing amino-acids. With small overdoses in well-nourished, healthy, people there is sufficient glutathione (a sulphur-containing amino-acid) to prevent the NABQI from causing serious damage to tissue. However, after large overdoses, or in patients who are more susceptible to the effects of overdosage than normal, then serious and sometimes fatal damage can occur.

The generation of NABQI, and the binding of NABQI to tissue proteins, take time. This means that there is some urgency to treat patients with significant poisoning. Antidotes exist (see below), but they become less effective as time goes by after 8 hours.

The damage done by paracetamol is usually not manifest for at least 24 hours, and is sometimes delayed for up to 72 hours. However, it would be exceptional not to find evidence of overdosage from laboratory tests of paracetamol concentration, or prothrombin time (a clotting test that depends on liver function, and is an early marker of liver damage) or creatinine concentration (a measure of kidney function) in a patient who had in fact taken a significant overdosage and was going to develop liver or kidney damage. Put another way, either the blood contains paracetamol, or the blood tests show evidence of impending organ damage.

14.2.1 The antidotes to paracetamol poisoning

The tissue damage caused by NABQI can be prevented by providing sufficient sulphur-containing amino acids to bind to the metabolite before it binds to cell proteins.

Two agents are used: methionine, which is a naturally occurring amino acid, and acetyl cysteine (N-acetylcysteine, 'Parvolex'), which is a modified amino acid. The former is usually given orally, and the latter is usually given intravenously in the United Kingdom (orally in the United States, where the intravenous preparation does not have a product licence).

Methionine tends to cause nausea and vomiting, which are anyway clinical features of significant paracetamol overdosage. This makes it rather less certain that the administered dose of antidote will be absorbed and therefore have a protective action. Methionine is not suitable for treating patients more than 8 hours after overdosage.

Acetylcysteine by intravenous infusion is a foul-smelling liquid that has to be diluted and administered in a dosage that depends on body weight. Errors in dilution are potentially serious, and patients who would not have died from paracetamol poisoning have occasionally died from an iatrogenic overdose of antidote (Mant *et al.* 1984).

The potentially dangerous adverse effect of acetylcysteine is that it can cause histamine release in about 10 per cent of patients. This is not usually serious, because the infusion can be stopped, the patient given antihistamines (and if necessary corticosteroids) and the reaction allowed to subside. The infusion can then be restarted at a lower rate.

Some (including the author) prefer to give acetylcysteine intravenously to all patients who are likely to have significant poisoning.

14.2.2 Significant poisoning

The definition of significant poisoning is largely agreed. It depends on three things: the concentration of paracetamol in the blood; the time from ingestion of the paracetamol to the taking of the blood sample; and the constitution of the patient.

For most patients, including children, treatment is based on a graph (usually referred to as the 'nomogram for paracetamol') of paracetamol concentration against the time from ingestion to sampling. Concentration-time points above the line are associated with a significant risk of serious liver damage in previously normal subjects. Concentrations which lie below the line at any given time are unlikely to be associated with serious damage.

In general, patients who were previously normal should be treated if the concentration lies on or above the line on the graph (and for pragmatic reasons if the concentration is just below the line). Some patients are at greater risk than normal (see below), but previously normal patients do not require treatment if the concentration is clearly below the line at the corresponding time from ingestion to sampling.

The graph starts at 4 hours after overdosage, since absorption can be assumed to be complete by then. The concentration in samples taken before 4 hours is uninterpretable.

Data after about 16 hours are lacking, and certainly by 24 hours the concentration of paracetamol can fall to low levels even after significant overdosage.

There are often ambiguities: if the overdosage is taken over several hours, for example, should the time elapsed between overdosage and sampling be counted from the beginning, middle, or end of the period over which the overdose was taken? It is, in practice, wisest to take the worst case.

It is important to know that the stated dose of paracetamol taken does not correspond well to the concentration measured some time afterwards. This may be due in part to vomiting or failure of absorption, in part to differences in individual rates of metabolism, and in part to the uncertainties in the patient's account. The concentration in blood, not the dose, is the determinant of damage.

Having said that the dose is not a good predictor of damage, it is clear that most patients who go on to develop serious features of paracetamol poisoning have in fact taken more than 150 milligrams per kilogram body-weight (that is, about 10 grams of paracetamol in an adult).

14.2.3 Patients at increased risk

The paracetamol 'nomogram' indicates risk for previously normal people. Some patients are at increased risk:

(1) patients who are malnourished, for example from AIDS or anorexia nervosa, and who therefore have depleted amino-acid stores to begin with;

(2) patients who have already taken an overdose of paracetamol within a few days prior to the current overdose, but have not been treated, since the original overdosage may have been enough to deplete amino-acid stores without itself causing serious liver damage; and

(3) patients who habitually drink heavily or who take anticonvulsant drugs, or other drugs that induce liver enzymes (increase the rate of metabolism catalysed by them), because the breakdown of paracetamol to NABQI is enhanced in such patients, who therefore produce larger amounts of NABQI for a given paracetamol concentration than do normal people.

Patients at increased risk should be treated at or above a concentration half as great as the concentration indicating risk in previously normal subjects at the same time between overdosage and sampling.

14.3 Forensic problems

Forensic problems related to paracetamol poisoning usually concern potentially negligent treatment.

CASE 14.1

A 23-year-old barmaid became depressed after her boyfriend died at sea. She had a Chinese meal and some alcohol one night, went home, and took an overdose of between 20 and 30 paracetamol tablets at about 3 a.m. She had subsequently vomited several times, and by 11.30 p.m. was sufficiently unwell that her mother telephoned the family's general practitioner. He advised fluids, and arranged to see the girl the next morning.

She was in fact seen by a partner, who arranged her admission to hospital. She became increasingly unwell, and died from liver failure in spite of care at a specialist liver unit.

The parents of the dead girl reported the general practitioner to the General Medical Council for serious professional misconduct.

The doctor argued that the dose was small, and some of the tablets had in fact been vomited back. He also argued that as 20 hours had already gone by, little active treatment could have been give to save the woman.

A dose of 30 tablets (15 grams) can certainly be lethal in a normal subject; and a barmaid might be expected to drink more than usual, and so be susceptible to paracetamol-induced damage.

It is true that the efficacy of specific antidotes to paracetamol poisoning wanes as the interval from overdosage increases above 8 hours. However, there is increasing evidence that acetylcysteine is safe after overdosage and can be helpful even in the late stages of poisoning. It is also the case that supportive care in hospital, with fluid replacement, attention to the blood glucose concentration and prophylactic (preventive) treatment for liver failure, might have been helpful.

The woman might have died even if given the best possible care, and the general practitioner was exonerated.

CASE 14.2

A 16-year-old girl, previously healthy, took about 20 paracetamol tablets one morning and was seen in a hospital casualty department soon afterwards. She was treated with activated charcoal (which can bind the drug in the stomach and prevent its absorption) and at 4 hours after overdose, a blood sample was taken that showed a concentration of 1.04 millimoles of paracetamol per litre.

The 'nomogram' line passes through 1.32 millimoles per litre (200 milligrams per litre) at four hours, so the measured concentration, 20 per cent below the line, was unlikely to be associated with severe liver damage. The girl was discharged into the care of her parents.

Unfortunately, she became unwell, and the general practitioner was contacted. Eventually, she was re-admitted to hospital, where she was found to be suffering from liver failure, and in spite of transfer to a specialist liver unit, she died.

There are several possible explanations for the events. These include an error in estimating the time of overdose, or deception as to the time of overdose; an error in taking the blood sample, mislabelling of the blood sample, or inaccurate analysis of the paracetamol concentration; and an extremely unusual and unsuspected susceptibility to paracetamol.

The dead girl's family was devastated by her potentially avoidable death, and by the difficulties of demonstrating negligence when the hospital doctor had apparently followed a set protocol for deciding on treatment.

14.4 Summary

Paracetamol is widely available: more widely than many realize, since many branded preparations contain the drug. When taken in overdosage, it has the potential to cause fatal liver damage. If prompt and competent treatment is given, then antidotal therapy is likely to be effective. However, if treatment is delayed, the outcome can be serious.

15

Anabolic androgens (anabolic steroids)

The paradigm anabolic androgen is the naturally occurring sex hormone testosterone, which exerts its actions through specific cellular receptors in the cytoplasm (intracellular fluid) of target cells (Lukas 1993). Testosterone is responsible for the development of male sexual characteristics *in utero* and for the changes that occur in male maturation: it is *androgenic*.

In eunuchoid ('eunuch-like') men, testosterone also helps to restore muscle mass: it is *anabolic* (Kenyon *et al.* 1938). This observation led to a hunt for related compounds that had anabolic properties without androgenic effects. An animal experimental model, the castrated rat, provided a test-bed (a 'guinea-pig'). The change in weight in the levator ani (a muscle whose name means 'anus-lifter') was compared with the change in weight of part of the prostate gland under the influence of the test drug (Kochackian 1976). In practice, all anabolic drugs are also androgenic.

The evidence that standard therapeutic doses of anabolic androgens increase muscle power in normal men is equivocal (Elashof *et al.* 1991); however, it seems that high doses may increase both muscle bulk and muscle power in weightlifters who are also training hard (Lukas 1993).

15.1 The drugs

The anabolic androgens, both naturally occurring and synthetic, can be divided into those that are orally active, and those that have to be given by injection in order to act. Testosterone itself is in the latter category, though a derivative, testosterone undecanoate, can be given by mouth. The drugs are listed in Table 15.1.

15.2 Therapeutic use of anabolic androgens

The only recognized uses of these drugs are:

1. To replace male sex steroids in men who have androgen deficiency. This could result, for example, from the loss of both testes.
2. The treatment of certain rare forms of aplastic anaemia (anaemia in which there is a lack of blood-forming cells in the bone marrow), which are, or may, be responsive to androgens.
3. Stanozolol is indicated in some rare conditions (hereditary angioedema and Behçet's disease); and in the palliation of itching from jaundice in terminal cancer. Nandrolone has been used to treat post-menopausal osteoporosis.

Table 15.1 Some anabolic-androgenic steroids

Orally active agents
    fluoxymesterone ('Testoral', 'Ultradren')
    mesterolone ('Pro-Viron'[a])
    methandienone ('Dianabol', 'Metanabol')
    methyltestosterone ('Primotest')
    oxandrolone ('Anavar')
    oxymetholone ('Anapolon'[a], 'Anasteron')
    stanozolol ('Stromba')
    testosterone undecanoate ('Restandol'[a])

Injectable agents
    methenalone enanthate ('Primobolan')
    nandrolone esters ('Deca Durabolin'[a], 'Durabolin'[a])
    testosterone ('Primoteston Depot'[a], 'Sustanon'[a], 'Virormone'[a])
    trenbolone ('Finajet'[b])

[a] Listed in the *British National Formulary*, 27th ed. 1994.
[b] Licensed as a veterinary product only.

These therapeutic uses create no major difficulties, except perhaps when 'androgen deficiency' is interpreted to mean any reduction in libido or potency for any reason, for example, depression, boredom, or old age.

15.3 Abuse of anabolic androgens

Although the evidence is lacking from controlled experiments of increased muscle bulk or power when taking anabolic androgens, there is no doubt that they are perceived as dramatically useful in improving athletic performance. After Ben Johnson's steroid-powered victory in the 1988 Olympic 100 metres final, even sceptics might be forgiven for thinking that controlled experiments are unnecessary (Ferner and Rawlins 1988).

The result is that body-builders (McKillop 1987), weightlifters, and athletes at all levels (Scarpino *et al.* 1990), including schoolchildren (Buckley *et al.* 1988) and non-competitive athletes, take anabolic androgens in order to increase muscle bulk and power.

Abusers often take enormous doses. *Stacking*, which is taking several different steroid preparations together; *pyramiding*, which describes the habit of increasing and then decreasing the dosage over a period of weeks; and *cycling*, alternating periods when the drugs are taken and not taken, are all common.

In body-building, the desiderata are to achieve muscle bulk and muscle definition, preferably accompanied by vascularity, that is, veins that stand out. Male and female practitioners go to enormous lengths to achieve these ends, taking bizarre diets and sometimes abusing diuretics ('water tablets'), thyroid hormones and growth hormones as well as anabolic androgens.

15.4 Physical adverse effects of high doses of anabolic androgens[1]

The anabolic androgens, especially in high dosages, cause severe adverse effects. Effects in women and men are somewhat different.

[1] From Ferner, R. E. *Anabolic steroids*. World Health Organization/International Program for Chemical Safety poisons information monograph, in press.

In women, anabolic androgens can cause virilization (the appearance of male characteristics). They can develop facial hair, male-pattern baldness, acne, deep male voices, atrophic (shrunken) breasts, and enlargement of the clitoris (Strauss *et al.* 1985). The changes are not reversible. The androgens also result in irregular periods.

In men, the early occurrence of prostatic enlargement and prostatic cancer have been described (Roberts and Essenhigh 1986). Although libido can increase initially, prolonged exposure to high doses leads to testicular atrophy (shrinkage), impotence, and infertility.

Adolescents are at risk of premature closure of the epiphyses (the growing centres in the long bones) which results in failure to achieve full height.

Both sexes can develop the following disorders:

1. Diseases of the heart and blood vessels: high blood pressure, left ventricular hypertrophy (enlargement of the main heart chamber), and premature disease of the coronary arteries, that can lead to myocardial infarction ('heart attack').
2. Diseases of the nervous system: stroke
3. Diseases of the liver: the orally active anabolic androgens can cause liver damage. This is most often seen as a change in the biochemical tests, but can result in obvious jaundice. Rare liver tumours have occasionally been described.
4. Skin disease: severe acne is a common consequence of anabolic androgen abuse.
5. Metabolic disease: anabolic androgens cause glucose intolerance (a stage in the development of 'sugar diabetes') and hypercholesterolaemia (an increase in the cholesterol level in the blood).

15.5 Psychiatric effects of anabolic androgens

The popularly imagined link between male sex hormones and aggression has experimental support. In a study where male volunteers were given methyltestosterone or placebo, the active drug resulted in more 'irritability, mood swings, violent feelings, and hostility' than the placebo (Su *et al.* 1993).

In another study, anabolic androgen abusers were compared with body-builders who did not use drugs. The abusers were significantly more likely to suffer episodes of disordered mood, for example, excitement or depression, than the non-users. Abusers also suffered sometimes from a distorted body image, believing that they were puny even though in fact they were large and muscular. The authors have coined the term 'reverse anorexia nervosa' for this distortion (Pope and Katz 1994).

Hallucination and delusion have been described in abusers (Pope and Katz 1994). Depression is a fairly common sequel to withdrawal from anabolic androgens.

15.6 The forensic importance of anabolic androgens

First, the use of anabolic androgens is banned in many sports, and so their use can lead to severe penalties for athletes who are caught.

The International Olympic Committee, the United Kingdom Sports Council (Badewitz-Dodd 1991), and other regulatory bodies lay down lists of banned substances and products, together with rules for detecting their use and action to be taken if results are positive.

Banned drugs include testosterone, anabolic steroids derived from it, and peptide hormones (notably gonadotrophin releasing hormone and human chorionic gonadotrophin) that cause its increased secretion[2].

The perceived advantages of taking anabolic androgens include an increase in muscle strength, a faster recovery from hard muscular exertion, and increased 'competitiveness', a synonym for aggression. The increase in aggression leads to the second forensic problem—that the aggression and changes in mood produced by anabolic androgens can precipitate violence. The behaviour usually takes the form of direct physical violence.

The impotence that can be caused by anabolic androgens is sometimes accompanied by morbid jealousy.

CASE 15.1

A 29-year-old bar doorman ('bouncer') and former boxer took oral and injectable anabolic androgens in large doses to improve his physique. He found that they made him 'snappy' (bad-tempered), where previously he had been placid. At first, his libido had increased, but he later found that he had difficulty in maintaining erections. He returned home one night and accused his girlfriend of seeing other men while he had been at work. She had in fact been at home. He went berserk, smashing her in the face repeatedly with an ash-tray and then stabbing her in the chest. She required urgent thoracic surgery to save her life and plastic surgery to repair her damaged face.

He was remanded on a charge of attempted murder. While he was on remand in prison, his girlfriend decided to marry him, and refused to give evidence against him. The charge of murder was dropped but he was still charged with wounding with intent to cause grievous bodily harm, under Section 18 of the Offences against the Person Act 1861. The defence sought to establish in mitigation that the jealousy and the aggressive outburst were the result of the anabolic androgens. This may indeed have been so, though the issue was never tested in court as the accused was shot dead shortly before his trial.

The aggressive behaviour can sometimes be manifest as a change in personality, with criminal behaviour related to a loss of control, but not taking the form of 'lashing out'.

CASE 15.2 (SCHULTE *ET AL.* 1993)

A 19-year-old college athlete took intramuscular testosterone and oral methandrostenolone (yet another orally active anabolic androgen) over a period of 4 months. He became increasingly aggressive with his wife and child. After he had scalded the child's buttocks with boiling water, he stopped taking anabolic androgens, and his violence and aggression resolved within 2 months.

The drug-taker can also suffer as the result of impulsiveness and aggression against himself. Coroners at inquest are required to form a judgement as to when, where, and by what means the deceased has met his death, and drug-taking can have an influence on the verdict.

CASE 15.3

A 36-year-old man had for many years held a firearms certificate for a revolver. One day, after he had been ill with a chest infection, he had a trivial argument with his wife about buying catfood, went upstairs and shot himself dead with the revolver. His general practitioner was called soon afterwards and discovered some pills which he had not prescribed, but which it transpired were taken by the deceased for body-building, and which included anabolic androgens (anabolic steroids). The court heard that anabolic androgens cause both depression and unpredictable outbursts of aggression.

[2] Interestingly, neither alcohol nor marijuana is banned by the International Olympic Committee.

The coroner found that the deceased had taken his own life 'whilst the balance of his mind was disturbed by the anabolic steroids'.

A third forensic problem concerns the supplying of anabolic androgens. Supplying and trafficking in anabolic androgens is likely to become a criminal offence in the United Kingdom (Travis, 1994). The Home Secretary is to make the offence punishable by up to 5 years in prison, with an unlimited fine. Possession for personal use will not be an offence.

15.7 Summary

Anabolic androgens have only a few recognized therapeutic uses, and their forensic importance lies in their susceptibility to abuse, sometimes in enormous doses, and their liability to cause severe adverse effects. The adverse effects encountered in abusers include increased aggression, which entrains further forensic problems.

Appendix A Pharmacokinetic calculations

A.1 Some further details of the dosage of drugs

The amount of a drug is usually measured either in mass units (by 'weight') or in molar units. Certain substances, notably insulin and some vitamins, are measured in other, internationally agreed, units.

Measures of weight are usually based on the metric Système International (SI) unit, the kilogram. The most common measures in pharmacology are the gram (1/1000 of a kilogram), the milligram (1/1 000 000 of a kilogram) and the microgram (1/1 000 000 000 of a kilogram).

Molar units are based not on the weight of drug present, but on the number of molecules of drug. Since drugs work through the interactions of one molecule with another, pharmacological effects are determined by the number of molecules. In practice, the mass of a molecule of any particular chemical compound is constant, so a given weight of that compound always contains a fixed number of molecules.

The primary molar unit is the *mole*, the quantity which contains a particular number of molecules, Avogadro's number. This enormous number, 6.023×10^{23}, is the number of hydrogen atoms (H) which weigh 1 gram. A mole of hydrogen molecules (H_2) weighs 2 grams, because there are two hydrogen atoms in each molecule. The weights of Avogadro's number of atoms of each of the elements have been measured by experiment. These weights are called atomic weights. If the formula of a molecule is known, the weight of a mole, the gram molecular weight, can be calculated.

For example, the formula for ethanol (ethyl alcohol), is C_2H_5OH. The ethanol molecule contains 2 atoms of carbon, each of atomic weight 12 grams, 6 atoms of hydrogen, each with an atomic weight of 1 gram, and an oxygen atom of atomic weight 16 grams. One mole of ethanol therefore weighs:

carbon 2×12 = 24 +
hydrogen 6×1 =   6 +
oxygen 1×16 = 16
                              ——
                              46 grams.

A bottle of wine, which contains about 75 grams of ethanol, therefore contains 75/46 moles of ethanol, that is, 1.63 moles of ethanol. This is the same as saying that there are $1.63 \times$ Avogadro's number of ethanol molecules in the bottle, very nearly 10^{24}, or 1 000 000 000 000 000 000 000 000 molecules!

A.2 Concentration in calculations

A.2.1 Calculating amount from concentration

If the concentration of a compound and the total volume in which it is distributed are known, then the total amount of compound present can be calculated:

$$\text{total amount} = \frac{\text{concentration}}{\text{(amount per unit volume)}} \times \text{total volume.}$$

For example, if the concentration of ethanol in a particular wine is 100 grams per litre, then the total amount of ethanol in a glass whose volume is 180 millilitres (0.18 litres) is:

$$100 \times 0.18 = 18 \text{ grams.}$$

A.2.2 Calculating volume from concentration

The concept of concentration can also be used to determine an unknown volume. A known amount of a substance is introduced into the unknown volume, and mixed so that the concentration is uniform. Measuring the concentration then allows the volume to be calculated.

For example, to determine the volume of a bath of water, we could add 1 gram of red dye to the bathwater, mix it thoroughly, and then take a sample. Let us suppose that the concentration of dye in the sample is 25 milligrams per litre (which is 0.025 grams per litre). Then:

$$\frac{\text{the total volume}}{\text{of the bath}} \times \frac{\text{the concentration of}}{\text{dye per unit volume}} = \frac{\text{total amount of}}{\text{dye in the bath,}}$$

or

$$\text{total volume of bath in litres} \times 0.025 \text{ grams per litre} = 1 \text{ gram,}$$

or

$$\text{total volume of bath} = 1/0.025 = 40 \text{ litres}$$

Clearly, the greater the unknown volume, the smaller the concentration that we find after mixing in a given amount of dye.

A.3 Calculations using volume of distribution

A.3.1 Using volume of distribution and concentration to estimate dose

Consider an injection of a known amount of a particular drug into the bloodstream. The concentration of drug in the blood falls after injection, partly because of distribution of the drug out of the bloodstream and into the tissues, and partly because the drug is being changed by metabolic processes or being excreted by the kidney and other organs.

When mixing and distribution have occurred, but before any elimination has taken place:

$$\frac{\text{volume of distribution}}{\text{(units of volume)}} \times \frac{\text{concentration}}{\text{(amount per unit volume)}} = \frac{\text{dose.}}{\text{(amount)}}$$

After some elimination has taken place, the total quantity of drug in the body is less than the dose, but the concentration in blood has also fallen, and the ratio between total amount of drug and the amount in the blood stays constant:

volume of distribution × concentration in blood = quantity in body.

That is, the volume of distribution also represents the ratio between the total amount of drug in the body and the amount in one unit volume of blood.

A.3.2 A forensic example

The volume of distribution of a drug can provide useful forensic information.

CASE A.1

A 3-week-old baby died 15 hours after being given a dose of medicine. Post-mortem examination revealed severe brain damage, probably due to violent shaking, and the father was charged with murder.

The defence discovered that the mother could not read, and that there was a bottle of 'Phenergan' syrup in the house. 'Phenergan' is the sedative antihistamine promethazine. The baby's blood at death contained 30 micrograms of promethazine per litre. The baby weighed 4 kilograms.

Had the baby been given an overdose of promethazine, which might have caused or contributed to its death?

To answer this, it is first necessary to determine how much promethazine was in the baby's body at the time it died. Promethazine has a volume of distribution in adults of approximately 13 litres per kilogram body-weight. It is much greater than the physical volume of the body, because promethazine is readily taken up into fat. Babies have a higher proportion of body fat than adults, so their volume of distribution for promethazine may be even higher per kilogram than that of adults.

As an approximation, take the baby's volume of distribution for promethazine to be 13 litres per kilogram. Since the baby weighed 4 kilograms,

$$\text{the volume of distribution} = 13 \text{ (litres/kilogram)} \times 4 \text{ (kilograms)}$$
$$= 52 \text{ litres}$$

The concentration of promethazine, which is the weight of promethazine in 1 litre of blood, was 30 micrograms. Therefore, the weight of promethazine in the baby's body was:

$$\text{amount (micrograms)} = \text{weight in 1 litre} \times \text{volume in litres}$$
$$= 30 \times 52 \text{ micrograms}$$
$$= 1560 \text{ micrograms}$$
$$= 1.56 \text{ milligrams.}$$

The minimum dose of promethazine that the baby could have received was 1.56 milligrams. Because only a fraction of the oral dose is absorbed into the body and since a proportion of the absorbed drug would have been eliminated over the 15 hours since the dose was given, the amount administered must in fact have been higher. (Consideration of this case is continued on p. 189.)

A.4 The calculations of drug disposition

A.4.1 First-order kinetics

Basic calculations

At any given instant, the rate of disappearance of a drug that undergoes first-order disposition depends upon the concentration of the drug at that instant. Such processes are also called exponential[1], because the concentration C_t at some time t can be related to the initial concentration C_0 by an equation in the form;

$$C_t = C_0.e^{-k.t}$$

or, taking logarithms,

$$k.t = \ln C_0/C_t.$$

The parameter k is the *rate constant*, which is one of the characteristics of an exponential process. The rate constant is related to the proportional change in concentration in unit time. It is in fact the (natural) logarithm of the ratio of the concentrations at the beginning and end of a unit time-period, say C_0 and C_1 respectively. It is related to the *half-life*, which is the time taken for the concentration to change by 50 per cent.

Exponential growth is illustrated by the tale of the good sultan and his grand vizier, who advised him how to confound the bad sultan: 'take a chess-board, Oh Master, and ask him to place one grain of rice on the first square, two on the second square, four on the third square, and so on, doubling the number of grains from one square to the next'. The good sultan followed the grand vizier's advice, and the bad sultan laughed; but he soon found that there was not enough rice in his whole kingdom to cover the chess-board.

The number of grains of rice on successive squares increases very rapidly, and on the sixty-fourth square there are 2^{63} grains, or nearly $10\,000\,000\,000\,000\,000\,000$.

The disappearance of many drugs proceeds exponentially.

Calculations from the elimination rate constant

We have discussed on p. 21 the disposition of paracetamol, whose concentration in blood falls by 16 per cent per hour. So it would fall from 160 to 84 to 71 to 59 milligrams per litre in successive hours.

In this example, the rate constant, k, is:

$$k = \ln C_0/C_1 = \ln 100/84 \, (= \ln 84/71 = \ln 71/59 = \ln 59/50)$$
$$= 0.17$$

The ratio of the concentrations can be derived from the rate constant by transforming the equation:

$$C_0/C_1 = e^k = 1.19 : 1.$$

---

[1] An 'exponent' is a 'power'. For example, in the expression $3^2=9$, the exponent is 2; in $3^3=27$, the exponent is 3. The mathematical symbol 'e' is the sum of a series called the exponential series, the basis for natural logarithms:

$$e^x = 1 + x + \frac{x^2}{2.1} + \frac{x^3}{3.2.1} + \frac{x^4}{4.3.2.1} + \ldots.$$

A forensic example using first-order kinetics

CASE A.1 (CONTINUED)

In this case, discussed in Section A.3.2, the concentration of promethazine in the baby's blood 15 hours after he was brought to hospital was 30 micrograms per litre. No promethazine was given while the baby was in hospital. What was the promethazine concentration when the baby was admitted?

The elimination rate constant, k, for promethazine is approximately 0.058 per hour in normal adults. So,

$$\ln C_0/C_t = k.t$$
$$= 0.058 \times 15 = 0.87$$

and,

$$C_0/C_t = 2.4$$

and,

$$C_0 = 2.4 \times C_t$$
$$= 2.4 \times 30$$
$$= 72 \text{ micrograms per litre.}$$

The concentration of promethazine on admission was 72 micrograms per litre, assuming that the elimination rate constant is the same in a baby who is seriously ill as in an adult.

In considering how large a dose the child received, we previously calculated that the dose was at least 1.56 milligrams. On the basis of the present calculation, the amount in the baby's body when he arrived at hospital was 2.4 times as great, that is:

amount of promethazine in the body on admission = $2.4 \times 1.56 = 3.7$ milligrams

It becomes increasingly likely that the baby was deliberately given the drug, as one tea-spoonful of the paediatric syrup contains 5 milligrams of promethazine.

Appendix B Detailed aspects of measurement of ethanol and calculations based on ethanol concentration

B.1 Peak-height ratios in gas chromatography

This Section explains the quantitation of gas chromatograms referred to in Section 7.1.2. Peak-height is an approximation for peak area, and the latter is now generally used. By way of example, consider the case where an unknown solution is compared with solutions of concentration 50 milligrams per 100 millilitre, and 200 milligrams per 100 millilitre. If the ratio of the peak areas of the calibration samples to the peak areas of the internal standards are, say 0.73:1 and 2.92:1, then we can calculate that an ethanol peak with the same area as the peak of internal standard would be equivalent to an ethanol concentration of 50/0.73 or 200/2.92, that is, 68.5 milligrams of ethanol per 100 millilitres. The two calibration readings give the same result, showing that the system is linear between 50 and 200 milligrams per 100 millilitres. This means that there is a simple straight-line relationship between peak area and ethanol concentration in this range: double the peak area indicates double the ethanol concentration.

If the two results do not agree, the system is not linear, and it is not possible to be sure of the unknown concentration. If the unknown concentration is outside the range which is known to be linear, then the sample should be diluted or the concentration of the calibration samples changed, since it cannot be assumed that the system is still linear outside the calibration range.

Let us say that the unknown ethanol peak area is 1.5 that of the internal standard. Then the concentration of ethanol in the unknown is $(50/0.73) \times 1.5 = 102.7$ milligrams per 100 millilitres.

The unknown has been mixed with internal standard and may have been diluted. Time has gone by, and ethanol may have evaporated. To be sure that the result truly represents the ethanol concentration in the original sample, it is usual to assay a second sample (duplicate sample or duplicate), and to check that the results for the two samples agree.

B.2 Watson's equations for total body water (TBW) in human subjects

Ethanol is distributed in body water, and the percentage of water for an individual can be calculated. Useful equations based on over 700 people aged between 17and 86 were derived by Watson *et al.* (1980):

In men:

mean TBW = 2.45 + (0.107 × height) + (0.336 × weight) − (0.0952 × age).

In women:

mean TBW = −2.10 + (0.107 × height) + (0.247 × weight),

where TBW is the total body water in litres, and age is measured in years, height in centimetres and weight in kilograms.

B.3 The use of Watson's formula and the Widmark equation

CASE B.1

A man aged 34 years, who was 168 centimetres (5 feet 6 inches) tall and weighed 118 kilograms (18 stones 8 pounds), had a blood ethanol concentration of 150 milligrams per 100 millilitres of blood when arrested by the police beside his motor-car. How much ethanol was in his body at the time of his arrest ?

First, his TBW is given by Watson's regression equation (Section B.2) as:

TBW $= 2.45 + (0.107 \times 168) + (0.336 \times 118) - (0.0952 \times 34)$
$= 56.8$ litres
$= 568$ decilitres (1 decilitre $= 100$ millilitres).

Concentration of ethanol in water $=$ concentration in blood / fraction of water in blood
$= 150/0.8$ milligrams per 100 millilitres
$= 187.5$ milligrams per 100 millilitres of water.

So,

total amount of ethanol in the body

$=$ concentration in water $\times$ volume of water
$= 187.5 \times 568$ milligrams
$= 106500$ milligrams
$= 106.5$ grams.

This is equivalent to about a third of a bottle of whisky.

The standard calculation, using a Widmark factor r of 0.68, gives the weight of ethanol in the body as 120.4 grams, 13 per cent more than the calculation based on total body water.

B.4 Back-calculation of ethanol concentration

Back-calculation is illustrated by the following cases:

CASE B.2

The 35–year–old manager of a public house drank some beer and a whisky between 7 p.m. and 9 p.m. one night. At 11.30 p.m., he was involved in a motor-car accident, and at 12.30 a.m. his blood ethanol concentration was measured at 56 milligrams per 100 millilitres of blood. What was his ethanol concentration at the time of the accident?

Over 2 hours had passed between the last drink and the accident, so it is reasonable to assume complete ethanol absorption. One hour passed between the accident and the estimation of blood ethanol concentration. On the assumption that the subject metabolized ethanol at the average rate,

amount removed in 1 hour = 18.7 milligrams per 100 millilitres,

therefore,

blood concentration at the time of the accident

$$= \text{concentration 1 hour later} + \text{amount removed in 1 hour},$$
$$= 56 + 18.7 \text{ milligrams per 100 millilitres}$$
$$= 74.7 \text{ milligrams per 100 millilitres}$$

which is below the legal limit of 80 milligrams per 100 millilitres.

In fact, he might have had either very fast, or less likely, very slow ethanol metabolism. Using the fastest and slowest rates of ethanol removal yields the boundaries for the likely ethanol concentration 1 hour before:

lowest likely concentration $= 12.5 + 56$
$$= 68.5 \text{ milligrams per 100 millilitres}$$

highest likely concentration $= 25 + 56$
$$= 81 \text{ milligrams per 100 millilitres}$$

We can be reasonably confident that the true ethanol concentration in blood at the time of the accident was between 69 and 81 milligrams per 100 millilitres; in an average man, it would have been 75 milligrams per 100 millilitres.

The interval between the accident and the ethanol analysis was quite short in this example, but the extreme estimates none the less lie on either side of the permitted ethanol concentration for a driver.

CASE B.3

In another case (Brahms 1988b; Dyer 1988b), a man named Gumbley drank until 10.45 p.m., and was involved in a motor-car accident at 11.15 p.m. in which his brother was killed. Afterwards he felt sick, and vomited, and was then taken to hospital. As a result, a specimen for blood ethanol concentration was not taken until 4 hours 20 minutes after the accident, when it was 59 milligrams per 100 millilitres blood.

Is it likely that the blood ethanol concentration was above the legal limit, which is 80 milligrams per 100 millilitres, 4 hours and 20 minutes prior to the measurement of 59 milligrams per 100 millilitres? Let us assume that the concentration was in fact exactly 80 milligrams per 100 millilitres. Then, if all the ethanol already consumed was absorbed by the time of the accident, the least amount that could have been eliminated (if the concentration were 80 milligrams per 100 millilitres) was

$80 - 59 = 21$ milligrams per 100 millilitres.

Provided all the ethanol which had been drunk had already been absorbed, we can calculate the elimination rate which would have just been enough to reduce the blood ethanol concentration from 80 to 59 milligrams/100 millilitres in 4.3 hours (4 hours and 20 minutes), as

rate $= (80–59)/4.3 = 21/4.33 = 4.8$ milligrams per 100 millilitres per hour.

It is beyond reasonable doubt that the true rate was higher than this, because there is a 95 per cent chance that it lies between 12.5 and 25 milligrams per 100 millilitres per hour.

B.5 Calculations in the hip-flask defence

The following case illustrates the calculations.

CASE B.4

A man who weighed 76 kilograms (12 stones), reportedly drank 2 pints of Newcastle Scotch Beer (3.6 per cent ethanol by volume) between 4.15 p.m. and 5.15 p.m., and then drove to his grand-mother's house, where he was struck down with diarrhoea, and his brother provided him with the family remedy for this condition: three double measures of a mixture of brandy and port wine. He was followed to the house by a policeman, who subsequently arrested him for driving with excess ethanol in the breath. A sample taken at 6 p.m. in the police station gave a reading of 73 micro-grams ethanol per 100 millilitres breath. 'We need to know if, when   driving his car at 17.15 hours, our client would have been under the limit, and whether the reading of 73 micrograms per 100 millilitres could have been the result of the combination of Scotch beer, brandy and port', wrote the instructing solicitor.

The steps in the calculations are as follows:

1. *Determine the volume of distribution of ethanol for the subject.* If only the weight is known, then Widmark's formula may have to be used:

volume in which ethanol is distributed = $r \times$ body weight (in kilograms)

The average of Widmark's r for a man = 0.68, with upper and lower limits of $\pm$ 25 per cent. The conversion factor for stones to kilograms = 6.25,

so body weight $= 12 \times 6.25 = 76$ kilograms
and volume of distribution $= 0.68 \times 76$ litres in the average case
$= 52$ litres.

The highest value is 25 per cent greater than this, that is, 65 litres.

If the age and height of the subject are known, Watson's formula is likely to be better. Let us assume that he was 40 years old and 68 inches (173 centimetres) tall. Then

TBW $= 2.45 + (0.107 \times 173) + (0.336 \times 76) - (0.0952 \times 40)$
$= 42.7$ litres.

Converting this to the equivalent volume of blood:

equivalent volume of blood $=$ TBW/proportion of water in blood
$= 42.7/0.8 = 53.4$ litres

The upper limit is approximately 10 per cent higher, that is 58.7 litres, and the lower limit 48.1 litres.

2. *From the volume of distribution, the maximum blood ethanol concentration after an ethanol load can be calculated.* In this case, the 2 pints of beer were drunk over 1 hour, and it is reason-able to assume that there would be no 'overshoot' in blood ethanol concentration due to very rapid absorption accompanied by slow distribution to the water in tissues. Therefore,

the peak ethanol concentration, C_{max}, will be less than, or equal to, dose/volume of distribution:

C_{max} = dose of ethanol/volume of distribution.

The dose of ethanol =	volume	× proportion by volume	× relative density
(in grams)	(millilitres)	of ethanol	(grams/millilitre)
		(% by volume)	

2 pints   = 2 × 568 = 1136 millilitres beer
volume of ethanol   = 1136 × 3.6/100 = 40.9 millilitres
weight of ethanol   = 40.9 × 0.791 = 32.6 grams.

So, C_{max} = 32.6/53.4 = 0.61 grams per litre of blood, or
                               = 610 milligrams per litre, or
                               = 61 milligrams per 100 millilitres.

Only a small proportion of the population is 'average', and by definition approximately half will have smaller than average volumes of distribution for ethanol, and therefore higher peak ethanol concentrations. However, using the smallest likely volume of distribution from Watson's formula, 48.1 litres, yields:

highest likely C_{max} = 32.6/48.1 = 0.678 grams/litre
                               = 67.8 milligrams per 100 millilitres.

So the conclusion from this part of the calculation is that if the subject was an average man who had only drunk 2 pints of beer with an ethanol concentration of 3.6 per cent by volume, then his blood ethanol concentration would not have exceeded 61 milligrams per 100 millilitres, and even in the extreme case of a very small volume of distribution, it would not have exceeded 68 milligrams per 100 millilitres.

3. *Establish whether the breath ethanol concentration that was actually observed was compatible with the drinking history.* Two sources of ethanol have to be considered, the beer and the mixed diarrhoea remedy. The assessment of the effect of the remedy is made more difficult by the short time between drinking it and having a breath sample taken. The assumption cannot be made that the ethanol was all absorbed before the test was taken, since at most 45 minutes elapsed between drinking and being tested. This has two effects. The ratio between breath ethanol and blood ethanol concentration is unlikely to have reached the equilibrium value of 2300:1, and the blood ethanol concentration may be less than the expected peak, because the concentration is still rising, or greater than the expected peak because the diarrhoea has been associated with rapid gastric emptying, the absorption has been rapid, and distribution of ethanol into tissue water has been relatively slow.

4. *Calculate the contribution from the mixture of brandy and port.* Let us assume that the mixture contained three measures of brandy (40 per cent ethanol by volume) and three measures of port (20 per cent ethanol by volume), equivalent to a mixture of six measures containing 30 per cent ethanol by volume. 1 measure was a sixth of a gill, which is a quarter of a pint, so 1 measure was one 24th of a pint, or 568/24 = 23.7 millilitres. (It is now defined as 25 millilitres.) The density (ratio of weight to volume) of ethanol is 0.791 grams per millilitre, so

dose $= 6 \times 23.7 \times (30/100) \times 0.791 = 34.0$ grams ethanol,

and

C_{max} $= 34.0/53.4 = 0.636$ grams per litre
$= 63.6$ milligrams per 100 millilitres,

assuming an average volume of distribution.

5. *Find the amount of ethanol remaining from beer drunk previously.* We have calculated that the maximum concentration after drinking the beer would have been 61.6 milligrams per 100 millilitres, given an average volume of distribution. This peak is calculated on the assumption that no ethanol is eliminated before complete absorption has taken place, but in practice the two processes will have been occurring simultaneously, and ethanol will have been removed from the circulation throughout the time of drinking. Even if we allow for a lag before the ethanol concentration begins to rise, as would be reasonable for beer, or if the subject had eaten, the lag is unlikely to have been more than 30 minutes. Therefore we can assume that ethanol has been disappearing at a constant rate from 4.45 p.m. to 6 p.m.; that is, over 1 hour and 15 minutes.

The rate at which the ethanol has been disappearing can, for practical purposes, be taken to be Widmark's β. An average value of 18.7 milligrams per 100 millilitres per hour gives the fall in blood ethanol concentration to be:

Fall in concentration $=$ rate of fall $\times$ time
$= 18.7 \times 1.25$
$= 23.4$ milligrams per 100 millilitres.

Using the upper value of 25 milligrams per 100 millilitres per hour yields a value of 31.3 milligrams per 100 millilitres, and a lower value of 12.5 milligrams per 100 millilitres per hour, a minimum fall of 15.6 milligrams per 100 millilitres.

So, the likely fall in ethanol concentration was 23 milligrams per 100 millilitres, but it could reasonably have been between 16 and 31 milligrams per 100 millilitres.

The peak concentration due to the two different drinking episodes is given by the sum of the two values for C_{max}, this was:

$= 61.0 + 63.6$
$= 125$ milligrams per 100 millilitres (with a margin of $\pm$ 10 per cent).

The likely blood concentration at the time of testing was therefore:

C_t $= C_{max} -$ fall
$= 125 - 23 = 102$ milligrams per 100 millilitres.

The highest value which might reasonably occur would result from the lowest reasonable volume of distribution and the lowest reasonable elimination rate, so

highest reasonable C_t $= 137 - 15.6$
$= 121$ milligrams per 100 millilitres.

6. *Consider the relationship between breath ethanol and blood ethanol concentration.* At equilibrium, a value of 80 000/35 (approximately 2300:1) is assumed. Using this ratio, the likely breath ethanol concentrations are:

average $= 102 \times 35/80\,000 = 44.6$ micrograms per 100 millilitres

highest $= 121 \times 35/80\,000 = 53$ micrograms per 100 millilitres.

If the measured breath ethanol of 73 micrograms per 100 millilitres corresponded to a blood ethanol concentration of 121 milligrams per litre, the blood:breath ethanol concentration ratio would have been 1668:1. This value is not compatible with any reasonable assumptions about a post-absorptive sample, but IS compatible with the stated drinking history and a sample taken during the absorptive phase, when the blood:breath ratio may be even lower than 1668:1.

B.6 Calculations in the lacing defence

The calculations for (or against) the lacing defence follow a similar pattern.

CASE B.5

A typical passage from a solicitor's letter of instruction reads: 'Our client is aged 52 years, is 6 feet 3 inches tall, and weighs 14 stone ... our client was in the Public House all evening drinking lime juice and soda water. We have obtained a statement from one of the customers who confirms that whisky was poured into our client's drink.'

A customer admitted that 'two double whiskies', that is, a sixth of a pint of whisky, were added to the man's drink. The client in question was arrested, and a breath test gave a reading of 69 micrograms per 100 millilitres. The defence solicitors wanted to know whether the lacing of their client's drink could account for such a high breath reading.

The question can be answered by calculating the smallest amount of ethanol which is likely to have led to such a reading, or alternatively, by calculating the highest reading which could have resulted from the stated amount of ethanol. The approach in an individual case might be determined by whether the expert has been retained by the prosecution, when he or she will be keen to show that much more ethanol than the stated amount has been drunk, or by the defence, when it may be possible to argue that at the extreme, the result could be compatible with the story.

1. *Calculation of the volume of distribution for ethanol.* In this case, Watson's formula for a man of 52 years, height 75 inches (190 centimetres), weight 14 stone (88.9 kilograms), gives an average value of

$$\text{TBW} = 2.45 + (0.107 \times 190) + (0.336 \times 88.9) - (0.0952 \times 52)$$
$$= 47.7 \text{ litres}$$

so,

$$\text{equivalent volume of blood} = 47.7/0.8$$
$$= 60 \text{ litres}.$$

The smallest likely volume is 10 per cent less than this, that is 54 litres.

2. *Relationship between breath and blood ethanol level.* No information was given on the time of drinking in relation to the time of the breath test. If the subject had absorbed all the ethanol, the average ratio would be $80\,000/35$, and a breath ethanol of 69 micrograms per 100

millilitres of breath would be equivalent to a blood ethanol concentration of 158 milligrams per 100 millilitres of blood.

3. *Amount of ethanol in the body.* The amount of ethanol in the body = the concentration in blood × the volume of distribution (in decilitres of blood). So,

amount   = $158 \times 600 = 94\,800$ milligrams = 95 grams.

4. *Equivalent volume of spirits.* The weight of ethanol is 95 grams, and relative density 0.791, so the volume would be:

volume   = 95/0.791 millilitres
                      = 120 millilitres of pure ethanol.

If the ethanol is diluted to make up a solution of 40 per cent by volume, as is usual for spirits, then 120 millilitres represents only 40 per cent of the total volume of spirits, and

volume of spirits = $120 \times 100/40$
                      = 300 millilitres.

This is equivalent to over half a pint of spirits.

There may be some difficulty for the defence in arguing that a man could drink over half a pint of spirits in lime juice and soda water without realizing that something was amiss. In any event, the 'friend' in this case claimed to have added only four measures of spirits (one-sixth of a pint) to the defendant's drink.

B.7 The ethanol content of alcoholic drinks

Calculations of the quantity of ethanol consumed require a knowledge of the ethanol concentration in various drinks. Some relevant concentrations are tabulated in Table B.1, but the expert would usually wish to know the particular values for the drinks involved in any specific case. Concentrations in beer are sometimes different in draught beer, bottled beer, and canned beer carrying the same name; and drink bought duty-free or abroad can have a different concentration from the locally marketed product. Fitzgerald and Hume (1987*b*) give a table for drinks in the United States.

Table B.1   Examples of the ethanol content of various drinks

		Ethanol content (% by volume)
Beers		
Stout		
Beamish	can	4.3
Guinness	bottle	4.3
Guinness	can	4.3
Mackeson	can	3
Murphy	can	4.0
Lager—low alcohol		
Kaliber	can	0.05
Swan Light	can	0.9
Tennant's LA	can	1.0

Table B.1 *Continued*

		Ethanol content (% by volume)
Lager		
Carling Black Label		4.1
Carlsberg Special		9.0
Forster's		4.0
Hofmeister Special		9.0
Hofmeister		3.4
Kestrel Super		9.0 (previously 9.5)
Labbat's		4.0
McEwan's		4.0
Stella Artois		5.2 (previously 5.0)
Tennent's Extra		4.8
Tennent's Super		9.0
Tennent's Pilsner		3.4
Bitter, mild, etc.		
Banks's bitter	can	3.8
Banks's mild	can	3.5
Bass	can	4.4
Guinness draught bitter	can	4.4
John Smith's draught bitter	can	4.0
McEwan's Export	can	4.5
Newcastle Brown Ale	can	4.7
Sam Smith's strong pale ale	bottle	5.0
Sam Smith's bitter	can	3.8
Tetley Bitter	can	3.6
Webster's Yorkshire Bitter	can	3.8
Whitbread White Label	can	1.0
Worthington Best Bitter	can	3.8
Cider		
Blackthorn	bottle	5.0
Bulmer's original	can	6.0
Copperhead	can	5.0
Diamond White	can	8.2
Ice Dragon	can	8.2
Strongbow super	can	8.0
Strongbow	can	5.3
Woodpecker	can	3.5
White wines		
Château Liot Barsac 1988		14
Sainsbury's Liebfraumilch		9.5
Sainsbury's Sancerre		11
Wine Society Mâcon Villages		13
Red wines		
Bulgarian Cabernet Sauvignon Sainsbury		12
Ch. Villadiere Lussac-St-Emilion 1990		12.5
Côtes de Beaune Villages Louis Latour		13
Lambrusco light Sainsbury		3.0
Lambrusco Sainsbury		8.0

Table B.1 *Continued*

	Ethanol content (% by volume)
Minervois Safeway	12
Penfold's Cabernet Sauvignon Bin 707	13.5
Wyndham Australian Shiraz	12.5
Sparkling wines	
Freixenet Cordon Negro Cava	11.5
Pommery 1987 Champagne	12.5
Veuve Clicquot Champagne	12
Fortified wines	
Cockburn's Ruby Port	20
Croft Original Sherry	17.5
Emva Cream Cyprus Sherry	15
Garvey Extra Dry Sherry	16
Gonzalez Byass Elegante Sherry	15.5
Harvey's Club Amontillado	17.5
QC British Cream Sherry	15
Stone's Green Ginger Wine	13.5
Aperitifs, etc.	
Campari	23.6
Cinzano	14.7
Dubonnet	14.7
Martini bianco	14.7
Martini rosso	14.7
Noilly Prat	17
Pimms No 1 cup	25
Punt è Mes	16
Spirits	
Beefeater gin	40
Bell's whisky	40
Chartreuse Green	55
Cointreau	40
Drambuie	40
Glenfiddich malt whisky	40
Glenmorangie malt whisky	40
Gordon's dry gin	37.5 (duty free: 47.3)
Grand Marnier	40
Hine VSOP cognac	40
Lamb's Navy rum	40
Marquis de Senac armagnac	40
Ricard Pastis	40 (duty free: 45)
Smirnoff vodka	37.5
Southern Comfort	40
Vladivar vodka	37.5

Concentrations refer to drinks bought in England, and may be different for duty-free or imported drink, even when it has the same trade name, and may differ from time to time.

Appendix C Brief details of some drugs of forensic importance

C.1 Introduction

This section contains brief details of several drugs used in medicine that are of forensic importance. The approved name of the drug is given, and this is followed by the trade name of one or more of the most common forms available in England. A résumé of the uses and usual doses follows, together with a note of some of the most common or most important side-effects. The licensed indications for a drug, that is, the conditions for which the manufacturer may promote its use, are laid down in the product licence, and also in the product data sheet. Many products are widely used outside their licensed indications, which anyway change from time to time. The reader is referred to the current ABPI *Data sheet compendium*, or the manufacturer's updated data-sheet if one exists, for definitive information on the licensed indications.

There are several sources of basic information on medicines, including the *British National Formulary* (Prasad 1994); the ABPI *Data sheet compendium* (ABPI 1993–4a); and others (Gilman *et al.* 1990; Dollery 1991–4; Reynolds 1992); and on their laboratory analysis (Stead and Moffat 1983; Paterson 1985; Moffat 1986; Baselt 1989; Widdop and Caldwell 1991). The *British National Formulary* is updated twice a year, and the ABPI *Data sheet compendium* is republished annually.

The pharmacokinetics of each agent is described in rather more detail, and references are given to some of the more important original work or to useful reviews.

The notes are not in any way intended as a guide to prescribing the drugs, and must not be relied on to provide accurate or sufficient information for the safe use of the agents described.

C.2 Amitriptyline
('Lentizol','Tryptizol' and as a component of 'Limbitrol' and
'Triptafen')

Amitriptyline is a sedating tricyclic antidepressant, which is indicated for the treatment of depression, 'especially where sedation is required', and in nocturnal enuresis (bed-wetting) where organic pathology is excluded. It is also used to treat chronic pain including atypical facial pain, and as prophylaxis against migraine.

The drug is usually given orally in doses up to 150 milligrams per day; a parenteral preparation exists for intramuscular injection, up to the same daily dose.

Amitriptyline has marked antimuscarinic anticholinergic effects (it inhibits the action of the nerve transmitter substance acetylcholine at sites in the parasympathetic nervous system).

These effects cause the common adverse reactions of a dry mouth, constipation, blurred vision, and difficulty in passing urine. Somnolence is common. Overdosage causes convulsions and disturbances of heart rhythm. It is commonly encountered as an agent of overdosage with serious or fatal consequences (Braithwaite 1995).

Pharmacokinetics of amitriptyline

Amitriptyline is extensively metabolized in the liver, and has an active metabolite, nortriptyline. At least 17 other metabolites are known (Koppel *et al.* 1992). The elimination half-life of the parent compound varies greatly between individuals, with a range of about 10–30 hours; and 15–40 hours after overdosage (Hulten *et al.* 1992). The distribution volume is large—around 10–20 litres per kilogram body-weight.

Total tricyclic concentrations (amitriptyline + metabolites) between 120 and 240 micrograms per litre are effective in the treatment of depression (Montgomery *et al.* 1979).

C.3 Amylobarbitone (Amobarbital in the United States)
('Amytal' , 'Sodium Amytal' , and as a component of 'Tuinal')

Amylobarbitone is a long-acting barbiturate sedative. It is still prescribable 'for the treatment of severe, intractable insomnia', but is rarely prescribed since the advent of the benzodiazepines. Injectable preparations have been used to treat status epilepticus (prolonged epileptic fitting) and can still be obtained. The standard oral dosage in insomnia is 60–200 milligrams at bedtime; tolerance to the hypnotic effect occurs after several doses. An intramuscular dose of up to 1 gram can be given in status, provided no more than 200 milligrams is given at any one site (ABPI 1993–4*i*).

The most important acute adverse effect of amylobarbitone is central nervous system depression, with drowsiness and unsteadiness, which is potentiated by ethanol and other central nervous system depressants. Paradoxical excitement can occur. Repeated usage easily induces dependence so that physical and psychiatric symptoms occur on withdrawing treatment.

Pharmacokinetics of amylobarbitone

Amylobarbitone is metabolized in the liver to inactive metabolites, with a half-life of 20–24 hours. The therapeutic plasma concentration is between 2 and 12 milligrams per litre. The width of the therapeutic range reflects the fact that habitual users become tolerant to the drug (Parker *et al.* 1970).

C.4 Buspirone
('Buspar')

Buspirone is a non-benzodiazepine anxiolytic drug, said to be largely lacking in sedative, anticonvulsant, or muscle relaxant actions (Reynolds 1992) The drug is recommended for use in adults at doses up to 45 milligrams per day (60 milligrams a day in the United States). It is recommended only for short-term treatment in elderly patients, in whom the recommended maximum dosage is 30 milligrams per day; and should not be used in patients with severe hepatic or renal impairment.

Dizziness, excitement, and sleep disturbance are the common adverse effects. Dependence might occur, but has not been documented unequivocally with this new agent.

Pharmacokinetics of buspirone

Buspirone is extensively metabolized in the liver, though many of the metabolites are uncharacterized. The plasma elimination half-life is said to be around 2½ hours, but with a range of 2–33 hours in volunteers in several studies (Gammans *et al.* 1986). The volume of distribution is apparently 5 litres per kilogram body-weight (Mayol *et al.* 1985).

C.5 Chlordiazepoxide
('Librium' and a component of 'Limbitrol')

Chlordiazepoxide is a benzodiazepine sedative, indicated for the short-term treatment of symptoms of anxiety, for relieving muscle spasm, and for palliating the effects of ethanol withdrawal. It is available orally and the maximum recommended daily dose in adults is 30 milligrams for muscle spasm or insomnia with anxiety, 100 milligrams for anxiety states, and 200 milligrams for ethanol withdrawal.

The adverse effects are the same as those of diazepam (q.v.)

Pharmacokinetics of chlordiazepoxide

Chlordiazepoxide is metabolized in the liver to desmethylchlordiazepoxide, desmethyl-diazepam, oxazepam, and other active metabolites. The parent drug has an elimination half-life of about 15 hours and a volume of distribution of about 0.5 litres per kilogram. The active metabolites have substantially longer half-lives than the parent drug. The half-life may be longer in women than in men, and longer in women who take the oral contraceptive pill than in those who do not (Roberts *et al.* 1979).

C.6 Chlormethiazole
('Heminevrin' , 'Hemineurin' in the United States)

Chlormethiazole is a sedative hypnotic which is structurally unrelated to the benzodiazepines. It is indicated for the treatment of agitation and insomnia in the elderly and in relieving the symptoms of ethanol withdrawal. The intravenous preparation can also be used to stop fits in status epilepticus (prolonged epileptic fits). There is the potential for confusion over the dosage of chlormethiazole, since capsules contain 192 milligrams of chlormethiazole base, and this is equivalent to the 250 milligrams of chlormethiazole edisylate that is contained in 5 millilitres of chlormethiazole syrup. The recommended dose of the drug for treating insomnia in the elderly is up to 2 capsules or 10 millilitres of syrup at night. The maximum recommended dose in treating ethanol withdrawal is 12 capsules or 60 millilitres of syrup in 24 hours.

The intravenous preparation of chlormethiazole, which is often used to control the fits and agitation that can occur during ethanol withdrawal, and can also be used to treat prolonged fits of any cause, is difficult to use safely. Patients differ in their response to the drug, and an infusion rate which is appropriate in the initial treatment of a patient may no longer be safe after the treatment has continued for some time. The intravenous preparation should therefore only be used where the patient can be monitored closely.

The danger of the intravenous preparation is that it can induce fatal respiratory depression or cardiac arrhythmia. Both oral and intravenous preparations cause sneezing and headache.

Pharmacokinetics of chlormethiazole

Chlormethiazole is extensively metabolized. The plasma elimination half-life is about 4 hours in the young, and 8 hours in the elderly. The volume of distribution is about 9 litres per kilogram body-weight in the young, and 13 litres per kilogram body-weight in the elderly (Burgess *et al.* 1979; Wendkos, 1979; Dollery 1991–4).

Plasma concentrations of chlormethiazole above about 10 milligrams per litre are associated with unconsciousness.

C.7 Chlorpromazine
('Largactil', 'Thorazine')

Chlorpromazine is the classical phenothiazine neuroleptic drug, principally used to treat patients with schizophrenia or other serious psychotic illnesses. It is also used to control seriously disturbed, violent or dangerously impulsive patients (the 'chemical strait-jacket'). The drug has a number of secondary uses, including the control of nausea, the relief of hiccups, and the palliation of the severe abdominal pain of acute porphyria.

Chlorpromazine is available as tablets, a syrup and a suspension for oral use, and as a solution for intramuscular injection or intravenous infusion. The recommended initial adult dose in schizophrenia is 75 milligrams in a day, but some patients 'may require up to 1 gram daily' (ABPI, 1993–4c). The initial daily dose in elderly or debilitated patients should be 25 or 50 milligrams.

Major adverse effects include sudden death, especially after high doses of parenteral chlorpromazine, in patients with pre-existing cardiac disease, in the elderly, in Afro-Caribbean patients, and in those also taking tricyclic antidepressant drugs. The neuroleptic malignant syndrome, in which there is disturbed consciousness, muscular rigidity, an increase in core body temperature, and disturbances of the regulation of blood pressure, pulse rate, and breathing, is a known complication of treatment with phenothiazines, including chlorpromazine, and of several other drugs (see Section 11.3). Agranulocytosis (a fall in the white-cell count) occurs rarely.

Movement disorders are common, and can take the form of acute dystonic reactions (in which there are writhing movements of the limbs, or stiffness of the muscles with arching of the neck and back, and abnormal eye movements); acute akathisia, an exaggerated form of restlessness; and chronic syndromes including parkinsonism, when the patient has difficulty in moving combined with a resting tremor, and oro-facial dyskinesia, in which the patient incessantly moves the lips and tongue, often licking the lips (see Section 11.1). A rash on skin exposed to sunlight is fairly common in patients on long-term chlorpromazine therapy.

Pharmacokinetics of chlorpromazine

Chlorpromazine is difficult to analyse and some analytical methods are unable to distinguish between the parent drug and its metabolites. Its 'metabolism is exceedingly complex: 168 possible metabolites have been postulated, and at least 20 of them have been isolated' (Baselt 1989). Conversion between chlorpromazine and its metabolites can occur during analysis (Hubbard *et al.* 1985). The rate and route of metabolism are different in the same individual from one time to another, and between different individuals. Individuals also differ in their responses to a given plasma concentration of the drug. For these reasons, the pharmacokinetic parameters, and their relevance to therapy, are ill-defined.

Baselt (1989) quotes the range for chlorpromazine elimination half-life in different individuals from different studies to be between 7 and 119 hours. Elsewhere the more modest range of 8–35 hours, based on the mean values from several studies, is quoted (Vincent and Emery 1978; Dollery 1991–4). The volume of distribution seems likely to lie between 7 and 35 litres per kilogram body-weight. Perhaps more practically useful information comes from the study by Phillipson *et al.* (1978) in which chlorpromazine concentrations were measured in 17 patients when they stopped taking chlorpromazine after chronic treatment. Twenty-four hours after treatment ceased, median chlorpromazine concentration was 45 micrograms per litre of plasma (range 0–263 micrograms per litre), and three patients had detectable chlorpromazine concentrations for up to 6 days.

C.8 Clozapine
('Clozaril')

Clozapine is an antipsychotic drug which has a benzodiazepine-like chemical structure. It is indicated for the treatment of schizophrenia in patients who have not responded to treatment with at least two other ('conventional') antipsychotic agents. The restrictions on the use of clozapine are necessary because it can cause agranulocytosis, a failure of production of granulocyte white blood cells. All patients undergoing treatment have to be registered with a monitoring service run by the manufacturer (Sandoz) as a condition of the product licence.

Clozapine is only available orally. The maximum recommended daily dose is 900 milligrams, and most patients require no more than 450 milligrams.

Adverse effects besides agranulocytosis include drowsiness, cardiac damage, and cardiac or respiratory arrest.

Pharmacokinetics of clozapine

Clozapine is extensively metabolized, and the major metabolites norclozapine and clozapine-*N*-oxide have little or no therapeutic activity (Balant-Gorgia and Balant 1987). The median elimination half-life is said to be 12 hours (range 6–26 hours) (ABPI 1993–4*e*); four studies gave mean values from 9 to 17 hours (Jann *et al.* 1993).

A study of clozapine kinetics in 17 patients found a mean serum clozapine concentration of 250 micrograms per litre[1], but with a 'standard deviation' of 130 micrograms per litre[1], and a ratio of clozapine concentration to dose of 80 ± 46[1] micrograms per litre:milligrams per kilo-

---
[1] The distribution must be skewed, and not Gaussian.

gram. This means that the concentration was very variable, and did not depend strongly on the dose of clozapine. The same was true for norclozapine and for clozapine-N-oxide, the major metabolites, and for the sum of the three clozapine compounds (Centorrino *et al.* 1994*a*, *b*).

C.9 Dexamphetamine, D-amphetamine
('Dexedrine')

Dexamphetamine is the dextro-isomer of amphetamine, a synthetic sympathomimetic amine (an amine that stimulates the sympathetic nervous system). Its main action is as a central nervous system stimulant. The approved indications are narcolepsy, a condition in which the patient can fall asleep without warning; and 'attention deficit hyperkinetic states' ('hyper-activity') in children. Only oral preparations are available for therapeutic use. The usual start-ing dose is 2.5 milligrams daily in young children, 5 milligrams daily in older children and the elderly, and 10 milligrams daily in adults. Tolerance occurs with repeated dosing, and doses up to 60 milligrams daily may be necessary.

Only the oral route is used to administer dexamphetamine therapeutically, but dexam-phetamine and related drugs are also abused orally or intravenously, alone or in combination with diamorphine ('speedball'). Some derivatives are smoked.

The adverse effects of insomnia, a dry mouth and an increase in heart rate are expected from the pharmacological actions. An increase in blood pressure occurs and can be severe enough to cause cerebral haemorrhage. A psychosis clinically indistinguishable from schizophrenia can be seen. High doses, and especially overdose, can precipitate hyperpyrexia (a dangerously high body temperature), muscle spasm and muscle breakdown that can lead to kidney failure and death.

Pharmacokinetics of dexamphetamine

Dexamphetamine undergoes metabolism in the liver, but in addition, 5–30 per cent is excreted unchanged in the urine, and the percentage depends on urinary pH. The elimination half-life is around 12 hours (Balon *et al.* 1987; Ananth *et al.* 1988; Dollery 1991–4), and the therapeu-tic concentration is said to lie between 20 and 100 micrograms per litre (Beckett *et al.* 1969).

C.10 Diamorphine, heroin

Diamorphine, also called heroin or 3,6-diacetylmorphine, is a semisynthetic derivative of mor-phine. It is rapidly taken up into brain tissue after an intravenous injection, and is then metab-olized to 6-monoacetylmorphine and morphine itself. Diamorphine has little or no intrinsic opioid activity, and its opioid effects are due to the actions of these metabolites. The rapid uptake into brain probably accounts for the intensity of the 'high' or 'rush' experienced with intravenous diamorphine injection, and so for its widespread abuse by addicts. It is no longer permitted in medicine in the United States, but is used in Britain, especially for the relief of pain in myocardial infarction ('heart attack') and in the terminal care of patients with cancer. It is also used in the emergency treatment of acute pulmonary oedema, a condition in which the airspaces of the lungs fill with fluid. Advantages over morphine include both higher solubility and greater potency, so that smaller injection volumes are needed. Diamorphine may also be more euphoriant than morphine. Discussion about the relative merits of morphine and diamorphine continues, though there is unlikely to be a large difference in efficacy between the two drugs (Levine *et al.* 1986).

Diamorphine for pharmaceutical use is available as powder for injections. A slow intravenous injection of 5–10 milligrams is given to relieve the pain of acute myocardial infarction and to treat pulmonary oedema. The standard therapeutic dose of diamorphine by subcutaneous or intramuscular injection for pain in adults is 5–10 milligrams every 2–4 hours. A continuous subcutaneous or intravenous injection of diamorphine is often given to palliate pain in terminal cancer.

Adverse reactions are similar to those of morphine. Diamorphine is thought to be more addictive.

Pharmacokinetics of diamorphine

Diamorphine (3,6–diacetylmorphine) is rapidly hydrolysed in the body to 6-monoacetylmorphine and morphine. The metabolites are responsible for the drug's opioid actions, and both are further metabolized to inactive glucuronides which are excreted in the urine.

The plasma half-life of diamorphine is 3 minutes (range 1.7–5.3 minutes), and the effective half-life of the opioid activity is about 3–4 hours since it depends on the half-lives of 6-monoacetylmorphine and morphine (Inturrisi *et al.* 1984; Portenoy *et al.* 1992).

During continuous infusion of diamorphine at a rate of 112 micrograms per minute, the 2-hour concentrations of diamorphine, morphine, and 6-monoacetylmorphine were approximately 60, 30, and 15 micrograms per litre, respectively, in one patient with cancer (Inturrisi *et al.* 1984).

C.11 Diazepam
('Valium', 'Atensine', 'Diazemuls', 'Stesolid')

Diazepam is the most well-known of the benzodiazepine anxiolytic drugs, and is used to treat anxiety, insomnia, muscle spasm, and prolonged epileptic convulsion, and to ameliorate the symptoms of ethanol withdrawal.

The maximum dose recommended to treat anxiety or night terrors in children is 5 milligrams in a day; for elderly and debilitated patients with insomnia or anxiety it is 15 milligrams in a day; and for other adults, 30 milligrams in a day. Cerebral spasticity can be treated with higher doses: up to 40 milligrams daily in children, and up to 60 milligrams daily in otherwise fit adults. Intravenous diazepam is usually reserved for the treatment of fits, and the recommended dosage is 0.3 milligrams per kilogram body weight, up to a maximum of 3 milligrams per kilogram body-weight per day. Infusions containing up to 10 milligrams per kilogram body-weight per day can be needed in the treatment of tetanus (an infection marked by intense muscle spasm).

Intravenous diazepam can cause respiratory arrest, especially if the dosage is high, or the patient is elderly or has lung disease. Other major adverse effects include dependence, drowsiness, and dizziness. Diazepam and other benzodiazepines can impair the formation of memories, cause mental confusion, and provoke, in rare instances, paradoxical excitement.

Pharmacokinetics of diazepam

Diazepam is metabolized to desmethyldiazepam and temazepam, both of which are active benzo-diazepines. The pharmacokinetics, and the relationship between concentration and effect, are correspondingly difficult to disentangle. The elimination half)life of the parent drug is about 1½ days (range 1–5 days) and of the active metabolites up to about 9 days (Greenblatt *et al.* 1980, 1981).

The enzyme responsible for breaking down diazepam exists in genetically distinct forms. In three subjects who had inherited the 'poor metabolizer' form of the enzyme[2], the mean half-life of diazepam was 88 hours (range 69–101 hours), whereas in 13 'good metabolizers', the mean half-life was 40 hours (range 21–62 hours). The breakdown of desmethyldiazepam was also dramatically prolonged, with a mean half-life of 128 hours (range 102–147 hours) in the poor metabolizers, compared with 59 hours (range 32–83 hours) in the controls (Bertilsson *et al.* 1989). Women may metabolize diazepam more slowly than do men (Wilson 1984).

The volume of distribution is about 1 litre per kilogram body-weight (Braithwaite 1990).

Total benzodiazepine concentration was between about 0.5 and 3 milligrams per litre in 110 men taking the drug chronically, and the concentration of desmethyldiazepam was about 1.25 times the concentration of diazepam (range 0.2–3.2) (Greenblatt *et al.* 1981).

C.12 Fluoxetine
('Prozac')

Fluoxetine is the best-known of the newer, non-sedating antidepressants called 5-HT re-uptake inhibitors or selective serotonin-reuptake inhibitors (SSRIs). It is indicated for the treatment of depression and for patients with the eating disorder bulimia nervosa (a form of binge eating followed by self-induced vomiting or purging). It is marketed as a capsule for oral use.

The standard dose in depression is 20 milligrams daily, and higher doses increase the likelihood of adverse effects without increasing the therapeutic effect. The recommended dose of fluoxetine for bulimia nervosa is 60 milligrams daily.

The maximum antidepressant effect is no more than with conventional tricyclic antidepressants (Song *et al.* 1993), but the drug has been enveloped in hyperbolic mystique to the extent that it has been said to make normal people feel better and more assertive. A major protagonist is Kramer, who describes in his book *Listening to Prozac* (Kramer 1994) an architect called Sam, who 'drafted, thought and talked more fluently when on [fluoxetine]'; it made him feel 'better than well'.

Adverse effects of fluoxetine in therapeutic doses include gastrointestinal symptoms, especially nausea and diarrhoea, central nervous system symptoms including fits, headache and dizziness, loss of libido, mania, fever, and a severe skin rash due to vasculitis (inflammation of the blood vessels). Less serious rashes are common.

Fluoxetine is relatively safe in overdosage, and much less toxic in that situation than the older tricyclic antidepressants.

Pharmacokinetics of fluoxetine

Fluoxetine is metabolized to norfluoxetine in the liver. The metabolite has the same antidepressant activity as the parent drug. The half-life of fluoxetine after single doses in healthy

[2] Cytochrome P450 2C, also called CYP2C and *S*-mephenytoin hydroxylase.

volunteers is 3 days, and of norfluoxetine 7–9 days. The volume of distribution of the parent drug is large and variable: a range of 20–42 litres per kilogram body-weight is quoted.

C.13 Fluphenazine
('Moditen', 'Modecate', 'Permitil', 'Prolixin').

Fluphenazine is a phenothiazine neuroleptic drug related to chlorpromazine but about 50 times more potent (50 milligrams of chlorpromazine has the same effect as 1 milligram of fluphenazine). The drug is used to treat schizophrenia. Fluphenazine hydrochloride is water soluble, and can be given orally or by intramuscular injection. The fat-soluble enanthate and decanoate esters can be given as depot ('slow-release') intramuscular injections every 2–4 weeks, which makes it easier to ensure that patients receive their medicines.

Adverse reactions are similar to those of chlorpromazine (q.v.).

Pharmacokinetics of fluphenazine

Fluphenazine is metabolized to inactive metabolites, and only a small quantity of unchanged drug is excreted in the urine.

The plasma concentrations of fluphenazine depend largely on the dosage form and the route of administration. A study of radiolabelled fluphenazine in seven subjects, only one or two receiving any one treatment, gave these results (Curry *et al.* 1979):

Since the radioactive label is present on inactive metabolite as well as parent drug, such results

Preparation	Route	Apparent half-life
Fluphenazine hydrochloride	oral	12–19 hours
	IM	12–16 hours
Fluphenazine enanthate	IM	83–96 hours
Fluphenazine decanoate	IM	127–281 hours

are bound to be very imprecise. The low steady-state concentrations of parent drug have made more accurate studies difficult (Dahl 1986).

Radioimmunoassay measurement of plasma levels in 33 schizophrenic patients during long-term treatment with fluphenazine decanoate gave values between 0.88 and 16.8 micrograms per litre, and concentrations were only modestly correlated with daily dose (Wiles and Gelder, 1979). In another group of 12 patients, the range was from 0.6 to 14 micrograms per litre, and there was a tenfold variation in concentrations measured a few weeks apart in individual patients (Brown and Silver 1985). It is therefore perhaps surprising that a therapeutic range of 0.5–2 micrograms per litre has been suggested (Dahl 1986). Koreen *et al.* (1994) were unable to find any relationship between the concentration of fluphenazine and the response to treatment in patients treated during a first episode of schizophrenia.

C.14 Haloperidol
('Haldol', 'Serenace')

Haloperidol is a butyrophenone major tranquillizer, used to treat schizophrenia, paranoia, mania, and aggressive behaviour. It is also used to treat hiccups, to alleviate nausea and vomiting, and in the management of the Gilles de la Tourette syndrome of tics accompanied by impulsive and uncontrollable coprolalia (the use of foul language).

The free drug is available as tablets or an oral solution, and as a solution for intramuscular or intravenous injection. Haloperidol decanoate in sesame oil is available for depot (slow-release) administration as a deep intramuscular injection.

The recommended oral dose of haloperidol in adults is 3–9 milligrams a day for moderate symptoms, and 6–15 milligrams a day for severe symptoms. However, some schizophrenic patients apparently require doses up to 200 milligrams a day. The maximum dose in children is 10 milligrams daily.

The recommended dose for parenteral administration in severely disturbed psychiatric patients is up to 30 milligrams; and it is said that this may be given every 4–8 hours 'although it may be given every hour if necessary' (data sheet for 'Haldol' (ABPI 1993–4g)).

The initial dose of depot haloperidol decanoate is 50 milligrams every 4 weeks, though up to 300 milligrams every 4 weeks may prove necessary.

Adverse effects due to haloperidol include the neuroleptic malignant syndrome in which there is disturbed consciousness, muscular rigidity, an increase in core body temperature, and disturbances of the regulation of blood pressure, pulse rate, and breathing. Movement disorders are common, and can take the form of acute dystonic reactions (in which there are writhing movements of the limbs, or stiffness of the muscles with arching of the neck and back, and abnormal eye movements), acute akathisia, an exaggerated form of restlessness, and chronic syndromes including parkinsonism, when the patient has difficulty in moving combined with a resting tremor, and oro-facial dyskinesia, in which the patient incessantly moves the lips and tongue, often licking the lips.

Acute overdosage can cause respiratory depression and hypotension (an abnormally low blood pressure).

Pharmacokinetics of haloperidol

Haloperidol is extensively metabolized to reduced haloperidol and to propionic and acetic acid derivatives which are excreted in the urine. The elimination half-life is in the region of 15-25 hours, and the volume of distribution around 10–20 litres per kilogram body-weight, the wide ranges pointing to large interindividual differences in metabolism (Froemming *et al.* 1989). In one study, values for the elimination half-life in normal men after intravenous haloperidol ranged from 9 to 32 hours (Holley *et al.* 1983).

Smith *et al.* (1984) examined plasma haloperidol in 27 patients given between 10 and 25 milligrams daily, and found concentrations between 2 and 23 micrograms per litre 90 minutes after a dose. A therapeutic range has been proposed with lower and upper bounds of 4 and 55 micrograms per litre (Van Putten *et al.* 1991).

C. 15 Insulin

Here are some pharmacokinetic data for insulin, which is discussed in Chapter 9.

Units of measurement   1 Unit = approximately $\frac{1}{28}$th of a milligram, or 6.1 nanomoles
Molecular weight $c.5800$
Oral absorption   zero
Volume of distribution[1]   85-100 millilitres per kilogram body-weight
Plasma half-life[2]   3-5 minutes

Table C.1   Effects of subcutaneous injection

Tye of insulin	Time in hours		
	Onset	Peak	Duration
Soluble	½–1	4	8
Isophane Insulin zinc suspension }	1–2	4–14	up to 28
Protamine zinc insulin	4	10–20	up to 35

C.16 Lorazepam
('Ativan')

Lorazepam is a benzodiazepine, used orally as an anxiolytic and premedication before operations. An intravenous preparation is also available, and can in addition be used to treat status epilepticus (prolonged epileptic fits).

The maximum recommended dosage of oral lorazepam in adults is 4 milligrams daily; half the normal dose is recommended in the elderly. To treat epilepsy, up to 4 milligrams of lorazepam by intravenous injection can be given to adults, but only 2 milligrams is recommended in children and the elderly.

The adverse effects are the same as those of diazepam. It has the potential to induce dependence, and treatment should only last a short time: no more than 4 weeks.

Pharmacokinetics of lorazepam

Lorazepam was found to have a mean elimination half-life of 11 hours (range 8–24 hours) in six healthy volunteers (Greenblatt *et al.* 1988). In another study, the mean half-life was 16 hours in six healthy volunteers, and 28 hours in four subjects with renal failure needing dialysis.

C.17 Morphine
('Oramorph', 'Duramorph', 'MST Continus')

Morphine is an opiate analgesic isolated from the opium poppy, and used in the treatment of severe pain. It can be given orally, intramuscularly, intravenously, or rectally. Slow-release oral formulations of morphine are available.

[1] The volume of distribution is larger in patients with insulin antibodies.
[2] The half-life is longer in patients with insulin antibodies.

The daily dose is not well-defined, since chronic use causes tolerance to the effects of the drug, and very high doses can be taken. A common starting dose of morphine is 10 milligrams every 4 hours.

Adverse effects include respiratory depression or respiratory arrest, physical and psychological dependence, confusion, constipation, cough suppression, nausea, and vomiting. Morphine and other opiates can cause anaphylactoid reactions, that is reactions resembling anaphylactic reactions[3], but not immunologically mediated.

Pharmacokinetics of morphine

Morphine is metabolized in the liver mainly to inactive metabolites, but the active 6-glucuronide can accumulate in renal failure (Hanna et al. 1993; Osborne et al. 1993). The elimination half-life is about 3 hours in patients with cancer, and the volume of distribution around 2 litres per kilogram body-weight (Sawe et al. 1981). Morphine is eliminated more slowly in the newborn (Choonara et al. 1992) and the elderly, and in liver disease. The plasma concentration necessary to control pain varied from 110 micrograms per litre to 14 milligrams per litre (Aherne et al. 1979), perhaps because this early study relied on a relatively non-specific radioimmunoassay. Values between about 10 and 50 micrograms per litre are now accepted (Dollery 1991-4).

It was possible to detect morphine in the blood of those who died after diamorphine (heroin) overdose, when concentrations of 100–930 micrograms per litre were found in those who died within 3 hours. A concentration of 60 micrograms per litre was found some 3 days after poisoning in one patient (Garriott and Sturner 1973).

C.18 Pethidine (meperidine in the United States)

('Demerol' in the United States; and as an ingredient of 'Pamergan P100' in the United Kingdom)

Pethidine is an opioid analgesic used to treat moderate or severe pain. It is available as tablets for oral use and as solution for subcutaneous, intramuscular or intravenous injection. The maximum recommended single doses in adults are 150 milligrams orally, 100 milligrams subcutaneously or intramuscularly, and 50 milligrams intravenously. In elderly patients, the initial dose should not exceed 50 milligrams orally or 25 milligrams by injection; and in children, the initial dose should not exceed 2 milligrams per kilogram body-weight orally or intramuscularly.

The adverse effects are similar to those of morphine. There is no doubt that the drug is addictive (Rasor and Crecraft 1955). Convulsions can occur in patients with renal failure, or when high doses are used, as for example in patients with sickle-cell crisis (an extremely painful recurrent condition due to an inborn blood disorder), who receive large doses. The convulsions are due to a metabolite, norpethidine, which is usually excreted by the kidneys.

Pharmacokinetics of pethidine

The metabolism of pethidine is complex. Norpethidine, one of the major metabolites, has both opioid and pro-convulsant properties.

[3] An anaphylactic reaction takes the form of sudden wheezing, flushing, swelling of the lips and tongue, and circulatory collapse.

The elimination half-life of pethidine after intravenous administration was estimated as 190 minutes (standard deviation 50 minutes) in eight normal men (Klotz *et al.* 1974); and as 160 minutes (standard deviation 80 minutes) in nine pregnant women during labour (Husemeyer *et al.* 1982). In women during labour, the apparent elimination half-life was both longer, at 230 minutes, and more variable (standard deviation 110 minutes) after intramuscular injection (Husemeyer *et al.*, 1982). These authors also calculated the mean apparent elimination rate after epidural injection as 190 minutes in pregnant women, and 290 minutes in non-pregnant women. The results point towards a marked variation between individuals. The kinetics of epidural (but not intravenous) pethidine are altered in pregnancy.

The steady-state volume of distribution was around 4 litres per kilogram body-weight in normal man (Klotz *et al.* 1974).

The relationship between pain relief and blood pethidine concentration was examined in surgical patients by Austin *et al.* (1980). The minimum pethidine concentration for reliable analgesia was 460 micrograms per litre, equivalent to 0.46 micrograms per millilitre (standard deviation 0.18 micrograms per millilitre).[4]

C.19 Temazepam
('Normison', 'Temazepam Gelthix Capsules')

Temazepam is a benzodiazepine hypnotic, licensed for the short-term treatment of severe or disabling insomnia. It is available as tablets or as capsules containing a viscous gel intended to be difficult to aspirate from the capsule with a syringe and needle, and so difficult to abuse intravenously. The ingenuity of the manufacturers has, in practice, been more than matched by the ingenuity of the drug abusers.

The maximum recommended dose is 60 milligrams at night in adults, and 30 milligrams at night in the elderly.

The adverse effects are the same as those of diazepam. Intravenous, and especially, intra-arterial, injection of temazepam gel can cause severe damage to blood vessels and tissue.

Pharmacokinetics of temazepam

Temazepam is metabolized mainly to an inactive glucuronide metabolite, though small amounts of the active benzodiazepine oxazepam can also be detected.

The elimination half-life of temazepam appears to depend on sex and age, being longest in elderly women. Estimates of mean elimination half-life range from about 8 to about 16 hours (Bittencourt *et al.* 1979; Divoll *et al.* 1981; Jochemsen *et al.* 1983).

C.20 Thiopentone (thiopental in the United States)
('Intraval sodium', 'Pentothal')

Thiopentone is an ultra-short-acting barbiturate used intravenously to induce general anaes-thesia and to control convulsions in status epilepticus (prolonged epileptic fits). The usual dose is 4 milligrams per kilograms body-weight, but the necessary amount can be half this in the elderly and twice as much in children.

[4] Incidentally, this is misprinted as 0.46 ± 0.18 g/ml in the legend to one of the figures in the original paper.

Respiratory depression is expected, and adequate provision must be made to support the patient's breathing with artificial ventilation. Spasm of the vocal cords and related muscles can occur after thiopentone injection, and this has the serious consequence that the anaesthetist may be unable to pass a tube from the mouth into the trachea (the main windpipe carrying air to the lungs). Overdosage of thiopentone can result in prolonged unconsciousness and circulatory failure. The solution of thiopentone is very alkaline, with a pH above 10, and causes severe spasm of the blood-vessel if given into an artery, as sometimes occurs by mistake. The spasm can be sufficient to cause gangrene.

Pharmacokinetics of thiopentone

Thiopentone rapidly passes from the bloodstream into the brain tissues. Changes in the electroencephalogram (brain-wave recording) can be seen about 15 seconds after injection. The effect wears off quite rapidly as the drug is redistributed into other tissues, a process that occurs with a half-life of a few minutes. In one study in men, the values ranged from 1 to 7 minutes, being significantly longer in men aged 60–80 years than in men aged 20–30 years (Christensen *et al.* 1982). The elimination half-life after small intravenous doses is about 10 hours. Studies during long-term infusions demonstrate that thiopentone is broken down more slowly as the concentration rises above 30 milligrams per litre, because of saturable (Michaelis–Menten) kinetics. The volume of distribution at steady state is about 4 litres per kilogram body-weight (Turcant *et al.* 1985).

The mean plasma thiopentone concentration required to induce anaesthesia in 36 subjects was 40 micrograms per litre with a standard deviation of 12 micrograms per litre (Becker 1978).

C.21 Thioridazine
('Melleril')

Thioridazine is a phenothiazine neuroleptic which is used to treat schizophrenia and used to control agitated behaviour, especially in elderly or demented patients. It is also licensed for the treatment of children with severe behavioural problems such as self-mutilation or temper tantrums.

Only oral preparations are marketed. The maximum recommended dose of 800 milligrams daily is only suitable for treatment of severely disturbed patients with schizophrenia, in hospital, under specialist supervision, and for no longer than 4 weeks. It is very much greater than the starting dose of 25 milligrams at night that might be used in an elderly person. The recommended dose in children aged 1–5 years is 1 milligram per kilogram body-weight per day.

The adverse effects of thioridazine are generally similar to those of other phenothiazines such as chlorpromazine. It is particularly likely to cause changes in the electrocardiogram (see footnote, p. 164), with prolongation of the Q–T interval (Thomas 1994). This can be a precursor to serious heart rhythm disturbance. Thioridazine, in addition to sharing the problems of other phenothiazines, can cause blindness as a result of pigmentary changes in the retina.

Pharmacokinetics of thioridazine

Thioridazine is extensively metabolized in the liver by several routes. At least two of the metabolites are present in significant concentrations in blood, and are themselves active. One, thioridazine-2-sulphoxide (mesoridazine, 'Serentil') is marketed in the United States as a neuroleptic drug.

The mean elimination half-life of thioridazine is around 30 hours, but it is shorter in alcoholics and longer in the elderly and the obese. Axelsson and Martensson (1979) reviewed earlier studies and found individual values for elimination half-life to vary from 4 to 80 hours. The enormous variation may in part be due to the variable ability of different analytical methods to distinguish between thioridazine and its metabolites.

The volume of distribution is also uncertain; it probably lies between 10 and 20 litres per kilogram body-weight.

C.22 Triazolam
('Halcion')

Triazolam is a potent benzodiazepine hypnotic with a short half-life. It is no longer licensed for use in Britain, but a tablet was available until 1992 for use in a dose of 250 micrograms at night in adults, and 125 micrograms at night in the elderly.

The drug was withdrawn because of concern that triazolam could cause severe psychiatric adverse effects, especially in the elderly. It shares the other adverse effects of benzodiazepines such as diazepam. Volunteers treated with triazolam for 7–10 nights experienced rebound insomnia on abrupt cessation of active treatment (Greenblatt *et al.* 1987).

Pharmacokinetics of triazolam.

Triazolam is metabolized in the liver to active metabolites, though it is unlikely that they contribute substantially to the drug's action at therapeutic doses. A review of the pharmacokinetics of triazolam (Pakes *et al.* 1981) suggests that the elimination half-life of the parent drug is 2–3 hours, and of the active metabolites about 4 hours. The volume of distribution in healthy subjects is approximately 1 litre per kilogram body-weight.

C.23 Vincristine
('Oncovin')

Vincristine is a naturally occurring alkaloid from the periwinkle, *Vinca rosea*, which is used as an anticancer agent, particularly in the treatment of leukaemia (malignancy of the white blood cell) and lymphoma (malignancy of the lymph nodes). The dosage regimes are complex and require careful calculation. Except for very small children, the dosage is based on body surface-area, and not body weight, so that both the height and weight of the patient need to be known. Doses are not given more frequently than once a week.

The drug is given intravenously, but may be part of a regime which includes other, intrathecally administered, drugs (drugs given into the cerebrospinal fluid surrounding the spinal cord). Intrathecal administration of vincristine IS USUALLY LETHAL, and the data sheet now contains clear warnings to this effect.

Vincristine, like other anticancer drugs, has a low therapeutic ratio: adverse effects occur close to or at the therapeutic dose. It causes hair loss. A more serious, dose-related effect is damage to the nerves that can cause weakness of the hands and feet, and severe pain. Liver damage, and damage to the bone marrow, are also important effects.

Pharmacokinetics of vincristine

Vincristine is metabolized in the liver and the metabolites are excreted in the bile. The elimination half-life is approximately 85 hours, and the volume of distribution is over 8 litres per kilogram body-weight.

Peak blood concentrations after a standard dose are approximately 350 micrograms per litre (Balis *et al.* 1983).

C.24 Warfarin (warfarin sodium)
('Marevan')

Warfarin is the most commonly used oral anticoagulant agent, and it reduces the formation of clotting factors in the blood by inhibiting the enzyme responsible for activating vitamin K, a co-factor necessary for the formation of the clotting factors II, VII, IX, and X.

Warfarin is used to make clotting less likely in patients who have had serious blood clots, for example pulmonary thrombosis or deep vein thrombosis, or who are at particular risk from them, such as patients undergoing prolonged surgical operations, those with the irregular heart rhythm atrial fibrillation, and those with artificial heart valves. It has also been used to prevent recurrent heart attacks, and continues to be used for this purpose in The Netherlands. The dosage is critically important, because individuals vary greatly in their sensitivity to the anticoagulant effects of warfarin, and because the degree of anticoagulation is very important: it should be sufficient to make clotting unlikely while not increasing the risk of major haemorrhage to an unacceptable degree. Since the risk to the patient is dependent on the illness, the desirable degree of anticoagulation is also dependent on the illness. The degree of anticoagulation is expressed as the international normalized ratio (INR), being 1.0 if the clotting is normal, and higher than this if the patient is anticoagulated. The recommended ranges are given in the *British National Formulary*, and include: INR 2.0–2.5, for prevention of deep vein thrombosis in surgical patients at high risk; INR 2.0–3.0, in patients with atrial fibrillation; and 3.0–4.5 in patients with mechanical prosthetic heart valves.

To ensure that the patient's INR falls within the desirable range, careful dosage adjustment is needed, and it has to be guided by measurement of the INR at frequent intervals; to maintain the INR in the correct range, it has to be checked every few weeks, even in patients who have been controlled on the same dose for some time. Most general hospitals run anticoagulant clinics for this reason.

Serious adverse effects are mainly due to haemorrhage, often into the brain to cause stroke. Warfarin can rarely induce an ulcerating necrotic skin rash.

Pharmacokinetics of warfarin (Hignite et al. 1980; Choonara et al. 1985)

Warfarin is metabolized in the liver, and the metabolism is very sensitive to the presence of certain other drugs. Cimetidine, omeprazole, sulphonamides including co-trimoxazole, keto-conazole and probably other related drugs, ciprofloxacin and other related drugs, phenylbuta-zone and azapropazone, erythromycin and clarithromycin, hormone-like drugs such as tamoxifen and flutamide, all reduce the metabolism of warfarin and make haemorrhage more likely. Drugs such as griseofulvin and aminoglutethimide can increase the metabolism of war-farin, reduce its anticoagulant effect, and increase the risk of clotting.

The elimination half-life of warfarin is around 36 hours, but it is different for the R- and S-isomers, and differs markedly between individuals. The volume of distribution is small, being around 0.1–0.25 litres per kilogram body-weight.

Warfarin concentrations in patients who are satisfactorily anticoagulated are between 0.3 and 3 milligrams per litre.

References

ABPI (1993–4*a*). *Data sheet compendium*. Datapharm Publications Limited, London.

ABPI (1993–4*b*). *Data sheet compendium*. p. 1064. Datapharm Publications Limited, London.

ABPI (1993–4*c*). *Data sheet compendium*. pp. 1266–8. Datapharm Publications Limited, London.

ABPI (1993–4*d*). *Data sheet compendium*. p. 1378. Datapharm Publications Limited, London.

ABPI (1993–4*e*). *Data sheet compendium*. pp. 1378–80. Datapharm Publications Limited, London.

ABPI (1993–4*f*). *Data sheet compendium*. pp. 160–1. Datapharm Publications Limited, London.

ABPI (1993–4*g*). *Data sheet compendium*. p. 693. Datapharm Publications Limited, London.

ABPI (1993–4*h*). *Data sheet compendium*. pp. 874–6. Datapharm Publications Limited, London.

ABPI (1993–4*i*). *Data sheet compendium*. pp. 874–6. Datapharm Publications Limited, London.

Aherne, G. W., Piall, E. M., and Twycross, R. G. (1979). Serum morphine concentrations after oral administration of diamorphine hydrochloride and morphine sulphate. *British Journal of Clinical Pharmacology*, **8**, 577–80.

Al-Lanqawi, Y., Moreland, A., McEwen, J., Halliday, F., Durnin, C. J., and Stevenson, I. H. (1992). Ethanol kinetics: extent of error in back-extrapolation procedures. *British Journal of Clinical Pharmacology*, **34**, 316–21.

Altman, D. G. (1991). *Practical statistics for medical research*. Chapman and Hall, London.

Anand, N. (1990). Contribution of Ayurvedic medicine to medicinal chemistry. In *Comprehensive medicinal chemistry*. Vol. 1. (ed. C. Hansch), pp. 113–31. Pergamon Press, Oxford.

Ananth, J., Edelmuth, E., and Dargan, B. (1988). Meige's syndrome associated with neuroleptic treatment. *American Journal of Psychiatry*, **145**, 513–15.

Anonymous (1978). *The Times*, 28 April.

Anonymous (1979). Good dispensing practice. *Pharmaceutical Journal*, Aug. 18, 157–8.

Anonymous (1981). Hunting rare adverse drug reactions. *British Medical Journal*, **282**, 342.

Anonymous (1985). Confusing drug names. *Drug and Therapeutics Bulletin*, **23**, 77–9.

Anonymous (1986*a*). *Medical Protection Society Annual Review*, 44.

Anonymous (1986*b*). *Medical Defence Union Annual Report*, 31.

Anonymous (1986*c*). The law tries to decide whether whooping cough vaccine causes brain damage: Professor Gordon Stewart gives evidence. *British Medical Journal—Clinical Research*, **292**, 1264–6.

Anonymous (1987*a*). *Medical Protection Society Annual Review*, 24.

Anonymous (1987*b*). *Medical Defence Union Annual Report*, 35.

Anonymous (1988). *Medical Protection Society Annual Review*, 28.

Anonymous (1991*a*). Cyanide poisonings associated with over-the-counter medication—Washington State, 1991. *Journal of the American Medical Association*, **265**, 1806–7.

Anonymous (1991*b*). Hospital drug overdose led to man's death. *Guardian*, 26 Sept.

Anonymous (1992). Draft guidelines on preventable medication errors. *American Journal of Hospital Pharmacy*, **49**, 640–8.

Anonymous (1994*a*). Reilly's challenge. *Lancet*, **344**, 1585.

Anonymous (1994*b*). European Medicines Evaluation Agency and the new licensing arrangements. *Drug and Therapeutics Bulletin*, **32**, 89–90.

Applebe, G. E. and Wingfield, J. (1994) *Dale and Applebe's pharmacy law and ethics*, (5th edn). Pharmaceutical Press, London.

Armitage, P. and Berry, G. (1987). *Statistical methods in medical research*, (2nd edn). Blackwell, Oxford.

Aronson, J. K. (1994). What's in a brand name? *British Medical Journal*, **308**, 1140–1.

Arthur, M. J. P., Lee, A., and Wright, R. (1984). Sex differences in the metabolism of ethanol and acetaldehyde in normal subjects. *Clinical Science*, **67**, 397–401.

Asher, R. (1951). Munchausen Syndrome. *Lancet*, **i**, 339–41.

Ashton, C. H. (1984). Benzodiazepine withdrawal: an unfinished story. *British Medical Journal*, **288**, 1135–40.

Austin, K. L., Stapleton, J. V. and Mather, L. E. (1980). Relationship between blood meperidine concentrations and analgesic response: a preliminary report. *Anesthesiology*, **53**, 460–6.

Autret, E., Sanyas, P., Chantepie, A., Gold, F., and Laugier, J. (1982). Poisoning by externally-administered ethanol in an infant, [in French]. *Archives Françaises de Pédiatrie*, **39**, 823–4.

Axelgaard, G., Skensved, H., and Asfeldt, V. H. (1986). Hypoglycemia during treatment with sulfonylurea preparations, [in Danish]. *Ugeskrift for Laeger*, **148**, 2155–8.

Axelsson, R. and Martensson, E. (1979). On the clinical pharmacokinetics of thioridazine and its metabolites. In *Biological psychiatry today*. (ed. J. Obiols, C. Ballus, E. Gonzales Monclus, and J. Pujol), pp. 955–8. Elsevier, Amsterdam.

Badewitz-Dodd., L. (ed.) (1991). *Drugs and sport*. Media Medica, Chichester.

Balant-Gorgia, A. E. and Balant, L. (1987). Antipsychotic drugs. Clinical pharmacokinetics of potential candidates for plasma concentration monitoring. *Clinical Pharmacokinetics*, **13**, 65–90.

Balis, F. M., Holcenberg, J. S., and Bleyer, W. A. (1983). Clinical pharmacokinetics of commonly used anticancer drugs. *Clinical Pharmacokinetics*, **8**, 202–32.

Balon, R., Berchou, R., and Han, H. (1987). Priapism associated with thiothixene, chlorpromazine, and thioridazine. *Journal of Clinical Psychiatry*, **48**, 216.

Barker, G. R. (1993). Roxiam® (Remoxipride)—reports of aplastic anaemia. Letter to Medical Practitioners, 11 October. 1993.

Barnes, T. R. E. (1988). Tardive dyskinesia. *British Medical Journal*, **296**, 1004.

Baselt, R. (1989). *Disposition of toxic drugs and chemicals in man*. (3rd edn). Year Book Medical Publishers, St Louis, Missouri.

Bayliss, C. R. (1993). A pseudo body packer. *Clinical Radiology*, **47**, 219.

Bayly, G. R., Braithwaite, R. A., Sheehan, T. M. T., Dyer, N. H., Grimley, C., and Ferner, R. E. (1995). Lead-poisoning from Asian traditional remedies in the West Midlands—report of a series of 5 cases. *Human and Experimental Toxicology*, **14**, 24–8

Becker, K. E. (1978). Plasma levels of thiopental necessary for anesthesia. *Anesthesiology*, **49**, 192–6.

Beckett, A. H., Salmon, J. A., and Mitchard, M. (1969). The relation between blood levels and urinary excretion of amphetamine under controlled acidic and under fluctuating urinary pH values using [14C] amphetamine. *Journal of Pharmacy and Pharmacology*, **21**, 251–8.

Bedford, P. D. (1954). Acute potassium intoxication. *Lancet*, **2**, 268–70.

Bennion, L. J. and Li, T.-K. (1976). Alcohol metabolism in American Indians and whites. *New England Journal of Medicine*, **294**, 9–13.

Bertilsson, L., Henthorn, T. K., Sanz, E., Tybring, G., Sawe, J., and Villen, T. (1989). Importance of genetic factors in the regulation of diazepam metabolism: relationship to S-mephenytoin, but not debrisoquin, hydroxylation phenotype. *Clinical Pharmacology and Therapeutics*, **45**, 348–55.

Betts, T. A. and Birtle, J. (1982). Effects of two hypnotic drugs on actual driving performance next morning. *British Medical Journal*, **285**, 852.

Bhatkhande, C. Y. and Joglekar, V. D. (1977). Fatal poisoning by potassium in human and rabbit. *Forensic Science*, **9**, 33–6.

Bidot-Lopez, P., Casellas, J. F., and Hulme, C. D. (1987). Hypoglycemia: factitious or felonious? *Hospital Practice—Office Edition*, **22**, 125, 128–32.

Binimelis, J., *et al.* (1987). Massive thyroxine intoxication: evaluation of plasma extraction. *Intensive Care Medicine*, 13, 33–8.

Birkinshaw, V. J., Gurd, M. R., Randall, S. S., Curry, D. E., and Wright, P. H. (1958). Investigation of a case of murder by insulin. *British Medical Journal*, 2, 463–9.

Bittencourt, P., Richens, A., and Toseland, P. A. (1979). Pharmacokinetics of the hypnotic benzo-diazepine temazepam. *British Journal of Clinical Pharmacology*, 8, 37S-38S.

Bixler, E. O., Kales, A., Manfredi, R. L., Vgontzas, A. N., Tyson, K. L., and Kales, J. D. (1991). Next-day memory impairment with triazolam use. *Lancet*, 337, 827–31.

Bland, M. (1987). *An introduction to medical statistics.* Oxford University Press, Oxford.

Bodeker, G. C. (1990). Ayur-Vedic medicine. *Lancet*, 336, 1260.

Bolan, G., Laurie, R. E., and Broome, C. V. (1986). Red man syndrome: inadvertent administration of an excessive dose of rifampicin to children in a day-care center. *Pediatrics*, 77, 633–5.

Bowers, R. V., Burleson, W. D., and Blades, J. F. (1942). Alcohol absorption from the skin in man. *Quarterly Journal of Studies on Alcohol*, 3, 31–3.

Brahams, D. (1985*a*). Damages for stroke after cholera and typhoid vaccination. *Lancet*, 2, 1372.

Brahams, D. (1985*b*). Deliberate taking of diazepam may provide a defence to a criminal charge. *Lancet*, 1, 356.

Brahams, D. (1985*c*). Pertussis vaccine and brain damage: two claims before the courts. *Lancet*, 2, 1137–8.

Brahams, D. (1986*a*). Does pertussis vaccine cause brain damage? *Lancet*, 1, 1284.

Brahams, D. (1986*b*). Dosage of gentamicin and monitoring of blood levels: an action fails. *Lancet*, 1, 1395–6.

Brahams, D. (1988*a*). Pertussis vaccine: court finds no justification for association with permanent brain damage. *Lancet*, 1, 837.

Brahams, D. (1988*b*). Back calculation of alcohol—the hip-flask defence. *Lancet*, 2, 1504.

Brahams, D. (1989). Uninsured pharmacists and illegible prescriptions. *Lancet*, 1, 510.

Brahams, D. (1990*a*). Benzodiazepine sex fantasies—acquittal of dentist. *Lancet*, 335, 403–4.

Brahams, D. (1990*b*). Benzodiazepines and sexual fantasies. *Lancet*, 335, 157.

Brahams, D. (1990*c*). Doctor cleared of murder of cancer patient. *Lancet*, 335, 718.

Braithwaite, R. A. (1990). The impact of pharmacokinetics. In *The anxiolytic jungle: where next?* (ed. D. Wheatley), pp. 37–47. John Wiley and Sons, Chichester.

Braithwaite, R. A. (1995). The toxicity of tricylic and newer antidepressants. In *Handbook of Clinical Neurology*, Vol. 21 (65), (ed. F. A. de Wolff), pp. 311–28. Elsevier Science, Amsterdam.

Breuning, S. E., Ferguson, D. G., and Cullari, S. (1981). Analysis of single, double-blind procedures, maintenance of placebo effects, and drug-induced dyskinesia with mentally retarded persons—a brief report. *Psychopharmacology Bulletin*, 17, 122–3.

British Herbal Medical Association Scientific Committee (1990). *British herbal pharmacopoeia.* British Herbal Medical Association, Bournemouth.

Brown A. S. J. M., *et al.* (1995). The effect of gastritis on human gastric alcohol-dehydrogenase activity and ethanol-metabolism. *Alimentary Pharmacology and Therapeutics*, 9, 57–61.

Brown, G. A., Neylan, D., Reynolds, W. J., and Smalldon, K. W. (1973). The stability of ethanol in stored blood. Part 1. Important variables and interpretation of results. *Analytica Chimica Acta*, 66, 271–83.

Brown, W. A. and Silver, M. A. (1985). Serum neuroleptic levels and clinical outcome in schizophrenic patients treated with fluphenazine decanoate. *Journal of Clinical Psychopharmacology*, 5, 143–7.

Bruce, J. M. (1899). *Materia medica and therapeutics: an introduction to the rational treatment of disease.* Cassell, London.

Buckley, W. E., Yesalis, C. E. 3rd, Friedl, K. E., Anderson, W. A., Streit, A. L., and Wright, J. E. (1988). Estimated prevalence of anabolic steroid use among male high school seniors. *Journal of the American Medical Association*, 260, 3441–5.

Burgess, K. R., Jefferis, R. W., and Stevenson, I. F. (1979). Fatal thioridazine cardiotoxicity. *Medical Journal of Australia*, 2, 177–8.

Burman, D. and Stevens, D. (1978). Munchausen family. *Lancet*, **2**, 456.

Caddy, B. *et al.* (1978) Alcohol breath tests: criterion times for avoiding contamination by 'mouth alcohol'. *Behaviour Research Methods and Instrumentation*, **10**, 814–8. (Quoted in Fitzgerald and Hume, 1987*a*).

Campbell, E. J. M., Campbell, D. M. E., and Roberts, R. S. (1994). Ability to distinguish whisky (uisge beatha) from brandy (cognac). *British Medical Journal*, **309**, 1686–8.

Canlin, J. P. (1991). Legal responsibilities of pharmaceutical physicians: the view of the Medicines Control Agency. In *Pharmaceutical medicine and the law.* (ed. A. Goldberg and I. Dodds-Smith) pp. 25–31. Royal College of Physicians, London.

Centorrino, F., Baldessarini, R. J., Kando, J. C., Frankenburg, F. R., Volpicelli, S. A., and Flood, J. G. (1994*a*). Clozapine and metabolites: concentrations in serum and clinical findings during treatment of chronically psychotic patients. *Journal of Clinical Psychopharmacology*, **14**, 119–25.

Centorrino, F., *et al.* (1994*b*). Serum concentrations of clozapine and its major metabolites: effects of cotreatment with fluoxetine or valproate. *American Journal of Psychiatry*, **151**, 123–5.

Chang, R. B., Smith, W. A., Walkin, E., and Reynolds, P. C. (1984). The stability of ethyl alcohol in forensic blood specimens. *Journal of Analytical Toxicology*, **8**, 66–7.

Charney, D. S., Kales, A., Soldatos, C. R., and Nelson, J. C. (1979). Somnambulistic-like episodes secondary to combined lithium-neuroleptic treatment. *British Journal of Psychiatry*, **135**, 418–24.

Chaturvedi, A. K., Rao, N. G., and Moon, M. D. (1986). Poisoning associated with potassium. *Human Toxicology*, **5**, 377–80.

Cherry, J. D. (1984). The epidemiology of pertussis and pertussis immunization in the United Kingdom and the United States: a comparative study. *Current Problems in Pediatrics*, **14**, 1–78.

Chesney, R. W. and Brusilow, S. (1981). Extreme hypernatremia as a presenting sign of child abuse and psychosocial dwarfism. *Johns Hopkins Medical Journal*, **148**, 11–13.

Choonara, I. A., Scott, A. K., Haynes, B. P., Cholerton, S., Breckenridge, A. M., and Park, B. K. (1985). Vitamin-K1 metabolism in relation to pharmacodynamic response in anticoagulated patients. *British Journal of Clinical Pharmacology*, **20**, 643–8.

Choonara, I., Lawrence, A., Michalkiewicz, A., Bowhay, A., and Ratcliffe, J. (1992). Morphine metabolism in neonates and infants. *British Journal of Clinical Pharmacology*, **34**, 434–7.

Chouinard, G. and Jones, B. D. (1979). Early onset of tardive dyskinesia: a case report. *American Journal of Psychiatry*, **136**, 1323–4.

Christensen, J. H., Andreasen, F., and Jansen, J. A. (1982). Pharmacokinetics and pharmacodynamics of thiopentone. *Anaesthesia*, **37**, 398–404.

Clouston, E. (1994). Safety second in high-grade heroin hunt. *Guardian* 22 February.

Coe, J. I. (1974*a*). Postmortem chemistries on blood with particular reference to urea nitrogen, electrolytes, and bilirubin. *Journal of Forensic Sciences*, **19**, 33–42.

Coe, J. I. (1974*b*). Postmortem chemistry: practical considerations and a review of the literature. *Journal of Forensic Sciences*, **19**, 13–32.

Cohen, M. R. (1987). Medication errors. *Nursing*, **17**, 9.

Coid, J. (1979). Mania a potu: a critical review of pathological intoxication. *Psychological Medicine*, **9**, 709–19.

Collins, D. B. (1991). Medical manslaughter. *New Zealand Medical Journal*, **104**, 318–9.

Committee on Safety of Medicines (1983). OSMOSIN (controlled release indomethacin). *Current Problems*, **11**, 1–2.

Committee on Safety of Medicines (1988). Benzodiazepines, dependence and withdrawal symptoms. *Current Problems*, **21**, 1–2.

Committee on Safety of Medicines (1993). Clozapine. *Current Problems*, **19**, 9.

Cook, M. and Ferner, R. E. (1993). Adverse drug reactions: who is to know? *British Medical Journal*, **307**, 480–1.

Cooper, B., Gerlis, L., and Jeannet, E. (1992). *A consumer's guide to over-the-counter medicines.* Hamlyn, London.

Cooper, W. E., Schwar, T. G., and Smith, L. S. (1979a). *Alcohol, drugs and road traffic.* Juta, Cape Town.

Cooper, W. E., Schwar, T. G., and Smith, L. S. (1979b). *Alcohol, drugs and road traffic*, p. 155. Juta, Cape Town.

Cortot, A., Jobin, G., Ducrot, F., Aymes, C., Giraudeaux, V., and Modigliani, R. (1986). Gastric emptying and gastrointestinal absorption of alcohol ingested with a meal. *Digestive Diseases and Sciences*, **31**, 343–8.

Couropmitree, C., *et al.* (1975). Plasma C-peptide and diagnosis of factitious hyperinsulinism. Study of an insulin-dependent diabetic patient with 'spontaneous' hypoglycemia. *Annals of Internal Medicine*, **82**, 201–4.

Creese, I. (1983). *Stimulants, neurochemical, behavioural and clinical perspectives.* Raven Press, New York.

Crow, K. E. and Batt, R. D. (ed.) (1988). *Human metabolism of alcohol*, Vol. 1. CRC Press, Boca Raton, Florida.

Curran, W. J. (1969). Law-medicine notes. Medical management and confessions to crime. *New England Journal of Medicine*, **280**, 1008.

Curry, S. H., Whelpton, R., de Schepper, P. J., Vranckx, S., and Schiff, A. A. (1979). Kinetics of fluphenzine after fluphenazine dihydrochloride, enanthate and decanoate administration to man. *British Journal of Clinical Pharmacology*, **7**, 325–31.

Dahl, S. G. (1986). Plasma level monitoring of antipsychotic drugs. Clinical utility. *Clinical Pharmacokinetics*, **11**, 36–61.

Dale, J. R. and Appelbe, G. E. (1989). *Pharmacy law and ethics*, (4th edn). The Pharmaceutical Press, London.

Dalt, L. D., Dall'Amico, R., Laverda, A. M., Chemollo, C., and Chiandetti, L. (1991). Percutaneous ethyl alcohol intoxication in a one-month-old infant. *Pediatric Emergency Care*, **7**, 343–4.

D'Arcy, P. F. and Griffin, J. P. (ed.) (1986a). *Iatrogenic diseases*, (3rd edn). Oxford University Press, Oxford.

D'Arcy, P. F. and Griffin, J. P. (ed.) (1986b). *Iatrogenic diseases*, (3rd edn), p. 19. Oxford University Press, Oxford.

D'Arcy, P. F. and Griffin, J. P. (ed.) (1986c). *Iatrogenic diseases*, (3rd edn), pp. 604–12. Oxford University Press, Oxford.

D'Arcy, P. F. and Griffin, J. P. (ed.) (1986d). *Iatrogenic diseases* (3rd edn), pp. 651–72. Oxford University Press, Oxford.

D'Arcy, P. F. and Griffin, J. P. (1994). Thalidomide revisited. *Adverse Drug Reactions and Toxicological Reviews*, **13**, 65–76.

Darragh, A., Kenny, M., Lambe, R., and Brick, I. (1985). Sudden death of a volunteer. *Lancet*, **1**, 93–4.

David, A. B. and Jalilian-Marian, A. (1986). DTP: drug manufacturers' liability in vaccine-related injuries. *Journal of Legal Medicine—Chicago*, **7**, 187–233.

Davidson, D. C. (ed.) (1982). *Alder Hey Book of Children's Doses*, (4th edn). Alder Hey Hospital, Liverpool.

Davies, D. M. (ed.) (1991a). *Textbook of adverse drug reactions*, (4th edn). Oxford University Press, Oxford.

Davies, D. M. (ed.) (1991b). *Textbook of adverse drug reactions*, (4th edn) pp. 2–3. Oxford University Press, Oxford.

Davies, D. M. (ed.) (1991c). *Textbook of adverse drug reactions*, (4th edn), pp. 5–17. Oxford University Press, Oxford.

Davies, D. M. (ed.) (1991d). *Textbook of adverse drug reactions*, (4th edn), p. 549. Oxford University Press, Oxford.

Davies, D. M. (ed.) (1991e). *Textbook of adverse drug reactions*, (4th edn), pp. 601–42. Oxford University Press, Oxford.

Davis, A. R. and Lipson, A. H. (1986). Central-nervous-system depression and high blood ethanol levels. *Lancet*, **1**, 566.

Dawling, S. and Widdop, B. (1988). Use and abuse of the Toxi-Lab TLC system. *Annals of Clinical Bio-chemistry*, **25**, 708–9.

DeFronzo, R. A., Bia, M., and Smith, D. (1982). Clinical disorders of hyperkalemia. *Annual Review of Medicine*, **33**, 521–54.

de Gaard, J. W. (1979). Alcohol. In *Alcohol, drugs and road traffic*, (ed. W. E. Cooper, T. G. Schwar, and L. S. Smith), pp. 67–81. Juta, Cape Town.

de Lange de Klerke, E. S. M., Blommers, J., Kuik, D. J., Bezemer, P. D., and Feenstra, L. (1994). Effect of homeopathic medicines on daily burden of symptoms in children with recurrent upper respiratory-tract infections. *British Medical Journal*, **309**, 1329–32.

Denney, R. C. (1990). Solvent inhalation and 'apparent' alcohol studies on the Lion Intoximeter 3000. *Journal of the Forensic Science Society*, **30**, 357–61.

Desani, G. V. (1972). *All about H. Hatterr*. Penguin Books, Harmondsworth, Middlesex.

de Smet, P. A. G. M. (1995). Should herbal medicine-like products be licensed as medicines? *British Medical Journal*, **310**, 1023–4.

Devlin, P. B. (1985). *Easing the passing. The trial of Dr John Bodkin Adams*. Bodley Head, London.

Dickson, S. J., Cairns, E. R., and Blazey, N. D. (1977). The isolation and quantitation of insulin in post-mortem specimens—a case report. *Forensic Science*, **9**, 37–42.

Dimond, B. (1994). *Legal aspects of midwifery*. Books for Midwives Press, London.

Dine, M. S. (1965). Tranquillizer poisoning: an example of child abuse. *Pediatrics*, **36**, 782–5.

Dine, M. S. and McGovern, M. E. (1982). Intentional poisoning of children—an overlooked category of child abuse: report of seven cases and review of the literature. *Pediatrics*, **70**, 32–5.

Di Padova, C., Roine, R., Frezza, M., Gentry, R. T., Baraona, E., and Lieber, C. S. (1992). Effects of ranitidine on blood alcohol levels after ethanol ingestion. *Journal of the American Medical Association*, **267**, 83–6.

Divoll, M., Greenblatt, D. J., Harmatz, J. S., and Shader, R. I. (1981). Effect of age and gender on disposition of temazepam. *Journal of Pharmaceutical Sciences*, **70**, 1104–7.

Dollery, C. (ed.) (1991–4). *Therapeutic drugs*. Churchill Livingstone, Edinburgh.

Dubowski, K. M. (1986). Recent developments in alcohol analysis. *Alcohol, Drugs and Driving*, **2**, 13–46.

Dukes, M. N. G. (ed.) (1992). *Meyler's side effects of drugs. An encyclopaedia of adverse reactions and interactions*, (12th edn). Elsevier, Amsterdam.

Dukes, M. N. G. and Swartz, B. (1988a). *Responsibility for drug-induced injury*. Elsevier Science Publishers, Amsterdam.

Dukes, M. N. G. and Swartz, B. (1988b). *Responsibility for drug-induced injury*, pp. 151–96. Elsevier Science Publishers, Amsterdam.

Dukes, M. N. G. and Swartz, B. (1988c). *Responsibility for drug-induced injury*, p. 180. Elsevier Science Publishers, Amsterdam.

Dukes, M. N. G. and Swartz, B. (1988d). *Responsibility for drug-induced injury*, p. 202. Elsevier Science Publishers, Amsterdam.

Dukes, M. N. G. and Swartz, B. (1988e). *Responsibility for drug-induced injury*, p. 340. Elsevier Science Publishers, Amsterdam.

Dukes, M. N. G. and Swartz, B. (1988f). *Responsibility for drug-induced injury*, p. 345. Elsevier Science Publishers, Amsterdam.

Duncan, C. (1994). *Monthly Index of Medical Specialities (MIMS)*, November. Haymarket Medical Press, London.

Dundee, J. W. (1990a). Fantasies during benzodiazepine sedation in women. *British Journal of Clinical Pharmacology*, **30**, 311P.

Dundee, J. W. (1990b). Sexual fantasies during midazolam sedation. *British Journal of Anaesthesia*, **65**, 281P.

Dundee, J. W. (1990c). Unpleasant sequelae of benzodiazepine sedation. *Anaesthesia*, **45**, 336.

Dunea, G. (1983). Death over the counter. *British Medical Journal*, **286**, 211–12.

Dyer, C. (1988*a*). Judge 'not satisfied' that whooping cough vaccine causes permanent brain damage. *British Medical Journal—Clinical Research*, **296**, 1189–90.

Dyer, C. (1988*b*). Back calculation of alcohol. *British Medical Journal*, **297**, 1566–7.

Edwards, J. G. (1992). Medicolegal aspects of benzodiazepine dependence. *Medical Journal of Australia*, **156**, 733–7.

Edwards, M. A., Giguiere, W., Lewis, D., and Baselt, R. C. (1986). Intoxilyzer interference by solvents. *Journal of Analytical Toxicology*, **10**, 125.

Elashof, J. D., Jacknow, A. D., Shain, S. G., and Braunstein, G. D. (1991). Effects of anabolic-androgenic steroids on muscular strength. *Annals of Internal Medicine*, **115**, 387–93.

Ellenhorn, M. J. and Barceloux, D. G. (1988). *Medical toxicology, diagnosis and treatment of human poisoning*. Elsevier, New York.

Ettinger, P. O., Regan, T. J., and Oldewurtel, H. A. (1974). Hyperkalemia, cardiac conduction, and the electrocardiogram: a review. *American Heart Journal*, **88**, 360–71.

Farmer, J. G., Benomran, F., Watson, A. A., and Harland, W. A. (1985). Magnesium, potassium, sodium and calcium in post-mortem vitreous humour from humans. *Forensic Science International*, **27**, 1–13.

Farnsworth, N. R. (1990). Plants and traditional medicine. In *Economic and medicinal plant research*, Vol. 4, (ed. H. Wagner and N. R. Farnsworth). Academic Press, London.

Fenna, D., Mix, L., Schaefer, O., and Gilbert, J. A. L. (1971). Ethanol metabolism in various racial groups. *Canadian Medical Association Journal*, **105**, 472–5.

Fenton, A. C., Wailoo, M. P., and Tanner, M. S. (1988). Severe failure to thrive and diarrhoea caused by laxative abuse. *Archives of Disease in Childhood*, **63**, 978–9.

Ferner, R. E. (1992). Errors in prescribing and giving medicines. *Journal of the Medical Defence Union*, **3**, 60–4.

Ferner, R. E. (1993). Paracetamol poisoning—an update. *Prescribers' Journal*, **33**, 45–50.

Ferner, R. E. (1994). Dispensing with prescriptions. *British Medical Journal*, **308**, 1316.

Ferner, R. E. and Rawlins, M. D. (1988). Anabolic steroids: the power and the glory? *British Medical Journal*, **297**, 877–8.

Ferner, R. E. and Whittington, R. M. (1994). Coroner's cases of death due to errors in prescribing or giving medicines or to adverse drug reactions: Birmingham 1986–1991. *Journal of the Royal Society of Medicine*, **87**, 145–8.

Fitzgerald, E. F. and Hume, D. N. (1987*a*). *Intoxication test evidence: criminal and civil*. The Lawyers Cooperative Publishing Co., Rochester, NY.

Fitzgerald, E. F. and Hume, D. N. (1987*b*). *Intoxication test evidence: criminal and civil*, p. 114. The Lawyers Cooperative Publishing Co., Rochester, NY.

Fitzgerald, E. F. and Hume, D. N. (1987*c*). *Intoxication test evidence: criminal and civil*, p. 121. The Lawyers Cooperative Publishing Co., Rochester, NY.

Fitzgerald, E. F. and Hume, D. N. (1987*d*). *Intoxication test evidence: criminal and civil*, pp. 23–4. The Lawyers Cooperative Publishing Co., Rochester, NY.

Fitzgerald, E. F. and Hume, D. N. (1987*e*). *Intoxication test evidence: criminal and civil*, pp. 35–7. The Lawyers Cooperative Publishing Co., Rochester, NY.

Fleisher, D. and Ament, M. E. (1977). Diarrhea, red diapers, and child abuse. *Clinical Pediatrics*, **17**, 820–4.

Fletcher, S. M. (1983). Insulin. A forensic primer. *Journal of the Forensic Science Society*, **23**, 5–17.

Fletcher, S. M., Richards, L., and Moffat, A. C. (1979). The detection of fatal insulin poisoning by tissue analysis. *Veterinary and Human Toxicology*, **21**, (Suppl.), 197–9.

Florence, A. T. and Salole, E. G. (ed.) (1990). *Formulation factors in adverse drug reactions*. Wright, London.

Forbes, D. A., O'Loughlin, E. V., Scott, R. B., and Gall, D. G. (1985). Laxative abuse and secretory diarrhoea. *Archives of Disease in Childhood*, **60**, 58–60.

Forrest, A. R. (1993). ACP Broadsheet no 137: April 1993. Obtaining samples at post mortem examination for toxicological and biochemical analyses. *Journal of Clinical Pathology*, 46, 292–6.

Frezza, M., di Padova, C., Pozzato, G., Terpin, M., Baraona, E., and Lieber, C. S. (1990). High blood alcohol levels in women. The role of decreased gastric alcohol dehydrogenase activity and first-pass metabolism. [Published errata appear in *New England Journal of Medicine*, 24 May 1990, 322, (21); 1540 and 23 August 1990, 323, (8); 553.] *New England Journal of Medicine*, 322, 95–9.

Froemming, J. S., Lam, Y. W., Jann, M. W., and Davis, C. M. (1989). Pharmacokinetics of haloperidol. *Clinical Pharmacokinetics*, 17, 396–423.

Gammans, R. E., Mayol, R. F., and LaBudde, J. A. (1986). Metabolism and disposition of buspirone. *American Journal of Medicine*, 80, 41–51.

Garriott, J. C. (ed.) (1988). *Medicolegal aspects of alcohol determination in biological specimens*. PSG Publishing, Littleton, Mass.

Garriott, J. C. and Sturner, W. Q. (1973). Morphine concentrations and survival periods in acute heroin fatalities. *New England Journal of Medicine*, 289, 1276–8.

Gay, W. A., Jr and Ebert, P. A. (1973). Functional, metabolic, and morphologic effects of potassium-induced cardioplegia. *Surgery*, 74, 284–90.

Geiling, E. M. K. and Cannon, P. R. (1938). Pathologic effects of elixir of sulfanilamide (diethylene glycol) poisoning. *Journal of the American Medical Association*, 111, 916–26.

Gentry, R. T., Baraona, E., and Lieber, C. S. (1994). Agonist: gastric first pass metabolism of alcohol. *Journal of Laboratory and Clinical Medicine*, 123, 21–6.

Gerber, N. and Apseloff, G. (1993). Death from a morphine infusion during a sickle cell crisis. *Journal of Pediatrics*, 123, 322–5.

Gherardi, R. K., Baud, F. J., Leporc, P., Marc, B., Dupeyron, J.-P., and Diamant-Berger, O. (1988). Detection of drugs in the urine of body-packers. *Lancet*, 1, 1076–7.

Gilman, A. G., Rall, T. W., Nies, A. S., and Taylor, P. (eds.) (1990). *Goodman and Gilman's The pharmacological basis of therapeutics*, (8th edn). Macmillan, New York.

Goldman, B. (1988). Pertussis vaccine: is the controversy nearly over? *Canadian Medical Association Journal*, 139, 1082–7.

Gomm, P. J., Osselton, M. D., Broster, C. G., Johnson, N. M., and Upton, K. (1991). Study into the ability of patients with impaired lung function to use breath alcohol testing devices. *Medicine, Science and the Law*, 31, 221–5.

Graham, I. F. M. (1995). A fundemental problem of consent—GMC prefers prudent patient test. *British Medical Journal*, 310, 936.

Graves, D. (1994). 13 child cancer patients given drug overdose. *Daily Telegraph*, 15 December.

Green, A. (1993). Disposal of unwanted medicines—the law. *Journal of the Medical Defence Union*, (4), 79–80.

Greenblatt, D. J., Allen, M. D., Harmatz, J. S., and Shader, R. I. (1980). Diazepam disposition determinants. *Clinical Pharmacology and Therapeutics*, 27, 301–12.

Greenblatt, D. J., Laughren, T. P., Allen, M. D., Harmatz, J. S., and Shader, R. I. (1981). Plasma diazepam and desmethyldiazepam concentrations during long-term diazepam therapy. *British Journal of Clinical Pharmacology*, 1, 35–40.

Greenblatt, D. J., Harmatz, J. S., Zinny, M. A., and Shader, R. I. (1987). Effect of gradual withdrawal on the rebound sleep disorder after discontinuation of triazolam. *New England Journal of Medicine*, 317, 722–8.

Greenblatt, D. J., Harmatz, J. S., Dorsey, C., and Shader, R. I. (1988). Comparative single-dose kinetics and dynamics of lorazepam, alprazolam, prazepam, and placebo. *Clinical Pharmacology and Therapeutics*, 44, 326–34.

Greenblatt, D. J., Harmatz, J. S., Shapiro, L., Engelhardt, N., Gouthro, T. A., and Shader, R. I. (1991). Sensitivity to triazolam in the elderly. *New England Journal of Medicine*, 324, 1691–8.

Greenstreet, R. L. (1984). Estimation of the probability that Guillain-Barré syndrome was caused by the swine flu vaccine: US experience (1976–77). *Medicine, Science and the Law*, 24, 61–7.

Griffith, A. H. (1978). Reactions after pertussis vaccine: a manufacturer's experiences and difficulties since 1964. *British Medical Journal*, 1, 809–15.

Grunberger, G., Weiner, J. L., Silverman, R., Taylor, S., and Gorden, P. (1988). Factitious hypoglycemia due to surreptitious administration of insulin. Diagnosis, treatment, and long-term follow-up. *Annals of Internal Medicine*, 108, 252–7.

Guandolo, V. L. (1985). Munchausen syndrome by proxy: an outpatient challenge. *Pediatrics*, 75, 526–30.

Guillausseau, P. J., Mosse, A., and Lubetzki, J. (1983). C-peptide in factitious hypoglycemia from sulfonylurea. *Diabetes Care*, 6, 314–315.

Gutsche, H., Hopker, W., and Boenicke, G. (1969). Causes and prevention of hypoglycemia due to glibenclamide [in German]. *Medizinische Welt*, 35, 1876–8.

Gwynne, A. L. (1986a). *Cautionary tales*, (revised edn), pp. 44–5. Medical Defence Union, London.

Gwynne, A. L. (1986b). *Cautionary tales*, (revised edn), p. 50. Medical Defence Union, London.

Haibach, H., Dix, J. D., and Shah, J. H. (1987). Homicide by insulin administration. *Journal of Forensic Sciences*, 32, 208–16.

Hall, R. C. W. and Zisook, S. (1981). Paradoxical reactions to benzodiazepines. *British Journal of Clinical Pharmacology*, 11, 99S–104S.

Hamilton, G. (1993). The nurses are innocent. *Canadian Nurse*, 89, 27–32.

Hanna, M. H., *et al.* (1993). Morphine-6–glucuronide disposition in renal impairment. *British Journal of Anaesthesia*, 70, 511–14.

Hasche, H., Bachmann, W., Haslbeck, M., and Mehnert, H. (1982). Self-inflicted hypoglycaemia (three cases) [in German]. *Deutsche Medizinische Wochenschrift*, 107, 625–8.

Hawkes, N. (1994). Old chinese cure or killer? *The Times*, 1 February.

Hayes, A. G. and Chesney, T. M. (1993). Necrosis of the hand after extravasation of intravenously administered phenytoin. *Journal of the American Academy of Dermatology*, 28, 360–3.

Hearn, W. L., Keran, E. E., Wei, H. A., and Hime, G. (1991). Site-dependent postmortem changes in blood cocaine concentrations. *Journal of Forensic Sciences*, 36, 673–84.

Henry, J. A. (1992). Ecstasy and the dance of death. *British Medical Journal*, 305, 5–6.

Herold, K. C., Polonsky, K. S., Cohen, R. M., Levy, J., and Douglas, F. (1985). Variable deterioration in cortical function during insulin-induced hypoglycemia. *Diabetes*, 34, 677–85.

Heyndrickx, A., van Peteghem, C., van den Heede, M., de Clerck, F., Majelyne, W., and Timperman, J. (1980) Insulin murders: isolation and identification by radio-immunoassay after several months of inhumation. In *Annual European Meeting of The International Association of Forensic Toxicologists*, Glasgow, 1979, (ed. J. S. Oliver). Croom Helm, London.

Higgitt, A. C., Lader, M. H., and Fonagy, P. (1985). Clinical management of benzodiazepine dependence. *British Medical Journal*, 291, 688–90.

Hignite, C., Utrecht, C., Tschanz, C., and Azarnoff, D. (1980). Kinetics of R and S warfarin enantiomers. *Clinical Pharmacology and Therapeutics*, 28, 99–105.

Hill, C. and Doyon, F. (1990). Review of randomized trials of homeopathy. *Revue d'Epidémiologie et de Santé Publique*, 38, 139–47.

Hill, G. (1990). The KCl killer. *Journal of the Medical Defence Union*, 6, (Spring), 10–11.

Hindmarch, I., Beaumont, G., Brandon, S., and Leonard, B. E. (ed.) (1990). *Benzodiazepines*. John Wiley and Sons, Chichester.

Hinman, A. R. (1986). DTP vaccine litigation. *American Journal of Diseases of Children*, 140, 528–30.

Hirsch, S. R. and Barnes, T. R. E. (1994). Clinical use of high-dose neuroleptics. *British Journal of Psychiatry*, 164, 94–6.

Hitch, M. E. and Marshall, C. F. (1935). *Ballière's Nurses' complete medical dictionary*, (5th edn), p. 287. Ballière, Tindall, and Cox, London.

Hoffman, R. G., Speelman, D. J., Hinnen, D. A., Conley, K. L., Guthrie, R. A., and Knapp, R. K. (1989). Changes in cortical functioning with acute hypoglycemia and hyperglycemia in type I diabetes. *Diabetes Care*, 12, 193–7.

Holford, N. H. G. (1987). Clinical pharmacokinetics of ethanol. *Clinical Pharmacokinetics*, 13, 273–92.

Holley, F. O., Magliozzi, J. R., Stanski, D. R., Lombrozo, L., and Hollister, L. E. (1983). Haloperidol kinetics after oral and intravenous doses. *Clinical Pharmacology and Therapeutics*, 33, 477–84.

Hood, I., Mirchandani, H., Monforte, J., and Stacer, W. (1986). Immunohistochemical demonstration of homicidal insulin injection site. *Archives of Pathology and Laboratory Medicine*, 110, 973–4.

Horrocks, A. W. (1992). Abdominal radiography in suspected 'body-packers'. *Clinical radiology*, 45, 322–5.

Hubbard, J. W., *et al.* (1985). Therapeutic monitoring of chlorpromazine I: Pitfalls in plasma analysis. *Therapeutic Drug Monitoring*, 7, 222–8.

Huchard, H. and Fiessinger, C. (1911). *La thérapeutique en vingt médicaments*. Maloine, Paris.

Hulten, B.-A., Heath, A., Knudsen, K., Nyberg, G., Svensson, C., and Martensson, E. (1992). Amitriptyline and amitriptyline metabolites in blood and cerebrospinal fluid following human overdose. *Journal of Toxicology–Clinical Toxicology*, 30, 181–201.

Husemeyer, R. P., Cummings, A. J., Rosankiewicsz, J. R., and Davenport, H. T. (1982). A study of pethidine kinetics and analgesia in women in labour following intravenous, intramuscular and epidural administration. *British Journal of Clinical Pharmacology*, 13, 171–6.

Iglehart, J. K. (1987). Compensating children with vaccine-related injuries. *New England Journal of Medicine*, 316, 1283–8.

Illingworth, R. N. and Proudfoot, A. T. (1980). Rapid poisoning with slow-release potassium. *British Medical Journal*, 281, 485–6.

Insley, J. (ed.) (1990). *A paediatric vade-mecum* (12th edn). Edward Arnold, London.

Inturrisi, C. E., Max, M. B., Foley, K. M., Schultz, M., Shin, S.-U., and Houde, R. W. (1984). The pharmacokinetics of heroin in patients with chronic pain. *New England Journal of Medicine*, 310, 1213–17.

Jackson, P. R., Tucker, G. T., and Woods, H. F. (1991). Backtracking booze with Bayes—the retrospective interpretation of blood alcohol data. *British Journal of Clinical Pharmacology*, 31, 55–63.

Jann, M. W., Grimsley, S. R., Gray, E. C., and Chang, W.-H. (1993). Pharmacokinetics and pharmacodynamics of clozapine. *Clinical Pharmacokinetics*, 24, 161–76.

Jarvie, D. R. and Simpson, D. (1986). Drug screening: evaluation of the Toxi-Lab TLC system. *Annals of Clinical Biochemistry*, 23, 76–84.

Jastak, J. T. and Malamed, S. F. (1980). Nitrous oxide sedation and sexual phenomena. *Journal of the American Dental Association*, 101, 38–40.

Jennings, A. M., Wilson, R. M., and Ward, J. D. (1989). Symptomatic hypoglycemia in NIDDM patients treated with oral hypoglycemic agents. *Diabetes Care*, 12, 203–8.

Jetter, W. W. (1959). Postmortem biochemical changes. *Journal of Forensic Sciences*, 4, 330–41.

Jochemsen, R., van Boxtel, C. J., Hermans, J., and Breimer, D. D. (1983). Kinetics of five benzodiazepine hypnotics in healthy subjects. *Clinical Pharmacology and Therapeutics*, 34, 42–7.

Johnson, B. F., Fowle, A. S. E., Lader, S., Fox, J., and Munro–Faure, A. D. (1973). Biological availability of digoxin from Lanoxin products in the United Kingdom. *British Medical Journal*, 4, 323–6.

Johnson, R. A., Noll, E. C., and Rodney, W. MacM. (1982). Survival after a serum ethanol concentration of 1½ per cent. *Lancet*, 2, 1394.

Johnson, R. G., Jr, Bauman, W. A., Warshaw, A., and Axelrod, L. (1987). Factitious hypoglycemia due to administration of human synthetic insulin: new diagnostic challenge. *Diabetes Care*, 10, 253–5.

Jones, A. W. (1984). Interindividual variations in the disposition and metabolism of ethanol in healthy men. *Alcohol*, 1, 385–91.

Jones, A. W. (1985). Evaluation of breath-alcohol instruments. III. Controlled field trial with Alcolmeter pocket model. *Forensic Science International*, 28, 147–56.

Jones, A. W. (1987). Reliability of breath-alcohol measurements during the absorption phase. *Clinical Chemistry*, 33, 2128–30.

Jones, A. W. (1991). Top ten defence challenges among drinking drivers in Sweden. *Medicine, Science and the Law*, 31, 229–38.

Jones, A. W. and Neri, A. (1985). Age-related differences in blood ethanol parameters and subjective feelings of intoxication in healthy men. *Alcohol and Alcoholism*, **20**, 45–52.

Jones, A. W., Lund, M., and Andersson, E. (1989). Drinking drivers in Sweden who consume denatured alcohol preparations: an analytical-toxicological study. *Journal of Analytical Toxicology*, **13**, 199–203.

Jones, A. W., Beylich, K. M., Bjorneboe, A., Ingum, J., and Morland, J. (1992). Measuring ethanol in blood and breath for legal purposes—variability between laboratories and between breath-test instruments. *Clinical Chemistry*, **38**, 743–7.

Jones, C. A. G. (1994). *Expert witnesses*. Clarendon Press, Oxford.

Jones, G. R. and Pounder, D. J. (1987). Site dependence of drug concentrations in postmortem blood—a case study. *Journal of Analytical Toxicology*, **11**, 186–90.

Jones, M. A. (1995). The legal position. *British Medical Journal*, **310**, 46–7.

Kalimo, H. and Olsson, Y. (1980). Effects of severe hypoglycemia on the human brain. Neuropathological case reports. *Acta Neurologica Scandinavica*, **62**, 345–56.

Karch, F. E., Smith, C. L., Kerzner, B., Mazzullo, J. M., Weintraub, M., and Lassagna, L. (1976). Adverse drug reactions—a matter of opinion. *Clinical Pharmacology and Therapeutics*, **19**, 489–92.

Karhunen, P. J., Penttila, A., and Panula, A. (1987). Detection of heroin 'body-packers' at Helsinki airport. *Lancet*, **1**, 1265.

Kaye, S. and Haag, H. B. (1957). Terminal blood alcohol concentration in 94 fatal cases of alcoholism. *Journal of the American Medical Association*, **165**, 451–2.

Keen, R. W., Deacon, A. C., Delves, H. T., Moreton, J. A., and Frost, P. G. (1994). Indian herbal remedies for diabetes as a cause of lead-poisoning. *Postgraduate Medical Journal*, **70**, 113–14

Kendall, M. J., *et al.* (1994). Lack of effect of H_2-receptor antagonists on the pharmacokinetics of alcohol consumed after food at lunchtime. *British Journal of Clinical Pharmacology*, **37**, 371–4.

Kennedy, I. and Grubb, A. (1994). *Medical law: text with materials*, (2nd edn). Butterworths, London.

Kenyon, A. T., Sandiford, I., Bryan, A. H., Knowlton, K., and Koch, F. C. (1938). Effects of testosterone propionate on nitrogen, electrolyte, water and energy metabolism in eunuchoidism. *Endocrinology*, **23**, 135–53.

Kew, J., Morris, C., Aihie, A., Fysh, R., Jones, S., and Brooks, D. (1993). Lesson of the week—arsenic and mercury intoxication due to Indian ethnic remedies. *British Medical Journal*, **306**, 506–7.

Kintz, P., *et al.* (1990). Fly larvae and their relevance in forensic toxicology. *American Journal of Forensic Medicine and Pathology*, **11**, 63–5.

Klaber, M. (1992). Methotrexate tablet confusion. *Lancet*, **339**, 683.

Kleijnen, J., Knipschild, P., and ter Riet, G. (1991). Clinical trials of homeopathy. *British Medical Journal*, **302**, 316–23.

Klotz, U., McHorse, T. S., Wilkinson, G. R., and Schencker, S. (1974). The effects of cirrhosis on the disposition and elimination of meperidine in man. *Clinical Pharmacology and Therapeutics*, **16**, 667–75.

Kochackian, C. D. (ed.) (1976). *Anabolic-androgens*. Springer-Verlag, New York.

Koppel, C., Weigreffe, A., and Tenczer, J. (1992). Clinical course, therapy, outcome and analytical data in amitriptyline and combined amitriptyline/chlordiazepoxide overdose. *Human and Experimental Toxicology*, **11**, 458–65.

Kopun, M. and Propping, P. (1977). The kinetics of ethanol absorption and elimination in twins and supplementary repetitive experiments in singleton subjects. *European Journal of Clinical Pharmacology*, **11**, 337–44.

Koreen, A. R., *et al.* (1994). Relation of plasma fluphenazine levels to treatment response and extrapyramidal side-effects in first-episode schizophrenic patients. *American Journal of Psychiatry*, **151**, 35–9.

Koren, G., Barzilay, Z., and Greenwald, M. (1986). Tenfold errors in administration of drug doses: a neglected iatrogenic disease in pediatrics. *Pediatrics*, **77**, 848–9.

Kosmidis, H. V., *et al.* (1991). Vincristine overdose: experience with 3 patients. *Pediatric Hematology and Oncology*, **8**, 171–8.

Kramer, P. D. (1994). *Listening to Prozac*. Fourth Estate Limited, London.

Kulshrestha, M., Newey, S. E., and Ferner, R. E. (1994). A radiological lead in lead poisoning. *Human and Experimental Toxicology*, **13**, 369–70.

Lader, M. (1987). Clinical pharmacology of benzodiazepines. *Annual Review of Medicine*, **38**, 19–28.

Lathome Browne, G. and Stewart, C. G. (1883). *Reports of trials for murder by poisoning; by prussic acid, strychnia, antimony, arsenic, and aconitia*. Stevens and Sons, London.

Laurance, J. (1993). Victim of whooping cough vaccine wins £2.75m award. *The Times*, 12 May.

Laurence, D. R. and Bennett, P. N. (1992a). *Clinical pharmacology*, (7th edn), p. 105. Churchill Livingstone, Edinburgh.

Laurence, D. R. and Bennett, P. N. (1992b). *Clinical pharmacology*, (7th edn), p. 265. Churchill Livingstone, Edinburgh.

Laurence, D. R. and Bennett, P. N. (1992c). *Clinical pharmacology*, (7th edn), p. 287. Churchill Livingstone, Edinburgh.

Laurence, D. R. and Bennett, P. N. (1992d). *Clinical pharmacology*, (7th edn), p. 318. Churchill Livingstone, Edinburgh.

Lesar, T. S. (1992). Common prescribing errors. *Annals of Internal Medicine*, **117**, 537–8.

Lester, D., Greenberg, L. A., Smith, R. F., and Carroll, R. P. (1951). The inhalation of ethyl alcohol by man: part I. *Quarterly Journal of Studies on Alcohol*, **12**, 167–78.

Levine, M. N., Sackett, D. L., and Bush, H. (1986). Heroin vs morphine for cancer pain? *Archives of Internal Medicine*, **146**, 353–6.

Levitt, M. D. (1994). Antagonist: the case against first-pass metabolism of ethanol in the stomach. [Published erratum appears in *Journal of Laboratory and Clinical Medicine*, June 1994, **123**, (6), 873.] *Journal of Laboratory and Clinical Medicine*, **123**, 28–31.

Lewis, M. J. (1986). Blood alcohol: the concentration-time curve and retrospective estimation of level. *Journal of the Forensic Science Society*, **26**, 95–113.

Ley, N. J. (1993a). *Drink driving law and practice*. Sweet and Maxwell, London.

Ley, N. J. (1993b). *Drink driving law and practice*, p. 72. Sweet and Maxwell, London.

Lieber, C. (1977). *Metabolic aspects of alcoholism*. MTP Press, Lancaster.

Lieber, C. S. (1994). Mechanisms of ethanol-drug-nutrition interactions. *Journal of Toxicology—Clinical Toxicology*, **32**, 631–81.

Lindquist, O. and Rammer, L. (1975). Insulin in post-mortem blood. *Zeitschrift für Rechtsmedizin—Journal of Legal Medicine*, **75**, 275–7.

Loeper, J., *et al.* (1994). Hepatotoxicity of germander in mice. *Gastroenterology*, **106**, 464–72.

Logan, B., Howard, J., and Kiessel, E. L. (1993). Poisonings associated with cyanide in over-the-counter cold medication in Washington-state, 1991. *Journal of Forensic Sciences*, **38**, 472–6.

Lorber, J. (1978a). Unexplained coma in a two-year-old. *Lancet*, **2**, 680.

Lorber, J. (1978b). Unexplained coma in a two-year-old. *Lancet*, **2**, 472–3.

Lorber, J., Reckless, J. P. D., and Watson, J. B. G. (1980). Nonaccidental poisoning: the elusive diagnosis. *Archives of Disease in Childhood*, **55**, 643–7.

Luchins, D. J., Sherwood, P. M., Gillin, J. C., Mendelson, W. B., and Wyatt, R. J. (1978). Filicide during psychotropic-induced somnambulism: a case report. *American Journal of Psychiatry*, **135**, 1404–5.

Ludman, P., Mason, P., and Joplin, G. F. (1986). Dangerous misuse of sulphonylureas. *British Medical Journal*, **293**, 1287–8.

Lukas, S. E. (1993). Current perspectives on anabolic-androgenic steroid abuse. *Trends in Pharmacological Sciences*, **14**, 61–8.

Lundquist, F. and Wolthers, H. (1958). The kinetics of alcohol elimination in man. *Acta Pharmacologica et Toxicologica (Copenhagen)*, **14**, 265–89.

Lunn, J. N. (1995). An anaesthetist's view. *British Medical Journal*, **310**, 47–8.

Lurie, Y., Gottesfeld, F., and Bass, D. D. (1990). Benzodiazepines and fantasy. *Lancet*, **336**, 576.

McClelland, H. A. (1990). The forensic implications of benzodiazepine usage. In *Benzodiazepines: current concepts*, (ed. I. A. Hindmarch), pp. 227–50. John Wiley and Sons, Chichester.

McKillop, G. (1987). Drug abuse in body builders in the west of Scotland. *Scottish Medical Journal*, 32, 39–41.

McKusick, V. A. (1992). *Mendelian inheritance in man*, (10th edn). Johns Hopkins University Press, Baltimore.

McNulty, H. and Spurr, P. (1979). Drug names that look or sound alike. *British Medical Journal*, 2, 836.

McSweeney, J. J. and Hoffman, R. P. (1991). Munchausen's syndrome by proxy mistaken for IDDM. *Diabetes Care*, 14, 928–9.

Maher, G. and Frier, B. M. (1993). Hypoglycaemia and criminal responsibility. In *Hypoglycaemia and diabetes*, (4th edn), (ed. B. M. Frier and B. M. Fisher), pp. 380–6. Edward Arnold, London.

Mahesh, V. K., Stern, H. P., Kearns, G. L., and Stroh, S. E. (1988). Application of pharmacokinetics in the diagnosis of chemical abuse in Munchausen syndrome by proxy. *Clinical Pediatrics*, 27, 243–6.

Maltby, J. R. (1975). Criminal poisoning with anaesthetic drugs: murder, manslaughter or not guilty? *Forensic Science*, 6, 91–108.

Mann, R. D. (1986). Drug-induced disorders of central nervous function. In *Iatrogenic disease*, (3rd edn), (ed. P. F. D'Arcy and J. P. Griffin), pp. 576–650. Oxford University Press, Oxford.

Mant, T. G. K., Temposka, J. H., Volans, G. N., and Talbot, J. C. C. (1984). Adverse reactions to acetylcysteine and effects of overdose. *British Medical Journal*, 289, 217–9.

Marks, J. (1985). In *The benzodiazepines, current standards and practice*, (ed. D. E. Smith and D. R. Wesson), pp. 67–86. MTP, Lancaster.

Martensson, E., Olofsson, U., and Heath, A. (1988). Clinical and metabolic features of ethanol-methanol poisoning in chronic alcoholics. *Lancet*, 1, 327–8.

Martin, E., Moll, W., Schmid, P., and Dettli, L. (1984). The pharmacokinetics of alcohol in human breath, venous and arterial blood after oral ingestion. *European Journal of Clinical Pharmacology*, 26, 619–29.

Mason, J. K. and Smith R. A. M. (1995). A fundemental problem of consent—GMC may not be entitled to conclude that assault occurred. *British Medical Journal*, 310, 936.

Mavromatis, F. (1965). Tetracycline nephropathy. *Journal of the American Medical Association*, 193, 191–4.

Mayefsky, J. H., Sarnaik, A. P., and Postellon, D. C. (1982). Factitious hypoglycemia. *Pediatrics*, 69, 804–5.

Mayol, R. F., Adamson, D. S., Gammans, R. E., and LaBudde, J. A. (1985). Pharmacokinetics and disposition of ^{14}C buspirone HCl after intravenous and oral dosing in man. *Clinical Pharmacology and Therapeutics*, 37, 210.

Meade, T. W. (1986). Does pertussis vaccine cause brain damage? *Lancet*, 2, 286.

Meadow, R. (1977). Munchausen syndrome by proxy. The hinterland of child abuse. *Lancet*, 2, 343–5.

Meadow, R. (1989). ABC of child abuse. Poisoning. *British Medical Journal*, 298, 1445–6.

Meadow, R. (1993). Non-accidental salt poisoning. *Archives of Disease in Childhood*, 68, 448–52.

Mello, N. K. and Mendelson, J. H. (1970). Experimentally induced intoxication in alcoholics: a comparison between programmed and spontaneous drinking. *Journal of Pharmacology and Experimental Therapeutics*, 173, 101–16.

Melrose, D. G. (1978). Elective cardiac arrest: historical perspective. In *Modern cardiac surgery*, (ed. D. B. Longmore), pp. 271–5. MTP Press, Lancaster.

Merrills, J. and Fisher, J. (1995). *Pharmacy law and practice*. Blackwell Science, Oxford.

Milne, H. B. (1979). Epileptic homicide. *British Journal of Psychiatry*, 134, 547–8.

Missliwetz, J. (1994). Die Mordserie im Krankenhaus Wein-Lainz [Serial homicide in the Vienna-Lainz hospital] [in German]. *Archiv für Kriminologie*, 194, 1–7

Mitchell, J. (1995). A fundamental problem of consent. *British Medical Journal*, 310, 43–6

Moffat, A. C. (ed.) (1986). *Clarke's isolation and identification of drugs in pharmaceuticals, body fluids and post-mortem material*. The Pharmaceutical Press, London.

Montgomery, S. A., McAuley, R., Rani, S. J., Montgomery, B. D., Braithwaite, R. A., and Dawling, S. (1979). Amitriptyline plasma concentrations and clinical response. *British Medical Journal*, 1, 230–1.

Moritz, A. R. (1981). Classical mistakes in forensic pathology. *American Journal of Forensic Medicine and Pathology*, 2, 299–308.

Morley, C. J. (1992). Experts differ over diagnostic criteria for Munchausen syndrome by proxy. *British Journal of Hospital Medicine*, 48, 197–8.

Morris, H. H., 3rd and Estes, M. L. (1987). Traveler's amnesia: transient global amnesia secondary to temazepam. *Journal of the American Medical Association*, 258, 945–6.

Morrison, J. T. (1930). *Poisons*. Ernest Benn, London.

Mortimer, A. (1991). Making sense of shoplifting. *Medicine, Science and the Law*, 31, 123–6.

Nadkarni, S., Faye, S., and Hay, A. (1987). Experience with the use of the Toxi-Lab TLC system in screening for morphine/heroin abuse. *Annals of Clinical Biochemistry*, 24, 211–12.

Nelson-Jones, R. and Burton, F. (1990a). *Medical negligence case law*, p. 305. Format Press, London.

Nelson-Jones, R. and Burton, F. (1990b). *Medical negligence case law*, p. 290. Format Press, London.

Neuteboom, W. and Jones, A. W. (1990). Disappearance rate of alcohol from the blood of drunk drivers calculated from two consecutive samples: what do the results really mean? *Forensic Science International*, 45, 107–15.

Nott, D. M., Chandrasekar, R., Enabi, L., Greaney, B. A. and Harris, P. L. (1993). Intra-arterial injection of temazepam in drug abusers. *European Journal of Vascular Surgery*, 7, 87–9.

Oliver, J. E. (1990). Aggressiveness, anxiety and drugs. *British Journal of Psychiatry*, 157, 300.

Olson, K. R. (ed.) (1990). *Poisoning and drug overdose*, (1st edn). Appleton and Lange, East Norwalk.

Orfila, M. (1852). *Traité de Toxicologie* (5th edn), Vol. 1. Labé, Paris.

Osborne, R., Joel, S., Grebenik, K., Trew, D., and Slevin, M. (1993). The pharmacokinetics of morphine and morphine glucuronides in kidney failure. *Clinical Pharmacology and Therapeutics*, 54, 158–67.

Paice, B., Gray, J. M., McBride, D., Donnelly, T., and Lawson, D. H. (1983). Hyperkalaemia in patients in hospital. *British Medical Journal—Clinical Research*, 286, 1189–92.

Pakes, G. E., Brogden, R. N., Heel, R. C., Speight, T. M., and Avery, G. S. (1981). Triazolam: a review of its pharmacological properties and therapeutic efficacy in patients with insomnia. *Drugs*, 22, 81–110.

Parker, K. D., Elliott, H. W., Wright, J. A., Nomof, N., and Hine, C. H. (1970). Blood and urine concentrations of subjects receiving barbiturates, meprobamate, glutethimide, or diphenylhydantoin. *Clinical Toxicology*, 3, 131–45.

Paterson, S. (1985). Drug levels found in cases of fatal self-poisoning. *Forensic Science International*, 27, 129–33.

Paterson, S. (1993). Drugs and decomposition. *Medicine, Science and the Law*, 33, 103–9.

Petursson, H. and Lader, M. (1981). Withdrawal from long-term benzodiazepine treatment. *British Medical Journal*, 283, 643–5.

Phillips, A. P., Webb, B., and Curry, A. S. (1972). The detection of insulin in postmortem tissues. *Journal of Forensic Sciences*, 17, 460–3.

Phillipson, O., Baker, J., Sebastianpillai, F., Sheppard, G., and Brook, P. (1978). Disappearance of chlorpromazine from plasma following drug withdrawal. *Psychological Medicine*, 8, 331–4.

Pickford, E., Buchanan, N., and McLaughlan, S. (1988). Munchausen syndrome by proxy: a family anthology. *Medical Journal of Australia*, 148, 646–50.

Pikaar, N. A., Wedel, M., and Hermus, R. J. J. (1988). Influence of several factors on blood alcohol concentrations after drinking alcohol. *Alcohol and Alcoholism*, 23, 289–97.

Pike, R. (1994). Prized Rottweiller poisoned at show. *Daily Telegraph*, 14 April.

Playford, R. J. (1992). Allegation of sexual assault following midazolam sedation in a man. *Anaesthesia*, 47, 818.

Pohorecky, L. A. and Brick, J. (1988). Pharmacology of ethanol. *Pharmacology and Therapeutics*, **36**, 335–427.

Ponce, S. P., Jennings, A. E., Madias, N. E., and Harrington, J. T. (1985). Drug-induced hyperkalemia. *Medicine*, **64**, 357–70.

Pope, H. G., Jr and Katz, D. L. (1994). Psychiatric and medical effects of anabolic-androgen steroid use. *Archives of General Psychiatry*, **51**, 375–82.

Poplack, D. G. (1984). Massive intrathecal overdose: 'check the label twice'. *New England Journal of Medicine*, **311**, 400–2

Portenoy, R. K., Thaler, H. T., Inturrisi, C. E., Friedlander-Klar, H., and Foley, K. M. (1992). The metabolite morphine-6–glucuronide contributes to the analgesia produced by morphine infusion in patients with pain and normal renal function. *Clinical Pharmacology and Therapeutics*, **51**, 422–31.

Pounder, D. J. and Jones, G. R. (1990). Post-mortem drug redistribution-a toxicological nightmare. *Forensic Science International*, **45**, 253–63.

Power, K. G., Jerrom, D. W. A., Simpson, R. J., and Mitchell, M. (1985). Controlled study of withdrawal symptoms and rebound anxiety after six week course of diazepam for generalised anxiety. *British Medical Journal*, **290**, 1246–8.

Pramming, S., Thorsteinsson, B., Theilgaard, B., Pinner, E. M., and Binder, C. (1986). Cognitive function during hypoglycaemia in Type I diabetes mellitus. *British Medical Journal*, **292**, 647–50.

Prasad, A. B. (ed.) (1994). *British National Formulary*. (27, March 1994 edn). British Medical Association and Royal Pharmaceutical Society, London.

Proudfoot, A. T. (1989) Poisoning in children. In *Paediatric forensic medicine and pathology*, (ed. J. K. Mason), pp. 256–68. Chapman and Hall, London.

Rasor, R. W. and Crecraft, H. J. (1955). Addiction to meperidine (Demerol) hydrochloride. *Journal of the American Medical Association*, **157**, 654–7.

Rawlins, M. D. (1995). Parmacovigilance—paradise lost, regained or postponed—the William Withering lecture 1994. *Journal of the Royal College of Physicians of London*, **29**, 41–9.

Rawlins, M. D. and Thompson, J. W. (1991). Mechanisms of adverse drug reactions. In *Textbook of adverse drug reactions*, (4th edn), (ed. D. M. Davies), pp. 18–45. Oxford University Press, Oxford.

Reilly, D., *et al.* (1994). Is evidence for homeopathy reproducible? *Lancet*, **344**, 1601–6.

Reynolds, J. E. F. (ed.) (1992). *Martindale: the extra pharmacopoeia*, (30th edn). Pharmaceutical Press, London.

Roberts, J. T. and Essenhigh, D. M. (1986). Adenocarcinoma of the prostate in a 40–year-old body builder. *Lancet*, **2**, 742.

Roberts, R. K., Desmond, P. V., Wilkinson, G. R., and Schencker, S. (1979). Disposition of chlordiazepoxide: sex differences and effects of oral contraceptives. *Clinical Pharmacology and Therapeutics*, **25**, 826–31.

Rogers, D., Tripp, J., Bentovim, A., Robinson, A., Berry, D., and Goulding, R. (1976). Non-accidental poisoning: an extended syndrome of child abuse. *British Medical Journal*, **1**, 793–6.

Rohrig, T. P. and Prouty, R. W. (1989). Fluoxetine overdose: a case report. *Journal of Analytical Toxicology*, **13**, 305–7.

Rolfe, S. and Harper, N. J. N. (1995). Ability of hospital doctors to calculate drug doses. *British Medical Journal*, **310**, 1173–4

Rosen, M. (1995). A fundemental problem of consent—fact sheets may be useful. *British Medical Journal*, **310**, 936–7.

Rouzioux, J. M. (1980). Résultats des analyses toxicologiques lors des autopsies médico-légales. *Acta Medicinae Legalis et Socialis*, **30**, 25–42.

Ruben, S. M. and Morrison, C. L. (1992). Temazepam misuse in a group of injecting drug users. *British Journal of Addiction*, **87**, 1387–92.

Samuels, A. (1987). Iatrogenic crime—medicinal therapy, prescribed drugs, and criminal behavior. *Medicine, Science and the Law*, **27**, 302–3.

Sawe, J., Dahlstrom, B., Paalzow, L., and Rane, A. (1981). Morphine kinetics in cancer patients. *Clinical Pharmacology and Therapeutics*, **30**, 629–35.

Saxena, K. (1988). Death from potassium chloride overdose. *Postgraduate Medicine*, **84**, 97–8, 101–2.

Scarpino, V., *et al.* (1990). Evaluation of prevalence of 'doping' among Italian athletes. *Lancet*, **336**, 1048–50.

Scheifele, D. W. (1988). Pertussis vaccine and encephalopathy after the Loveday trial. *Canadian Medical Association Journal*, **139**, 1045–6.

Schnaps, Y., Frand, M., Rotem, Y., and Tirosh, M. (1981). The chemically abused child. *Pediatrics*, **68**, 119–21.

Schulte, H. M., Hall, M. J., and Boyer, M. (1993). Domestic violence associated with anabolic steroid abuse. *American Journal of Psychiatry*, **150**, 348.

Schultz, J., Weiner, H., and Westcott, J. (1980). Retardation of ethanol absorption by food in the stomach. *Journal of Studies on Alcohol*, **41**, 861–70.

Scott, A. I. F. (1988). Attempted strangulation during phenothiazine-induced sleep-walking and night terrors. *British Journal of Psychiatry*, **153**, 692–4.

Seitz, H. K., Egerer, G., and Simanowski, U. A. (1990). High blood alcohol levels in women. *New England Journal of Medicine*, **323**, 58.

Sellers, E. M., Schneiderman, J. F., Romach, M. K., Kaplan, H. L., and Somer, G. R. (1992). Comparative drug effects and abuse liability of lorazepam, buspirone and secobarbital in non-dependent subjects. *Journal of Clinical Psychopharmacology*, **12**, 79–85.

Shah, A. K. (1988). Detection of drugs in the urine of body-packers. *Lancet*, **1**, 1458.

Shaw, E. D., Mann, J. J., Weiden, P. J., Sinsheimer, L. M., and Brunn, R. D. (1986). A case of suicidal and homicidal ideation and akathisia in a double-blind neuroleptic crossover study. *Journal of Clinical Psychopharmacology*, **6**, 196–7.

Sheard, M. H. (1984). Clinical-pharmacology of aggressive-behavior. *Clinical Neuropharmacology*, **7**, 173–83.

Shew, E. S. (1960). *A companion to murder. A dictionary of death by poison, death by shooting, death by suffocation and drowning, death by the strangler's hand 1900–1950*. Cassell, London.

Simpson, D., Jarvie, D. R., and Heyworth, R. (1989). An evaluation of six methods for the detection of drugs of abuse in urine. *Annals of Clinical Biochemistry*, **26** (Pt 2, Mar), 172–81.

Simpson, G. (1987*a*). Accuracy and precision of breath alcohol measurements for subjects in the absorptive state. [Published erratum appears in *Clinical Chemistry* Nov. 1987, **33**, (11), 2130–1]. *Clinical Chemistry*, **33**, 753–6.

Simpson, G. (1987*b*). Concerning accuracy and precision of breath-alcohol measurements—reply. *Clinical Chemistry*, **33**, 1703–6.

Simpson, G. (1987*c*). Reliability of breath-alcohol measurements during absorption phase—reply. *Clinical Chemistry*, **33**, 2129–30.

Sjöström, H. and Nilsson, R. (1972). *Thalidomide and the power of the drug companies*. Penguin Books Ltd, Harmondsworth.

Skegg, D. C. G., Richards, S. M., and Doll, R. (1979). Minor tranquillizers and road accidents. *British Medical Journal*, **1**, 917–19.

Smith, D. E. and Wesson, D. R. (ed.) (1985). *The benzodiazepines: current standards for medical practice*. MTP, Lancaster.

Smith, R. C., *et al.* (1984). Haloperidol. Plasma levels and prolactin release as predictors of clinical improvement: chemical v radioreceptor plasma level assays. *Archives of General Psychiatry*, **41**, 1044–9.

Smith, T., DeMaster, E. G., Furne, J. K., Springfield, J., and Levitt, M. D. (1992). First-pass gastric mucosal metabolism of ethanol is negligible in the rat. *Journal of Clinical Investigation*, **89**, 1801–6.

Sneader, W. (1990). Chronology of drug introduction. In *Comprehensive medicinal chemistry*, Vol. 1, (ed. C. Hansch), pp. 7–80. Pergamon Press, Oxford.

Somogyi, G., Buris, L., and Nagy, F. L. (1986). Changes in blood alcohol concentration in storage [in German]. *Blutalkohol*, **23**, 208–13.

Song, F., *et al.* (1993). Selective serotonin reuptake inhibitors: meta-analysis of efficacy and acceptability. *British Medical Journal*, **306**, 683–7.

Southern, D. A. and Read, M. S. (1994). Lesson of the week—overdosage of opiate from patient-controlled analgesia devices. *British Medical Journal*, **309**, 1002.

Spiegel, R. J., Cooper, P. R., Blum, R. H., Speyer, J. L., McBride, D., and Mangiardi, J. (1984). Treatment of massive intrathecal methotrexate overdose by ventriculolumbar perfusion. *New England Journal of Medicine*, **311**, 386–8.

Stead, A. H. and Moffatt, A. C. (1983). A collection of therapeutic, toxic and fatal blood drug concentrations. *Human Toxicology*, **2**, 437–64.

Stephens, M. D. B. (1988). *The detection of new adverse drug reactions*, (2nd edn). MacMillam Press, Houndmills, Basingstoke.

Stevenson, J. and Hume, M. A. (1991). Concealed rectal opiates presenting as respiratory arrest: the importance of rectal examination in IV drug users. *Scottish Medical Journal*, **36**, 148.

Stofer, A. R. (1984). Vol a l'étalage sous l'influence de médicaments psychopharmacologiques. *Revue Médicale de la Suisse Romande*, **104**, 925–8.

Strang, J., Seivewright, N., and Farrell, M. (1992). Intravenous and other novel abuses of benzodiazepines: the opening of a Pandora's box? *British Journal of Addiction*, **87**, 1373–5.

Strang, J., Griffiths, P., Abbey, J., and Gossop, M. (1994). Survey of use of injected benzodiazepines among drug users in Britain. *British Medical Journal*, **308**, 1082.

Strauss, R. H., Liggett, M., and Lanese, R. (1985). Anabolic steroid use and perceived effects in 10 weight-trained women athletes. *Journal of the American Medical Association*, **253**, 2871–3.

Sturner, W. Q. and Garriott, J. C. (1973). Deaths involving propoxyphene. *Journal of the American Medical Association*, **223**, 1125–30.

Su, T.-P., Pagliaro, M., Schmidt, P. J., Pickar, D., Wolkowitz, O., and Rubinow, D. R. (1993). Neuropsychiatric effects of anabolic steroids in male normal volunteers. *Journal of the American Medical Association*, **269**, 2760–4.

Sutker, P. B., Goist, K. C., Jr, Allain, A. N., and Bugg, F. (1987). Acute alcohol intoxication: sex comparisons on pharmacokinetic and mood measures. *Alcoholism*, **11**, 507–12.

Sutphen, J. L. and Saulsbury, F. T. (1988). Intentional ipecac poisoning: Munchausen syndrome by proxy. *Pediatrics*, **82**, 453–6.

Swayne, J. M. D. (1989). Survey of the use of homeopathic medicine in the UK health system. *Journal of the Royal College of General Practitioners*, **39**, 503–6.

Sweeney, G. D. (1990). High blood alcohol levels in women. *New England Journal of Medicine*, **323**, 58–9.

Tattersall, R. (1986). Hypoglycaemia and criminal responsibility: a guide to a lawyer's view of diabetes. *Diabetic Medicine*, **3**, 470–4.

Tattersall, R. B. (1995). Hypoglycaemic amnesia. *Lancet*, **345**, 1188.

Teahon, K. and Bateman, D. N. (1993). A survey of intravenous drug administration by preregistration house officers. *British Medical Journal*, **307**, 605–6.

Tenenbein, M. (1986). Pediatric toxicology: current controversies and recent advances. *Current Problems*, **16**, 185–233.

Tennant, F. S. (1973). Complications of propoxyphene abuse. *Archives of Internal Medicine*, **132**, 191–4.

Terrell, H. B. (1988). Behavioral dyscontrol associated with combined use of alprazolam and ethanol. *American Journal of Psychiatry*, **145**, 1313.

Tesh, D. E., Beeley, L., Clewett, A. J., and Walker, G. F. (1975). Errors of drug prescribing. *British Journal of Clinical Pharmacology*, **2**, 403–9.

Thomas, S. H. L. (1993). Paracetamol (acetaminophen) poisoning. *Pharmacology and Therapeutics*, **60**, 91–120.

Thomas, S. H. L. (1994). Drugs, QT interval abnormalities and ventricular arrhythmias. *Adverse Drug Reactions and Toxicological Reviews*, 13, 77–102.

Thompson, C. (1994). The use of high-dose antipsychotic medication. *British Journal of Psychiatry*, 164, 448–58.

Todd, J. (1976). Pharmacogenic shoplifting? *British Medical Journal*, 1, 150.

Toon, S., Khan, A. Z., Holt, B. I., Mullins, F. G., Langley, S. J., and Rowland, M. M. (1994). Absence of effect of ranitidine on blood alcohol concentrations when taken morning, midday, or evening with or without food. *Clinical Pharmacology and Therapeutics*, 55, 385–91.

Travis, A. (1994). Howard makes steroid supply a criminal offence. *Guardian*, 3 November.

Trimble, M. R. (ed.) (1983). *Benzodiazepines divided*. John Wiley and Sons, Chichester.

Troisi, J. R. 2nd, Evans, S. M., and Griffiths, R. R. (1992). Human studies of relative abuse liability of benzodiazepines and novel sedatives/anxiolytics. *Clinical Neuropharmacology*, 15, (suppl.) 1, 108A–109A.

Trott, R. J. (1992). Diminished responsibility and the drug scene. *British Journal of Addiction*, 87, 189–92.

Turcant, A., *et al.* (1985). Thiopental pharmacokinetics under conditions of long-term infusion. *Anesthesiology*, 63, 50–4.

Turner, P. (1987). Clinical-pharmacology in criminal cases—discussion paper. *Journal of the Royal Society of Medicine*, 80, 438–40.

Tyrer, J. H., Eadie, M. J., Sutherland, J. M., and Hooper, W. D. (1970). Outbreak of anticonvulsant intoxication in an Australian city. *British Medical Journal*, 4, 271–3.

Tyrer, P., Owen, R., and Dawling, S. (1983). Gradual withdrawal of diazepam after long-term therapy. *Lancet*, 1, 1402–6.

Urso, T., Gavaler, J. S., and van Thiel, D. H. (1981). Blood ethanol levels in sober alcohol users seen in an emergency room. *Life Sciences*, 28, 1053–6.

Van Putten, T., Marder, S. R., Wirshing, W. C., Aravagiri, M., and Chabert, N. (1991). Neuroleptic plasma levels. *Schizophrenia Bulletin*, 17, 197–216.

Vella, E. J. and Edwards, C. W. (1993). Death from pulmonary microembolization after intravenous injection of temazepam. *British Medical Journal*, 307, 26.

Vestal, R. E., McGuire, E. A., Tobin, J. D., Andres, R., Norris, A. H., and Mezey, E. (1977). Aging and ethanol metabolism. *Clinical Pharmacology and Therapeutics*, 21, 343–54.

Vincent, F. M. and Emery, S. (1978). Antidiuretic hormone syndrome and thioridazine. *Annals of Internal Medicine*, 89, 147–8.

von Wartburg, J.)P. (1989). Pharmacokinetics of alcohol. In *Human metabolism of alcohol*, Vol. 1, (ed. K. E. Crow and R. D. Batt), pp. 17–22. CRC Press, Boca Raton, Florida.

Wakasugi, C., Nishi, K., and Yamada, M. (1986). Sudden death in a patient taking neuroleptics. *American Journal of Forensic Medicine and Pathology*, 7, 165–6.

Walia, B. N. S., Sarin, G. S., Chandra, R. I., and Ghai, O. P. (1963). Preterminal and postmortem changes in serum potassium of children. *Lancet*, 1, 1187.

Walls, H. J. and Brownlie, A. (1985a). *Drink, drugs and driving*, (2nd edn). Sweet and Maxwell, London.

Walls, H. J. and Brownlie, A. (1985b). *Drink, drugs and driving*, (2nd edn), pp. 111–14. Sweet and Maxwell, London.

Walls, H. J. and Brownlie, A. (1985c). *Drink, drugs and driving*, (2nd edn), p. 113. Sweet and Maxwell, London.

Walls, H. J. and Brownlie, A. (1985d). *Drink, drugs and driving*, (2nd edn), p. 167. Sweet and Maxwell, London.

Walls, H. J. and Brownlie, A. (1985e). *Drink, drugs and driving*, (2nd edn), p. 193. Sweet and Maxwell, London.

Walls, H. J. and Brownlie, A. (1985*f*). *Drink, drugs and driving*, (2nd edn), pp. 30–36. Sweet and Maxwell, London.

Walls, H. J. and Brownlie, A. (1985*g*). *Drink, drugs and driving*, (2nd edn), p. 76. Sweet and Maxwell, London.

Walls, H. J. and Brownlie, A. (1985*h*). *Drink, drugs and driving*, (2nd edn), p. 84. Sweet and Maxwell, London.

Wardle, J. and Jackson, H. (1995). *The Psychologist*, April, 157–63

Watson, J. B. G., Davies, J. M., and Hunter, J. L. P. (1979). Nonaccidental poisoning in childhood. *Archives of Disease in Childhood*, 54, 143–4.

Watson, P. E. (1988). Total body water and blood alcohol levels: updating the fundamentals. In *Human metabolism of alcohol*, Vol. 1. (ed. K. E. Crow and R. D. Batt), pp. 41–55. CRC Press, Boca Raton.

Watson, P. E., Watson, I. D., and Batt, R. D. (1980). Total body water measurements for adult males and females estimated from simple anthropometric measurements. *American Journal of Clinical Nutrition*, 33, 27–39.

Wax, P. M. (1995). Elixirs, diluents, and the passage of the 1938 Federal Food, Drug and Cosmetic Act. *Annals of Internal Medicine*, 122, 456–61

Wehr, K. and Alzen, G. (1989). Perfektionertes professionelles body-packing. *Zeitschrift für Rechtsmedizin— Journal of Legal Medicine*, 103, 63–8.

Weller, M. and Somers, W. A. (1991). Differences in the medical and legal viewpoint illustrated by R v. Hardie [1984]. *Medicine, Science and the Law*, 31, 152–6.

Wells, F. (1991). New medicines—their introduction and regulation. *Medico-Legal Journal*, 59, 239–51.

Welti, C. V. and Davis, J. H. (1978). Fatal hyperkalemia from accidental overdose of potassium chloride. *Journal of the American Medical Association*, 240, 1339.

Wendkos, M. H. (1979). Death attributed to ventricular arrhythmia. *Canadian Medical Association Journal*, 120, 1058–60.

Wettstein, R. M. (1985). Legal aspects of neuroleptic-induced movement disorders. *Legal Medicine*, (1985), 117–79.

Whittington, R. M. (1977). Dextropropoxyphene (Distalgesic) overdosage in the West Midlands. *British Medical Journal*, 2, 172–3.

WHO (1972). *International drug monitoring: the role of national centres*. Technical Report Series No 498. WHO, Geneva.

Widdop, B. and Caldwell, R. (1991). The operation of a hospital laboratory service for the detection of drugs of abuse. In *The analysis of drugs of abuse*, (ed. T. A. Gough), pp. 429–51. John Wiley and Sons, Chichester.

Widmark, E. (1932). Die theoretischen Grundlagen und die praktische Verwendbarkeit der gerichtlisch-medizinischen Alkoholbestimmung. Urban and Schwarzenberg, Berlin (quoted in Pohorecky and Brick, 1980).

Wiles, D. H. and Gelder, M. S. (1979). Plasma fluphenazine levels by radioimmunoassay in schizophrenic patients treated with depot injections of fluphenazine decanoate. *British Journal of Clinical Pharmacology*, 8, 565–70.

Wilkinson, P. K., Sedman, A. J., Sakmar, E., Kay, D. G., and Wagner, J. G. (1977). Pharmacokinetics of ethanol after oral administration in the fasting state. *Journal of Pharmacokinetics and Biopharmaceutics*, 5, 207–24.

Williams, R. H. (1973). Potassium overdosage: a potential hazard of non-rigid parenteral fluid containers. *British Medical Journal*, 1, 714–5.

Wilson, K. (1984). Sex-related differences in drug disposition in man. *Clinical Pharmacokinetics*, 9, 189–202.

Yap, V., Patel, A., and Thomsen, J. (1976). Hyperkalemia with cardiac arrhythmia. Induction by salt substitutes, spironolactone, and azotemia. *Journal of the American Medical Association*, **236**, 2775–6.

Zarafonetis, C. J., *et al.* (1978). Clinically significant adverse effects in a Phase I testing program. *Clinical Pharmacology and Therapeutics*, **24**, 127–32.

Zedeck, M. S. (1990). High blood alcohol levels in women. *New England Journal of Medicine*, **323**, 59.

Zhang, Y.-G. and Huang, G. -Z. (1988). Poisoning by toxic plants in China. *American Journal of Forensic Medicine and Pathology*, **9**, 313–9.

Index